CASE FILES®
Medical Ethics and Professionalism

Eugene C. Toy, MD
Vice Chair of Academic Affairs
Director of Generalist Division
Department of Obstetrics and Gynecology
The Methodist Hospital
Houston, Texas
Clinical Professor and Clerkship Director
Department of Obstetrics and Gynecology
University of Texas Medical School
　at Houston
Houston, Texas
John S. Dunn Senior Academic Chair
Department of Obstetrics and Gynecology
St Joseph Medical Center
Houston, Texas

Susan P. Raine, MD, JD, LLM, MEd
Vice Chair of Global Health Initiatives
Associate Professor
Department of Obstetrics and Gynecology
Associate Professor
Center for Medical Ethics and Health Policy
Baylor College of Medicine
Houston, Texas

Thomas I. Cochrane, MD, MBA
Assistant Professor of Neurology
Harvard Medical School
Associate Neurologist, Senior Ethics
　Consultant
Brigham and Women's Hospital
Boston, Masssachusetts

New York　Chicago　San Francisco　Athens　London　Madrid
Mexico City　Milan　New Delhi　Singapore　Sydney　Toronto

Notice

Medicine is an ever-changing science. As new research and clinical experience broaden our knowledge, changes in treatment and drug therapy are required. The authors and the publisher of this work have checked with sources believed to be reliable in their efforts to provide information that is complete and generally in accord with the standards accepted at the time of publication. However, in view of the possibility of human error or changes in medical sciences, neither the authors nor the publisher nor any other party who has been involved in the preparation or publication of this work warrants that the information contained herein is in every respect accurate or complete, and they disclaim all responsibility for any errors or omissions or for the results obtained from use of the information contained in this work. Readers are encouraged to confirm the information contained herein with other sources. For example and in particular, readers are advised to check the product information sheet included in the package of each drug they plan to administer to be certain that the information contained in this work is accurate and that changes have not been made in the recommended dose or in the contraindications for administration. This recommendation is of particular importance in connection with new or infrequently used drugs.

This book was set in Goudy by Cenveo® Publisher Services.
The editors were Catherine A. Johnson and Cindy Yoo.
The production supervisor was Catherine Saggese.
Project management was provided by Hardik Popli, Cenveo Publisher Services.
The cover designer was Thomas De Pierro.
RR Donnelley was printer and binder.

This book is printed on acid-free paper.

Library of Congress Cataloging-in-Publication Data

Toy, Eugene C., author.
    Case files. Medical ethics and professionalism / Eugene C. Toy, Susan P. Raine, Thomas I. Cochrane.
        p. ; cm.
    Medical ethics and professionalism
    Includes bibliographical references and index.
    ISBN 978-0-07-183962-4 (alk. paper)—ISBN 0-07-183962-3 (alk. paper)
    I. Raine, Susan P., author.   II. Cochrane, Thomas I., author.   III. Title.   IV. Title: Medical ethics and professionalism.
    [DNLM: 1. Ethics, Medical—Case Reports.   2. Ethics, Medical—Problems and Exercises.   W 18.2]
    R724
    174.2—dc23
                                                                                                2014042257

To my wife Terri Ruth, with whom we celebrate 30 wonderful years of marriage this July (2015). You have been an unwavering support all these years and shown everyone around you the essence of professionalism, highest ethical practice, and compassion. You have made me a better doctor and person. You are my best friend.

—ECT

For my parents who always told me I could do anything.

—SR

With deep gratitude to my mentors and teachers in medical ethics.

—TIC

CONTENTS

Anitra Beasley, MD, MPH
Associate Residency Program Director
Assistant Director, Ryan Residency
   Program in Family Planning
Assistant Professor
Division of Gynecologic and Obstetric Specialists
Division of Health Law and Policy
Department of Obstetrics and Gynecology
Baylor College of Medicine
Houston, Texas
Medical Intervention Against Patient's Will

Jennifer Bercaw-Pratt, MD
Clerkship Director
Assistant Professor
Division of Pediatric and Adolescent Gynecology
Department of Obstetrics and Gynecology
Baylor College of Medicine
Houston, Texas
Confidentiality

David Brendel, MD, PhD
Leading Minds Executive & Personal Coaching
Belmont, Massachusetts
Social Media Ethics

Rebecca Weintraub Brendel, MD, JD
Director, Master's Degree Program in Bioethics
Assistant Professor of Psychiatry
Harvard Medical School
Massachusetts General Hospital
Boston, Massachusetts
Jurisprudence

Gizelle Brooks-Carter, MD
Assistant Professor of Obstetrics and Gynecology
Weill Cornell Medical College
Department of Obstetrics and Gynecology
Houston Methodist Hospital
Houston, Texas
Prescribing for Friends and Family Members

Stephen D. Brown, MD
Assistant Professor of Radiology
Boston Children's Hospital and Harvard Medical School
Institute for Professionalism and Ethical Practice
Boston Children's Hospital
Boston, Massachusetts
Communicating Bad News

Thomas I. Cochrane, MD, MBA
Assistant Professor of Neurology
Harvard Medical School
Associate Neurologist, Senior Ethics Consultant
Brigham and Women's Hospital
Boston, Massachusetts
Futility
Informed Consent
Physician-Assisted Suicide
End-of-Life Ethics
Withholding Life Support

Jennifer DiPace, MD
Associate Professor of Clinical Pediatrics
Weill Cornell Medical College
New York, New York
Parental Decision-Making

Paula J. Efird, RNC-OB
Director of Women's Services
St Joseph Medical Center
Houston, Texas
Interdisciplinary Issues: Team Conflict

Martha Jurchak, RN, PhD
Executive Director, Ethics Service
Brigham and Women's Hospital
Boston, Massachusetts
Ethics Committees and Consultation

Joseph S. Kass, MD, JD
Vice Chair for Education, Department of Neurology
Associate Professor of Neurology, Psychiatry & Medical Ethics
Baylor College of Medicine
Houston, Texas
Risk Management

Charlie C. Kilpatrick, MD
Residency Program Director
Associate Professor
Female Pelvic Medicine and Reconstructive Surgery
Division of Gynecologic and Obstetric Specialists
Department of Obstetrics and Gynecology
Baylor College of Medicine
Houston, Texas
Cross-Cultural Issues

Lyuba Konopasek, MD
Designated Institutional Official
Associate Professor of Pediatrics
Weill Cornell Medical College/New York Presbyterian Hospital
New York, New York
Parental Decision-Making

Babu Krishnamurthy, MD
Assistant Professor of Neurology
Harvard Medical School
Beth Israel Deaconess Medical Center
Boston, Massachusetts
Research Ethics

Adrienne LeGendre, MD
Resident Physician
Department of Obstetrics and Gynecology
Houston Methodist Hospital
Houston, Texas
Prescribing for Friends and Family Members

Laurence B. McCullough, PhD
Dalton Tomlin Chair in Medical Ethics and Health Policy
Professor of Medicine and Medical Ethics
Associate Director for Education
Center for Medical Ethics and Health Policy
Baylor College of Medicine
Houston, Texas
Patient Abandonment
Physician–Patient Relationship

Aisling McGuckin, BSN, MSN, MPH
Maternal Child Health Nurse Consultant – Healthy Texas Babies
Office of Title V & Family Health
Texas Department of State Health Services
Austin, Texas
Public Health Ethics
(The views expressed in this chapter are those of the authors and
should not be perceived as representing the Texas Department of State
Health Services.)

Ali Mendelson, MD
Resident in Neurology
University of Pennsylvania
Perelman School of Medicine
Philadelphia, Pennsylvania
Complementary, Alternative, and Integrative Medicine

Peter Movilla
Senior Medical Student
Weill Cornell Medical College
New York, New York
Maternal–Fetal Conflict

Jillian O'Donnell
Senior Medical Student
University of Texas Medical School at Houston
Houston, Texas
Addictive Behavior in a Colleague

Francisco J. Orejuela, MD
Associate Professor
Female Pelvic Medicine and Reconstructive Surgery
Division of Gynecologic and Obstetric Specialists
Department of Obstetrics and Gynecology
Baylor College of Medicine
Houston, Texas
Cross-Cultural Issues

Hillary Patuwo, MD, MBA
Chief Resident and Patient Safety Officer
Obstetrics and Gynecology Residency
Houston Methodist Hospital
Houston, Texas
Resource Allocation

Frank X. Placencia, MD
Assistant Professor
Section of Neonatology
Department of Pediatrics
Center for Medical Ethics and Health Policy
Baylor College of Medicine
Houston, Texas
Truthtelling and Withholding Information

Peter Pressman, MD
Clinical Instructor
Department of Neurology
University of California, San Francisco
San Francisco, California
Student Issues: Procedures on Patients

Susan P. Raine, MD, JD, LLM, MEd
Vice Chair of Global Health Initiatives
Associate Professor
Department of Obstetrics and Gynecology
Associate Professor
Center for Medical Ethics and Health Policy
Baylor College of Medicine
Houston, Texas
Patient Abandonment
Physician–Patient Relationship

Steven A. Ringer, MD, PhD
Associate Professor of Pediatrics
Harvard Medical School
Chief, Newborn Medicine
Brigham and Women's Hospital
Boston, Massachusetts
Neonatal Intensive Care Unit Ethics

Marwa Saleh, MD
Resident in Family Medicine
University of Texas Southwestern Medical School
Dallas, Texas
Caring for a Patient Infected with HIV

S. Andrew Schroeder, PhD
Assistant Professor of Philosophy
Claremont McKenna College
Claremont, California
Basic Ethical Principles

Stephen Scott, MD, MPH
Associate Dean for Student Affairs
Weill Cornell Medical College in Qatar
Doha, Qatar
Caring for a Patient Infected with HIV

Jo Shapiro, MD
Associate Professor of Otolaryngology
Harvard Medical School
Chief, Division of Otolaryngology
Director, Center for Professionalism and Peer Support
Brigham and Women's Hospital
Boston, Massachusetts
Disclosure and Apology

Patricia A. Smith, MD
Department of Obstetrics and Gynecology
Medical Faculty Associates
The George Washington University
Washington, D.C.
Professionalism

Blake Sonne, MD
Emergency Medicine Resident
Hackensack University Medical and Trauma Center
Hackensack, New Jersey
Clinical Dishonesty
Difficult Consultation

Julie Stagg, MSN, RN, IBCLC, RLC
Women's and Perinatal Health Nurse Consultant
Office of Title V & Family Health
Texas Department of State Health Services
Austin, Texas
Public Health Ethics
(The views expressed in this chapter are those of the authors and should
not be perceived as representing the Texas Department of State Health
Services.)

Debra Taubel, MD
Clerkship Director and Associate Professor
Department of Obstetrics and Gynecology
Weill Cornell Medical College
New York, New York
Maternal–Fetal Conflict

Allison L. Toy
Senior Nursing Student
Scott and White Nursing School
Belton, Texas
Interdisciplinary Issues: Team Conflict

Eugene C. Toy, MD
Vice Chair of Academic Affairs
Director of Generalist Division
Department of Obstetrics and Gynecology
The Methodist Hospital
Houston, Texas
Clinical Professor and Clerkship Director
Department of Obstetrics and Gynecology
University of Texas Medical School
at Houston
Houston, Texas
John S. Dunn Senior Academic Chair
Department of Obstetrics and Gynecology
St Joseph Medical Center
Houston, Texas
Organ Transplantation and Do Not Resuscitate Orders

Michael J. Toy
Masters of Divinity Candidate
Princeton Theological Seminary
Princeton, New Jersey
Student Cheating and Plagiarism

Veronica Tucci, MD, JD
Assistant Residency Director
Assistant Professor
Section of Emergency Medicine
Department of Medicine
Baylor College of Medicine
Houston, Texas
Clinical Dishonesty
Difficult Consultation

Teresa M. Walsh, MD
Fellow, Minimally Invasive Surgery
Department of Obstetrics and Gynecology
Baylor College of Medicine
Houston, Texas
Boundary Issues

ACKNOWLEDGMENTS

The curriculum that evolved into the ideas for this series was inspired by Philbert Yau and Chuck Rosipal, two talented and forthright students, who have since graduated from medical school. It has been a tremendous joy to work with my excellent coauthors, Dr Susan Raine, who is an extraordinary educator, patient advocate, and attorney, and Dr Thomas I. Cochrane, whose expertise in neurology and ethics is the perfect combination for this text. I am greatly indebted to my editor, Catherine Johnson, whose exuberance, experience, and vision helped to shape this series. I appreciate McGraw-Hill's believing in the concept of teaching through clinical cases. I am also grateful to Catherine Saggese for her excellent production expertise and Cindy Yoo for her wonderful editing. I cherish the ever-organized and precise Hardik Popli and Anupriya Tyagi, project managers, whose precision and talent I greatly value. I appreciate Linda Swagger for her sage advice and support. At Methodist, I appreciate Drs Judy Paukert, Marc Boom, and Alan Kaplan who have welcomed our residents. Without my dear colleagues Drs Konrad Harms, Priti Schachel, Gizelle Brooks Carter, and Russell Edwards, this book could not have been written. Most of all, I appreciate my ever-loving wife Terri, and our 4 wonderful children—Andy and his wife Anna, Michael, Allison, and Christina—for their patience and understanding.

Eugene C. Toy

Mastering the diverse knowledge and complicated approach to disciplines such as ethics, professionalism, and jurisprudence in medicine is a formidable task. It is even more difficult to draw on that knowledge, procure and filter through the clinical or relational situation, develop an understanding of the ethical, legal, and moral issues, and, finally, to reach a reasonable approach. To gain these skills, the student learns best at in real-life situations, guided and instructed by experienced experts, and inspired toward self-directed, diligent reading. Clearly, there is no replacement for education in the real world. Unfortunately, students are often not invited to participate in these situations, and ethics and professionalism issues have long been neglected in the medical student curriculum. Perhaps the best alternative is a carefully crafted cases designed to stimulate the proper approach and the decision-making process. In an attempt to achieve that goal, we have constructed a collection of vignettes to highlight relevant issues and dilemmas.

Most importantly, the explanations for the cases emphasize the major principles, rather than merely rote questions and answers. By contrast to other more clinical disciplines, the subjects addressed in this book require a student to read through the case in a quiet setting, to allow the concepts to percolate and be analyzed. Yet, this text is still organized in the usual case files format: allowing the student "with limited time" to go quickly through the scenarios and check the corresponding answers, and it allows the student who wants thought-provoking explanations to obtain them. The answers are arranged from simple to complex: the bare answers, an analysis of the case, an approach to the pertinent topic, a comprehension test at the end, key points for emphasis, and a list of references for further reading. The text is organized by related subjects such as *General, Student Issues, Team Issues,* etc, to allow for more complete mastery of an area. A listing of cases is included in Section III to aid the student who desires to test his or her knowledge of a certain area, or to review a topic, including basic definitions.

Approach to Ethics, Professionalism, and Jurisprudence in Medicine

Medical ethics is the practice of systematic analysis of the morals of decision-making in the realm of health care. Professionalism is the practice of putting the interest of the patient above his or her self-interest, and involves accountability, altruism, and pursuit of excellence, as well as a higher calling of duty, integrity, and respect for others. Medical jurisprudence illustrates how medical ethics and legal medicine are intertwined in fields such as medical malpractice, forensic medicine, competency and psychiatric commitment, and withdrawing lifesaving measures.

Medical students should strive to attain some degree of mastery of basic concepts involving these 3 disciplines: ethics, professionalism, and jurisprudence. They can do so by approaching medical situations in 8 different ways.

1. Identify the moral and legal issues of a medical situation.

2. Identify the key aspects of a valid informed consent or a valid refusal of treatment.

3. Describe how to determine competence to consent to or refuse treatment.

4. List the process to decide when it is legally and ethically justifiable to withhold information from a patient.

5. Describe when it is morally and legally justifiable to break patient confidentiality.

6. Describe how to approach the patient who refuses treatment.

7. Describe the legal and ethical issues surrounding patients with a poor prognosis, including those with a terminal condition.

8. List the professional duties that a physician has to the patient and to the health care team.

   I. **Identify the moral and legal issues of a medical situation.**
      Every encounter with a patient is not only a clinical encounter but also one that encompasses ethics, the law, and professionalism. Principles such as patient autonomy, informed consent, honesty to presenting information, and confidentiality are relevant. Typically, medical students and physicians sail through the patient encounter easily without hitting any of the potential jagged edges of morality or the law. Occasionally, however, an issue arises that takes the health care team by surprise (eg, the patient who refuses lifesaving treatment because of an "irrational belief"). How does the health care professional deal with this issue? How does one step back from the shock that a seemingly reasonable person would adopt an unreasonable path? The answer to these questions depends on an understanding of the basic moral and legal concepts that govern the patient encounter. Thus, the first step for the student is to understand and apply the basic ethical and legal principles in some common situations.

   II. **Identify the key aspects of a valid informed consent or a valid refusal of treatment.**
      Informed consent, or the flip side of the same coin "informed refusal," is a fundamental concept that every health care professional must have mastery. To respect a patient's right to autonomy (self-governance), the physician

must provide the patient with the relevant information on his or her medical condition, the proposed treatment and its likelihood of benefit, the alternatives, and the risks of the various options. More than a moral responsibility, the physician has a legal responsibility for this informed consent process. By contrast, patients also have the right for refusal of treatment. Patients must be "fully informed" and "in their right mind" (competent) for the consent process to be valid. Students should become experts at identifying the key aspects of this counseling process.

III. **Describe how to determine competence to consent to or refuse treatment.**
Because patients must be given the proper information to make health care decisions, they must "have the mental capacity to decide." This is a legal concept and is sometimes referred to as decision-making capacity. Competence is an "absolute" and specific, and the patient is either competent or not competent to make a certain decision. The 4 key elements to decision-making capacity are: (1) **understanding** the information presented, (2) **appreciate** the significance of the situation including the risks and benefits, (3) ability to **reason** in the current situation and context, and (4) **express** a choice (communicate a preference). Being competent is not synonymous to making good decisions. A competent person may make poor choices. Competence can be impaired due to issues of cognition (dementia, brain injury), emotion (mania, depression), or delusional thinking (schizophrenia). The student must be well versed in how to determine competence to ensure the patient can make valid decisions.

IV. **List the process to decide when it is legally and ethically justifiable to withhold information from a patient.**
A physician is obligated to promote a patient's welfare and respect his or her autonomy by providing truthful information. However, there are some rare circumstances when it is **appropriate to withhold information** from a patient. In general, the term "withholding information" does not apply to disclosure of mistakes. Valid reasons for nondisclosure of relevant medical information depend on the likelihood of "serious harm" to the patient. This is more than the patient becoming emotional or upset or even if requested by a family member. One example of a valid situation is if information provided to a depressed patient may cause him or her to become suicidal. Another example is if the patient explicitly asks not to be told about the medical condition or diagnosis but, instead, that a family member be told and make decisions on his or her behalf. In this situation, "informed preference" means the patient understands the full ramifications of not making decisions for himself or herself. Almost universally, the physician should provide information to the patient, albeit in many circumstances, in a sensitive and measured manner. Note that withholding information is not the same as lying to the patient. In this setting, the student should know how to deliver bad news and also when it is acceptable not to disclose information.

V. **Describe when it is morally and legally justifiable to break confidentiality.**
Patient confidentiality is one of the foundations of the physician–patient relationship. Because the information being discussed is personal by nature, and

perhaps may be embarrassing if it becomes public, the patient must be able to depend on the physician being confidential. The patient must trust his or her doctor with sensitive and truthful information so accurate diagnoses can be made. This confidentiality is both an ethical as well as legal responsibility. The main ethical and legal justification to break confidentiality is when a risk for imminent harm is identified. The student should be aware of the physician's duty to the patient (protect patient confidentiality) versus duty to the public or another person and be able to balance their duties.

VI. **Describe how to approach the patient who refuses treatment.**
As discussed in the preceding points, the student must have an understanding of whether the patient has decision-making capacity (competence) and is given the proper information to make decisions (informed consent). Patients may choose to refuse the recommended treatment. Some decisions are of little consequence, while others may be life threatening. The novice health care professional may become frustrated at the latter situation and believe that the patient must have "diminished decision-making capacity" or not understand the situation, and try harder to "convince" him or her of the proper course. This response involves prejudgment on the part of the physician, and rarely is fruitful. Some strategies that are helpful include (1) clarifying whether the patient is aware of the situation (ask the patient to describe the medical condition), (2) understanding their story (ask how the patient made his/her decision), (3) being aware and understanding their concerns, (4) exploring fears and concerns, and (5) trying to find a win–win solution. The student should be aware of his/her own biases, cultural and religious beliefs, and values, and how it may alter complex medical decision-making.

VII. **Describe the legal and ethical issues surrounding patients with a poor prognosis including those with a terminal condition.**
The physician's role in end-of-life care is a difficult one. Issues relevant to this area include physician-assisted suicide, such as intentional termination or assisting in termination of life of a terminally ill patient on his or her request. State legal requirements have much to bear about the latitude of the physician in this area; in fact, some states have strict legal ramifications for physicians participating in patient-assisted death, including jail time. Advance directives, provision of life support, and withdrawing life support also fall into this area. Sometimes, there is no advance directive and family members may not be very aware of the patient's wishes. These situations are particularly challenging. The student should be aware of the legal and moral principles and limitations in end-of-life care, and the process whereby life-sustaining treatment may be withdrawn.

VIII. **List the professional duties that a physician has to the patient and to the health care team.**
The physician has numerous professional duties to the patient, including maintaining professional competence, honesty, confidentiality, maintaining appropriate relations with patients, commitment to excellence by keeping current in medical knowledge, managing conflict of interest, and maintaining

a collaborative relationship with the health care team. Physicians have an unfair power advantage over patients, and they should never exploit that advantage in dating, sexual relations, personal financial gain, or other private purpose. Sometimes, grateful patients may even give personal gifts to their doctor; in general, any gift that is of more than very little value should not be accepted. Recently, the disruptive behavior of physicians has been found to interfere with the care of patients and harm the health care team. Many professional and hospital associations have taken steps to advocate a "no tolerance policy for the disruptive health care member." The student should be aware of the basic professional obligations of the physician.

KEY POINTS

▶ The doctor has a fiduciary relationship to the patient built on trust, confidentiality, honesty, and respect.

▶ The physician must be aware of how to provide informed consent and be able to assess patient decision-making capacity.

▶ A competent patient has the right to make poor decisions.

▶ When a patient refuses treatment, the physician should explore the reasons why and try to understand the patient's viewpoint.

▶ Patient information must not be disclosed unless there is risk of imminent harm or there is a legal requirement to do so.

▶ End-of-life ethics is complicated and often depends on the presence of an advance directive or family members who are intimately aware of the patient's wishes.

▶ The physician has a high professional duty to the patient and health care team and should never exploit that power advantage over the patient.

REFERENCES

American Board of Internal Medicine Foundation. *Understanding Medical Professionalism*. New York, NY: McGraw-Hill; 2014.

Fremgen B. *Medical Law and Ethics*. 4th ed. New York, NY: Prentice Hall; 2011.

Judson K. *Law and Ethics for the Health Professions*. New York, NY: McGraw Hill; 2012.

Jonson A, Siegler M, Winslade W. *Clinical Ethics: A Practical Approach to Ethical Decisions in Clinical Medicine*. 7th ed. New York, NY: McGraw-Hill; 2010.

Ethics Cases

While walking home on a quiet evening, you see a car driving erratically down the street toward you. The car veers off the road, striking a pedestrian before crashing into a lamppost one block away. You run to the injured pedestrian who appears to be about 30 years of age. He has a compound fracture of the left tibia that is bleeding profusely. No other significant injuries are evident. While working to stop the bleeding and stabilize the leg, you notice a prescription bottle for atazanavir in the pedestrian's pocket. The pedestrian is in pain and scared, and he begs you to stay with him. A bystander yells to you from the wrecked car. She reports that she has already called emergency medical services. The driver does not have any obvious injuries but is moaning incoherently.

▶ What further information would you like to know before deciding what to do?
▶ What ethical issues or concerns may arise as the scenario unfolds?

ANSWERS TO CASE 1:
Basic Ethical Principles

Summary: You are off duty walking home when you see a car veering off the road, striking a pedestrian before crashing into a lamppost. You attend to the pedestrian who has a compound fracture of the left tibia that is bleeding profusely. While working to stop the bleeding, you notice a prescription bottle for atazanavir in the pedestrian's pocket. He is scared and begs you to stay with him. A bystander has called 911. The driver does not have any obvious injuries but is moaning incoherently.

- **Further information:** The most important pieces of missing information can be divided into two categories. First, it would be helpful to know the consequences of each possible course of action. If you leave the pedestrian to attend to the driver, what will happen to the pedestrian? What aid would you be able to provide to the driver? Will the driver contract HIV from the pedestrian's blood if you treat her? Second, it is important to know the wishes of each party. Would the pedestrian still insist you stay with him if he knew the driver was in more critical need of care? Would he object to your revealing his HIV status to the driver? Would the driver consent to being exposed to HIV if that was necessary to treat her injuries?

- **Ethical issues or concerns may arise:** The issues include concerns relating to the relative value we should assign to different outcomes, fairness, equality, treatment withdrawal, harm, personal responsibility, informed consent, privacy, mental competence, and the limits of a physician's obligation to his or her patients.

ANALYSIS

Objectives

1. To identify some of the relevant ethical factors in a difficult case.

2. To appreciate how simple ethical principles can be very complex, both internally and when they interact with other principles.

Considerations

This case poses a number of ethical challenges. Briefly, two foundational ethical principles are relevant. We ought to be concerned with the consequences of our actions, aiming to produce the best overall outcome we can. We also have an obligation to respect the autonomy of others, giving them the right to make certain choices for themselves. As this case illustrates, each of these principles is complex. For example, how should we determine what makes one outcome better than another? Can a patient in shock truly offer informed consent? The ethical challenges of the situation increase when the principles come into conflict with one another. In the end, what you ought to do in this case will depend on the information you obtain as the situation unfolds. However, even without knowing those details, going through the process of identifying the ethically salient aspects of a situation can itself improve ethical decision-making.

> # APPROACH TO:
> ## Basic Ethical Principles

DEFINITIONS

CONCERN FOR CONSEQUENCES: The ethical concept that an important aim of our actions should be to bring about the best outcome that we can for all parties affected by our actions.

RESPECT FOR AUTONOMY: The ethical concept that people have a right to decide for themselves how their lives will go in certain respects.

CLINICAL APPROACH

To analyze this case, we should first review the medical aspects of the situation. You know that if you are able to stop the bleeding, the pedestrian has a good long-term prognosis. If he is positive for HIV infection, as suggested by the prescription bottle, there is an increased possibility of a serious infection. Having come into contact with the pedestrian's blood, you are at a very low (well < 1%) risk of HIV infection. You can significantly reduce that risk with postexposure prophylaxis (PEP) treatment, although PEP can cause a number of unpleasant adverse events. You know less about the situation of the driver. She may be okay until the ambulance arrives, but there is a chance she has injuries requiring immediate attention. Discovering her status would probably require examining her yourself, exposing her to the pedestrian's potentially HIV-positive blood.

Should you remain with the pedestrian, or should you leave him so that you can examine and potentially treat the driver? One obvious way to decide would be to compare the likely consequences of each action. If, for example, the pedestrian would die of blood loss if you left, and the driver was not in danger of any serious injury, then it would be ethically indefensible to leave the pedestrian. But, if the pedestrian would be medically stable without you, while the driver needed your immediate attention to avoid a serious injury, then you ought to attend to the driver. This concern for consequences is an important element of nearly all ethical systems. All else being equal, we ought to act to produce the best outcome we can for all people involved.

Of course, it is often difficult to predict the consequences of a given action. In this case, for example, it is hard to know how much you will be able to help the driver by leaving the pedestrian. This is a problem of decision-making in the face of uncertainty, and it is not distinctively an ethical problem. Distinctively ethical problems arise when trying to decide which of two known or predicted outcomes is *better*. Suppose, for example, you believed that by helping the pedestrian you could marginally reduce his risk of wound infection, but by helping the driver you could prevent a minor but permanent mobility impairment. Which of those outcomes is better? Or, suppose that by helping the pedestrian you could significantly reduce his extreme pain and also provide psychological comfort; however, by helping the driver you could decrease her stay in the hospital by a few days while also slightly increasing her risk of HIV infection. Which of those outcomes is better? In the end, evaluating the consequences of your action will involve considering what you could do to treat each victim's injuries, the psychological impact your departure might have on the pedestrian, the risk that you might expose the driver to HIV infection, and the discomfort associated with PEP treatment. You might also want to consider the broader consequences of your actions (eg, effects on you and on the bystander); however, in this case it does seem that the driver and the pedestrian are most significantly affected by your decision.

Although the goal of producing good consequences is taken by most people to be very important, few believe that it is all there is to ethics. In particular, many people think that additional factors can affect the moral weight we should assign to an outcome:

- In the present case, you have already spent some time with the pedestrian. If you judge that further aid would have equal benefit for either victim, then considerations of *fairness* might suggest that you treat the driver.

- Suppose that both victims are in pain, and you judge that you could provide some pain relief to either victim. Many ethicists have argued that, if the benefit provided would be similar, then it should first go to the person who is worse off. In this case, providing relief to the person in more severe pain would be a way of *equalizing* the situation of the two victims.

- It might seem important that you have already begun treating the pedestrian. Many people believe that *withdrawing* treatment, once begun, is harder to justify than merely not starting treatment. This is perhaps why it seems more serious to remove someone from a respirator, than to fail to put her on a respirator in the first place. Therefore, it might be especially bad for you to leave a patient you have already begun treating.

- If you were to treat the driver, then you would be exposing her to HIV infection. Thus, you would potentially be *harming* her. Intuitively, this is an important moral consideration, as seen in the common bioethical injunction, "First, do no harm." Accordingly, it might seem that you ought to weigh the possible harm to the driver more heavily than whatever benefits you could provide to her.

- Questions of *responsibility* could be relevant. It was the driver who caused the pedestrian's injuries. If her erratic driving was the result of, say, intoxication, perhaps you should err on the side of treating the true victim, the pedestrian. Although this kind of moral adjudication is for good reason usually not regarded as appropriate in medical contexts, reflections of it can be seen in some policies on organ transplantation.

So far, we have looked at the consequences of your action under the principle that, all else being equal, you should aim to produce the best possible outcome. We then looked at a number of factors—fairness, equality, withdrawal of treatment, harm, and responsibility—that might affect the way in which you weigh the *value* of different consequences. However, another central ideal in bioethics takes a very different approach. Sometimes actions that produce good results can be morally unjustified because of the way in which those results were produced. For example, performing surgery on a patient who is mentally competent and refuses treatment is not ethically acceptable, even if doing so ends up being best for the patient. Conducting medical experiments on unsuspecting populations is not justified, even if those experiments produce important results that, overall, make their consequences good. The ends do not always justify the means. Accordingly, in addition to having a concern for consequences, it is ethically important to act in a way that *respects autonomy*, allowing people to make their own decisions about how their lives will go in certain respects. People have the right to decide for themselves whether to undergo surgery or participate in medical research. Unfortunately, however, applying this clear ideal in practice is not always straightforward.

In the case at hand, considerations of autonomy do not appear to tell you which victim to treat, at least assuming that both individuals at the scene want your help. But they do speak to *how* you should treat them. Respect for autonomy is usually taken to give individuals control over their medical records. We think that people should have the right to decide when and whether private personal information is released. In this case, that means that you need the pedestrian's permission to divulge his HIV status. But respect for autonomy is also usually taken to require that informed consent be obtained prior to any medical procedure. That means that the driver would need to be informed of the risk of HIV infection before you could examine her.

Therefore, respecting autonomy may sometimes lead to conflicting instructions. If the driver needs your help, then respect for her autonomy requires explaining the risk of HIV infection. But, respect for the pedestrian's autonomy does not permit you to divulge that information without his consent. Apparently, then, just as aiming for good consequences required us to make difficult comparisons (eg, between improving one patient's recovery time and alleviating another's pain), respect for autonomy also requires us to evaluate the importance of conflicting factors—in this case, the privacy right of the pedestrian versus the right to information of the driver.

Considerations of autonomy can also be more complex than they first appear. In this case, you might wonder whether the pedestrian and the driver are capable of giving or withholding consent. Agreeing to something requires understanding the matter under consideration. This is why we do not let children or people in impaired mental states enter into most legal contracts. If the victims are in shock, then are they really capable of rationally assessing their options and reaching an informed conclusion?

Or, suppose you explain to the driver that the pedestrian is HIV positive and that there is accordingly a small risk that she could contract HIV infection if you treat her. Most people overestimate the likelihood of transmission by an order of magnitude. Many people also still incorrectly view HIV infection as a death sentence. Although you might explain the truth to the driver, in this chaotic, hurried situation she may not have time to process and assess that information. If the driver refuses your help out of the doubly false belief that accepting it carries a high likelihood of a quick and agonizing death, then does that really count as an *informed* refusal? Does respecting a person's autonomy require accepting a judgment she hurriedly makes based on misinformation?

These are a few of the ethical issues that come up when thinking about how to respect the autonomy of the driver and the pedestrian. But the ideal of autonomy also applies to you. Like a patient, a physician also has certain rights to direct his or her own life. To this point, we have been assuming that your two choices are to stay with the pedestrian or to help the driver. But there is a third choice: you could leave both to minimize your exposure to HIV infection. Doing so would straightforwardly appear wrong if either individual was in urgent need of medical treatment. A marginal reduction in your risk of contracting HIV infection would clearly not justify putting either person's life in danger. Here, the bad consequences are clearly more significant than your right to make a decision for yourself. But suppose that both patients were medically stable, and so the only benefit you could provide would be psychological comfort to the pedestrian. In such a case, it is worth asking whether it might be permissible for you to withdraw from the situation to minimize your exposure to HIV infection should you want to. Of course, in making such a decision it would be important to ensure that your judgment was not being clouded by the stigma still associated with HIV infection.

Summary

In analyzing the scenario, we have looked at two guiding principles in ethics: (1) that when we act we should aim to produce the best outcome we can, and (2) that we should properly respect individual autonomy. With each principle, we have seen how what looks like a simple idea is actually quite complex. Determining what counts as a "better" outcome can be ethically challenging. First, we must weigh the relative significance of the two health states, and then we must assess whether any additional factors, such as fairness, equality, withdrawal of treatment, harm, or responsibility, affect the moral significance of those outcomes. Respect for autonomy directs us to let people decide for themselves how they will be treated. But, the privacy concerns of the pedestrian may conflict with the driver's claim to information about the risks to which she may be exposed. It is also not clear, ethically, what counts as legitimate consent. Does an impaired mental state or a lack of information give us license to discount someone's explicit wishes, on the grounds that they don't reflect her true will?

With so many factors in play, how should you go about making a decision? Different ethicists propose different methods, some of which will be explored in the later chapters of this book. However, the most common approach is recognizing that each factor potentially carries some ethical weight. To reach a decision, one must take into consideration all of the factors discussed previously, as well as (most likely) several more, and critically reflect on them. In the case at hand, which are legitimate ethical concerns? And then, looking at those legitimate concerns, where does the ethical weight seem to lie? Doing this can sometimes be fairly simple, although many situations are complex.

We have not yet directly answered the question with which we began: Should you remain with the pedestrian or leave him to treat the driver? That is because the case is seriously underdescribed. What you ought to do will depend on many factors that have not yet been specified: the details of the driver's condition, whether the pedestrian's bleeding is under control, whether the pedestrian consents to your revealing his HIV status, and so forth. But the type of analysis we have performed here is nevertheless important. The first step toward making an informed medical decision is to determine what medical possibilities are in play and then to use that to identify what further information you should gather. Similarly, the first step toward making an informed ethical decision is to determine what ethical factors are in play, and then to identify what further information you need. In addition, the list of considerations we have discussed—good consequences (including concerns of fairness, equality, withdrawal of treatment, harm, and responsibility) and autonomy (including issues related to consent, privacy, and competence)—can serve as a jumping off point for ethical analysis. Many ethical errors come from ignorance or from a failure to consider certain values. Keeping in mind these factors, along with the many additional ones that will be discussed later in this book, can help us to avoid making ethical mistakes.

COMPREHENSION QUESTIONS

1.1 The use of which of the following is most directly supported by considerations of autonomy?

A. Advance directives

B. Triage policies in emergency departments

C. Palliative care

D. Hospital ethics committees

1.2 Which of the following pieces of information would be most useful to you when aiming to produce the best outcome in a situation in which resources are limited?

A. Determining which patient has the most serious injuries

B. Determining which patient's injuries can be effectively treated

C. Determining what treatment plan each patient wants

D. Being aware of which patient has been waiting the longest

1.3 Ethical dilemmas can seem especially intractable when respecting autonomy conflicts with producing good consequences, because it is difficult to know how to compare such distinct values. Which of the following cases illustrates such a conflict?

A. A patient with Alzheimer disease requests the same medical treatment that she previously stated in an advance directive that she would not want.

B. A charitable organization has funds it can allocate to either distributing insecticide-treated bednets to guard against malaria or to school-based deworming programs.

C. An accident victim arrives in the emergency department, unconscious and in critical condition. A conservative approach would likely save her life but would leave her with permanent cognitive impairments. Aggressive treatment might prevent cognitive impairment, but it carries an increased risk of death.

D. A father refuses to authorize any vaccinations for his children.

ANSWERS

1.1 **A.** Advance directives allow a patient to express how he or she would like to be treated at a time when he or she may not be able to communicate his or her wishes. Thus, they allow patients to exercise their right to self-determination. Triage policies are generally designed to ensure that the most critical patients are treated first; therefore, their primary aim appears to produce good outcomes. Palliative care can be justified through autonomy-based considerations if a patient has requested such care, but it can also be justified through a concern for consequences, because relieving pain constitutes a good outcome. Hospital ethics committees exist to address ethical questions of all sorts, including those involving autonomy, good consequences, and other ethical values.

1.2 **B.** If our goal is to produce the best overall outcome, then it is critical that we first know which injuries we are able to treat. Which patient has the most serious injuries may be relevant to our choice, because we may decide to give extra weight to the needs of the most seriously injured. But that will only matter if we are actually able to treat the seriously injured. Similarly, considerations of fairness may dictate that, if all else is equal, we ought to focus on those who have been waiting longer—but only if their injuries are treatable. What treatment plan each patient wants is primarily a consideration of autonomy.

1.3 **D.** Parents are generally given the responsibility to make decisions for their children, so respect for a father's autonomy means giving him the right to determine what medical treatments his children will receive. However, in this case, the best outcome is one in which the children are protected against serious illnesses. Therefore, respect for autonomy suggests abiding by the father's wishes, whereas a concern for good consequences might mean looking for ways to vaccinate the children anyway (eg, pressuring the father, or advocating for a law mandating certain vaccinations). In the case of Alzheimer disease, we have a conflict primarily within autonomy: which expresses the true will of the patient, her earlier directive or her present request? The charitable organization must decide which outcome is better, saving a number of people from a potentially deadly illness or protecting a much larger group from the effects of parasitic worms. Finally, the case in the emergency department seems difficult primarily because the consequences of aggressive treatment are uncertain.

KEY POINTS

▶ The first step in making an informed ethical decision is to determine what ethical factors are potentially relevant.

▶ A number of ethical values, including a concern for consequences and respect for autonomy, are relevant to the case provided.

▶ A concern for consequences directs us to do what will result in the best overall outcome. Many people believe that factors such as fairness, equality, withdrawal of treatment, harm, and responsibility can influence how good or bad an outcome is.

▶ Respect for autonomy directs us to allow people to make certain decisions for themselves about how their lives will go.

▶ Even if we do not have a precise "recipe" for determining the right course of action, keeping in mind a list of ethical factors that are potentially relevant can improve ethical decision-making.

REFERENCES

Beauchamp TL, Childress JF. *Principles of Biomedical Ethics*. 7th ed. New York, NY. Oxford University Press; 2012.

Zalta EN, ed. *The Stanford Encyclopedia of Philosophy*.Stanford, CA. Center for the Study of Language and Information, Stanford University. http://plato.stanford.edu. Published 2014. Accessed June 2014.

WS is a third-year medical student on his core clerkship in pediatrics. He has missed several mandatory orientation activities for the clerkship and did not attend several of the formal teaching sessions that are held weekly at his assigned site. In the process of collecting midclerkship feedback, it was revealed that only a few residents and attending physicians had worked with WS. He had told his residents on the inpatient service that he was leaving Thursday afternoons to attend his preceptor's clinic; however, it became apparent that the preceptor never had met WS. When WS was confronted with his attendance issues, he admitted that he was taking days off to take care for his sick child (WS is married with 2 small children; his wife works full-time). He explained that he did not attend his mandatory clerkship activities because he believed that his absence would not be noticed. Similar behaviors and unexcused absences were noted on his previous clerkship rotation of psychiatry. This was verbally shared to the psychiatry clerkship director, but no written documentation of this behavior exists and no one specifically addressed WS on his absences.

▶ What are the breaches in professionalism exhibited by WS?
▶ Although WS is not directly responsible for patient care, why is his pattern of behavior important to note?

ANSWERS TO CASE 2:
Professionalism

Summary: A medical student on his required pediatric rotation has had a pattern of not meeting obligations to attending mandatory activities during the clerkship and was dishonest about his whereabouts. This behavior was apparently observed in his last rotation, but there was no documentation or action taken.

- **Breaches in professionalism:** WS has demonstrated a pattern of not attending mandatory activities in his role as a medical trainee. In addition, he has demonstrated a lack of integrity because he has not been truthful and straightforward regarding his absences.

- **Why this pattern of behavior important to note:** There is evidence demonstrating that certain behaviors exhibited by trainees early in medical education are predictive of unprofessional behavior later in the physician's career; therefore, it is crucial that these behaviors are identified, documented, and remediated.

ANALYSIS

Objectives

1. Describe the meaning of profession and characteristics of a professional.
2. List the fundamental principles of medical professionalism.
3. Describe the importance of patterns of unacceptable behaviors exhibited early in the learner/trainee's medical career.

APPROACH TO:
Professionalism

"Profession" and "professional" come from the Latin word *professio*, which means a public declaration with the force of a promise. The Roman physician Scribonius defined professionalism as "a commitment to compassion or clemency in the relief of suffering." He linked it to the act and the tradition of professing inherent in the Hippocratic oath.

Professions are groups that declare in a public way that their members promise to act or behave in certain ways for social benefit, and the society accepts the profession, expecting it to serve an important societal role. Therefore, a profession has a contract with society.

Failure for the member to act or behave in expected ways may cause the group and society to discipline those who fail to do so. The profession usually issues a code of ethics that states standards by which its members can be judged. Members of a profession regulate themselves. The traditional professions are medicine, law, education, and the clergy.

The hallmarks of a profession include the following:

- Competence in a specialized body of knowledge and skill

- An acknowledgment of specific duties and responsibilities toward the individuals it serves and toward society

- The right to train, admit, discipline, and dismiss its members for failure to sustain competence or observe the duties and responsibilities

Professionalism in a physician requires that the practitioner strive for excellence in several areas (Table 2–1).

The professional behavior of physicians and trainees has received increasing attention from medical educators, the medical community as a whole, and society at large. There is general agreement among medical educators that professionalism must be taught and evaluated as a specific topic. In the past, professionalism as a subject was largely implicit and primarily based on modeling, but it is now required that professionalism must be taught in medical education. In 1999, the Accreditation Council for Graduate Medical Education implemented 6 general core competencies in which each resident is evaluated across all specialties during training. It is expected that all residents attain minimum competency prior to graduation. One of the 6 core competencies is professionalism.

In 2002, the American Board of Internal Medicine Foundation, the American College of Physician Foundation, and the European Federation of Internal Medicine published *Medical Professionalism in the New Millennium: A Physician Charter*. Subsequently, most of the specialty and subspecialty groups in US medicine have endorsed the charter. The professionalism charter lays out 3 fundamental principles of professionalism as the following:

- **Primacy of patient welfare:** This principle focuses on altruism, trust, and patient interest.

- **Patient autonomy:** This principle incorporates honesty with patients with the need to educate and empower patients to make appropriate medical decisions.

Table 2–1 • CHARACTERISTICS OF PROFESSIONALISM OF PHYSICIANS	
Altruism	A physician is obligated to attend to the best interest of patients rather than his or her self-interest.
Accountability	Physicians are accountable to their patients, to society on issues of public health, and to their profession.
Excellence	Physicians are obligated to make a commitment to life-long learning.
Duty	A physician should be available and responsive when "on call," accepting a commitment to service within the profession and the community.
Honor and integrity	Physicians should be committed to being fair, truthful, and straightforward in their interactions with patients and the profession.
Respect for others	A physician should demonstrate respect for patients and their families, other physicians, medical trainees, and all members of the medical team regardless of role and background.

- **Social justice:** This principle addresses physician societal contract and distributive justice (ie, considering available resources and the needs of all patients while taking care of an individual).

The charter lists 10 categories of responsibilities of physicians with regard to their professionalism:

1. Maintain professional competence

2. Be honest with patients

3. Respect patient confidentiality

4. Avoid inappropriate relations with patients

5. Advance scientific knowledge

6. Fulfill the obligations imposed by membership of the profession

7. Improve the quality of care

8. Improve access to care

9. Promote the just distribution of resources

10. Maintain trust by managing conflicts of interest

This increasing emphasis on professionalism in medical education over the last 20 years coincides with increasing evidence that unprofessional behaviors in medical school are associated with future problems, including subsequent disciplinary action by state medical boards. A 2005 study examined individuals who graduated from 3 US medical schools from 1970 to 1999 and found that 235 had been disciplined by a US state medical board between 1990 and 2003. Two control groups were selected from the same graduating class ensuring that one of the controls practiced in the same specialty as the disciplined physician. Information was gathered on student grades, standardized test scores, demographic characteristics, and unprofessional behavior, including information from letters of recommendation, evaluations, and letters from the deans. Results of the study showed that students who exhibited unprofessional behavior in medical school were 3 times more likely to be disciplined by a medical board than those students who did not have behavioral issues in medical school. Particularly, the behavior code of "severe irresponsibility"—meaning the documentation of irresponsible behavior occurring in the files at least 3 times—had an odds ratio of 8.5 and the code of "diminished capacity for improvement"—meaning a lack of improvement despite counseling—had an odds ratio of 3.1. Attitudes of apathy and poor initiative in medical school also correlated with later disciplinary actions.

The need to teach professionalism and the need for medical professionals to demonstrate professionalism is undeniable. Explicit discussions of professionalism and a mandate to meet all expectations throughout medical training and beyond have replaced the "hidden curriculum," whereby medical trainees were expected to learn proper professionalism behaviors through observation and role modeling. It is imperative that society be able to rely on the professionalisms of medical personnel entrusted with their care and safety.

COMPREHENSION QUESTIONS

2.1 An obstetrics/gynecology resident was involved in a double breech vaginal delivery during her rotation. She was very excited about her recent clinical experience and shared her thoughts via social media, reporting that she "had an awesome day at work today…was in on a vaginal delivery of BREECH TWINS!!! Probably won't see too many of those for sure!" Her social media profile denotes that she is a resident physician at Hospital X.

Why is this resident's action a breach of professionalism?

A. Physicians should never use social media because it violates the social contract with the public.

B. Her post may have violated patient privacy because it provided sufficient information to identify the patient.

C. Her post demonstrates an inappropriate relationship with the patient.

D. Her post clearly demonstrates that her supervising physician violated the duty owed to the patient.

2.2 Which of the following medical student characteristics is the most predictive of future disciplinary action by a state medical board?

A. Younger age at entrance of medical school

B. Disadvantaged social economic status

C. Irresponsible behavior in medical school

D. Low USMLE step 1 and 2 scores

ANSWERS

2.1 **B.** Just as in the hospital or ambulatory setting, patient privacy and confidentiality must be protected at all times, especially on social media and social networking websites. These sites have the potential to be viewed by many people, and any breaches in confidentiality could be harmful to the patient and in violation of federal privacy laws, such as Health Insurance Portability and Accountability Act (HIPAA). Although physicians may discuss their experiences in nonclinical settings, they should never provide any information that could be used to identify patients. Physicians should never mention patient room numbers, refer to them by code names, or post their picture. If others outside the hospital were able to view pictures of patients, such an occurrence may constitute a serious HIPAA violation. Because a breech vaginal delivery of twins is an uncommon event and the resident is known to work at a particular hospital, this disclosure of information can easily identify the patient. This is a clear violation of professionalism.

2.2 **C.** Numerous studies have demonstrated that students who exhibit unprofessional behavior in medical school are 3 times more likely to be disciplined than those who have not to undergo disciplinary action.

KEY POINTS

▶ Professionalism is no longer implicit in the training of physicians; it is explicitly taught and evaluated as a core competence is mandated in medical education.

▶ Problems in unprofessional behavior exhibited early in medical training are predictive of unprofessional behavior later in residency and in practice.

REFERENCES

Accreditation Council for Graduate Medical Education. *General Competencies*. Chicago, IL: ACGME; 1999. http://www.acgme.org/outcome/comp/comFull.asp#5. Accessed March 20, 2014.

Cruess RL, Cruess SR, Steinert Y. *Teaching Medical Professionalism*. Cambridge University Press; 2009.

Jonsen AR, Braddock CH, Edwards KA. Professionalism: ethical topics in medicine. Published 1998. http://depts.washington.edu/bioethx/topics/profes.html. Accessed March 15, 2014.

Kirk LM. Professionalism in medicine: definitions and considerations for teaching. *Baylor Univ Med Cntr Proceed*. 2007;20:13-16.

Medical Professionalism Project. Medical professionalism in the new millennium: a physician charter. ABIM Foundation. ACP Foundation. European Federation of Internal Medicine. *Ann Intern Med*. 2002;136:243-246.

Papadakis MA, Teharani A, Banach MA, et al. Disciplinary action by medical boards and prior behavior in medical school. *N Engl J Med*. 2005;353:2673-2682.

MA is a 70-year-old woman who came to your local hospital emergency department with her daughter after she became dizzy and lost her balance at an afternoon family function. She has had a 1-month history of weight loss, a feeling that her stomach seemed larger to her and "full," and increasing abdominal pain that has now become excruciating. She had all but stopped eating and drinking due to poor appetite because she was fearful doing so would make her pain worse. She had previously been healthy and active but had stopped engaging in outside activities. MA's diagnostic evaluation included computed tomography, which revealed a large pancreatic mass suggestive of widely metastatic disease to her liver and peritoneum. She was admitted to the hospital for further evaluation and for symptomatic management. Biopsy confirmed stage 4 widely metastatic adenocarcinoma of the pancreas. She was given a poor prognosis but was given the options of palliative interventions and participation in a phase 2 clinical trial. She was discharged from the hospital on a narcotic pain medication regimen. The next day, she made a same-day appointment with her primary care physician (PCP). At the appointment, MA told her PCP that she no longer wished to live if she was going to die anyway and asked her PCP to either inject her with a "lethal dose" or give her a prescription for enough medication to "just get this over with." She told her PCP that she was ready to die and that there was nothing further to discuss.

▶ What are the guiding principles of medical ethics related to end-of-life care?
▶ What legal principles guide physician conduct when patients request to end their lives?
▶ What strategies can physicians use to address potential conflicts between the law and principles of medical ethics?

ANSWERS TO CASE 3:

Jurisprudence

Summary: An elderly woman who had been in previously excellent health has had a 1-month history of excruciating pain, difficulty eating, weight loss, and dizziness. She has been diagnosed with stage 4 widely metastatic adenocarcinoma of the pancreas. She has a poor prognosis but was given the options of palliative interventions and participation in a phase 2 clinical trial. She was discharged from the hospital on a narcotic pain medication regimen. At the follow-up appointment with her PCP, the patient stated she no longer wished to live and asked her PCP to inject her with a "lethal dose" of some medication. She indicated that she was ready to die and that there was nothing further to discuss.

- **Guiding principles from medical ethics related to end-of-life care:** The guiding principles are the physician's dual responsibilities of (1) doing no harm, and (2) relieving suffering. With the goal of medicine to treat illness and promote health, death as an end in itself is traditionally equated with harm. Therefore, according to traditional medical ethics reasoning, deliberately causing death is unethical. Medical ethics also recognizes patient autonomy, but that autonomy is limited when it is inconsistent with the physician's fiduciary responsibility to the patient (eg, physician acts contrary to his or her ethical responsibility by intentionally causing death).

- **Legal principles:** Most states do not have laws permitting physicians to assist in a patient's request to end his or her life. In these states, assisting patients in ending their lives may subject the physician to regulatory discipline by the licensing authority, ethics sanctions by professional organizations, and criminal prosecution. However, beginning with Oregon, a small number of states, including also Washington and Vermont, have explicitly legalized the practice and ballot initiatives and other steps to legalize the practice in additional states are occurring. Though these laws protect physicians from actions by licensing bodies and criminal prosecution in the applicable state, the individual may still be subject to ethics action by professional organizations.

- **Strategies physicians use to address potential conflicts between the law and principles of medical ethics:** The physician must understand the motivation, concerns, hopes, and fears behind the patient's request. Doing so may allow the physician to work with the patient to generate alternative approaches that respond to the patient's core considerations and autonomy interest. Physicians in states permitting physician-assisted suicide (PAS) may grant the patient's request but are not ethically or legally obligated to do so.

ANALYSIS

Objectives

1. Understand the ethical framework surrounding physician roles and responsibilities in end-of-life care.

2. Learn the legal framework guiding decisions about end-of-life care and, specifically, PAS.

3. Distinguish between death-causing end-of-life interventions, most particularly euthanasia and PAS and other interventions that may cause death including palliative care and palliative sedation.

4. Appreciate the complexities surrounding ethical and legal analysis and practice in providing end-of-life care such that the discourse continues to evolve.

Considerations

This case illustrates how medicine and law approach end-of-life decisions from distinct theoretical positions. Medicine—particularly organized medicine—approaches end-of-life decision-making from the standpoint of the professional and ethical framework of doing no harm and alleviating suffering while also considering patient autonomy. The law approaches end-of-life decision-making from the standpoint of the relative rights of the individual balanced against the well-established right of the state to preserve life. These starting points lead to divergent conclusions in how to approach PAS, as well as using a lethal dose of prescription medication at the request of a terminally ill patient, so that the patient could end his or her life. From the standpoint of organizations such as the American Medical Association (AMA), this practice is incompatible with established professional and ethical standards. From the legal standpoint, this practice could be acceptable provided that individual states determine that a balance between individual and state rights warrants legalizing the practice through the legislative and judicial processes.

APPROACH TO:

Jurisprudence

DEFINITIONS

EUTHANASIA: The administration of a lethal agent by another person to relieve intolerable and incurable suffering.

JURISPRUDENCE: The science of law that functions to ascertain the principles on which legal rules are based to classify those rules in their proper order, to show the relation in which they stand to one another, and to settle the manner in which new or doubtful cases should be brought under the appropriate rules.

PHYSICIAN-ASSISTED SUICIDE: The practice in which a terminally ill patient requests a prescription of a life-ending dose of medication from a physician, and the physician provides the patient with the prescription to obtain the medication for use at a future time. The physician does not administer the medication.

CLINICAL APPROACH

End-of-life care raises many ethical considerations. Many of these topics, including informed consent or refusal, autonomy, and nonmaleficence, are implicated in a host of medical treatment settings. However, end-of-life care has been the subject of significant attention from the medical ethics and legal communities. In addition, in the case of PAS, there is significant divergence in the analysis between legal approaches and organized medicine. In this chapter, we begin with a discussion of the traditional principles of medical ethics informing end-of-life care, followed by an introduction to the evolution of legal thought related to end-of-life decisions. Finally, this chapter addresses how, in practice, physicians may bridge this divide to provide sound care to patients who are terminally ill .

In medical ethics terms, the duty of the physician to the patient has historically included both positive and negative components. *Primum non nocere*, or first do no harm, is the negative expression of physician responsibility. But the responsibilities to restore health, alleviate suffering, or both are also key components of the profession. With advances in medical care, particularly life-sustaining care, there are situations in which the positive and negative tenets come into conflict. For example, aggressive efforts, such as in the case of MA, to prolong life in the setting of advanced malignancy may lead to greater suffering due to the adverse events of cancer treatment.

Against this backdrop, modern medical ethics also recognizes the broad autonomy interests of patients, such as MA, to refuse any and all medical interventions, provided the patient is competent to make this decision—in other words, she is capable of providing informed refusal. Under the principle of autonomy, patients have the right to be free from unwanted medical interventions, even when refusing these interventions may lead to death sooner than if the interventions were initiated or continued. So, in the case of MA, whether or not treatment would extend her life significantly over palliative care, autonomy would nonetheless permit her to refuse treatment so long as she had the requisite ability (capacity) to give informed refusal.

However, there are also limits on patient autonomy. Physicians have no ethical obligation to provide care that is futile. The AMA defines futility as "care that, in [physicians'] best professional judgment, will not have a reasonable chance of benefiting their patients." Restated, this means that patients should not be given treatments simply because they demand them. There are also limits on patient autonomy regarding the ability to control their deaths. From the standpoint of medical ethics (and consistent with universal legal prohibition in all US states and territories), physicians are prohibited from ending a patient's life or performing euthanasia. Euthanasia is broadly defined by AMA as "the administration of a lethal agent by another person to a patient for relieving the patient's intolerable and incurable suffering." This prohibition draws on a variety of ethical concepts, including nonmaleficence and respect for persons and life. The AMA classifies euthanasia as an ethical problem in itself, terming it "fundamentally incompatible with the physician's role as healer" but also cites concerns that euthanasia would be "difficult or impossible to control, and would pose serious societal risks." These latter rationales seem more practical and cautionary than ethical in themselves.

By contrast to euthanasia, PAS, also termed physician-assisted death, is a practice by which physicians assist patients who are terminally ill in obtaining lethal means to end their lives but do not actually administer those means. In practice, PAS is characterized by a physician giving a patient medication (eg, barbiturates) intended to be lethal. From an ethical perspective, PAS might be seen as less ethically problematic because it still requires the patient's independent action to cause death. In addition, proponents of PAS argue that it is respectful of autonomy given that its practice is, at the time of publication, limited to patients who are terminally ill and that patients themselves have the best self-knowledge and awareness about when the balance between prolonging life and relieving suffering tips in favor of ending life.

However, these arguments address the fundamental question of the legitimacy of the medical profession's intentional contribution to causing a patient's death, which has been a concern of the AMA. As such, the AMA opinion on PAS mirrors its position on euthanasia, classifying the practice as "fundamentally incompatible with the physician's role as healer." Framed in terms of the positive obligations of physicians, the AMA instead guides physicians to stand by their patients at the end of life and continue to provide care, including emotional support, comfort care, adequate pain control, and respect for patient autonomy. Although the AMA opinion considers its prohibition on PAS consistent with respect for patient autonomy, as above, the prohibition is clearly an imposition on the autonomy interest of the terminally ill patient, such as MA, to control the timing and manner of her death.

Several additional concepts warrant the introduction of a discussion of end-of-life care. First, the notion that physicians can never contribute to or hasten death would be overstated. The perhaps most widespread example of this principle is the doctrine of secondary effect, or the administration of palliative interventions that, while alleviating symptoms such as pain or air hunger in the case of morphine, also predictably lead to central nervous system and respiratory depression that secondarily hasten death. This practice is well accepted within clinical medicine, but it is also the subject of analyses in the medical ethics literature regarding whether the doctrine is substantively distinct from other interventions that hasten death such as PAS. Finally, terminal, palliative sedation is the sedation of a patient who is terminally ill to the point of unconsciousness to relieve suffering, and it is generally accepted as ethically permissible in practice, including by the AMA. As for the doctrine of secondary effect, it is beyond the scope of this chapter to further elucidate if there are and whether any distinctions justify treating palliative sedation to unconsciousness any differently than PAS beyond raising the question.

From the standpoint of the law, jurisprudence as described by *Black's Law Dictionary* is "the science of law, namely, that science which has for its function to ascertain the principles on which legal rules are based, so as not only to classify those rules in their proper order, and show the relation in which they stand to one another, but also to settle the manner in which new or doubtful cases should be brought under the appropriate rules." From the legal perspective, the permissibility or entitlement of MA's request from her physician that she either euthanized (inject me request) or have access to lethal means to end her own life (PAS) begin with an analysis of the central legal concepts.

From a legal perspective, the 1990 US Supreme Court decision in the *Cruzan v Director* case set the stage for how legal analyses of individual rights regarding end-of-life care would progress. Although this case is cited for the proposition that individuals have broad rights of autonomy to make decisions about their care, including the withdrawal of life-prolonging or sustaining care, the fundamental analysis in the case rests not on medical reasoning and ethics but on the relative balance between individual autonomy as derived from notions of privacy, on the one hand, and the state's historical well-defined legitimacy and interest in the preservation of life, on the other. In essence, the Court decided that the patient and subject of the case, Nancy Cruzan, a young woman in a persistent vegetative state following a motor vehicle collision, had the right to autonomy, including withdrawal of nutrition and hydration, but that Missouri, where she was hospitalized, had the right to require clear and convincing evidence that she would have wanted this treatment withdrawn as an expression of the state's countervailing interest in the preservation of life.

The legal—as opposed to ethical—prohibition on euthanasia in every US jurisdiction, then, easily flows from this well-recognized legitimate state interest of preserving life—in this instance, by prohibiting one private citizen from killing another citizen. Therefore, MA, both legally as well as ethically, has no claim that she has an entitlement to be euthanized by her—or any—physician. The bright-line nature of this prohibition on killing has led to criminal prosecution of physicians who have participated in active euthanasia (eg, Jacob "Jack" Kevorkian in Michigan).

However, the legal framework set forth in the *Cruzan* case regarding the appropriate analysis of individual versus state interests in end-of-life care left the door open for the next logical question. If patients have broad autonomy interests regarding withdrawal of life-sustaining care, then do patients who are terminally ill have the right to control the timing and manner of their own deaths? This question was the subject of the 1997 US Supreme Court companion cases of *Washington v Glucksberg* and *Vacco v Quill*. Both cases sought to assert through the complementary legal concepts of due process (liberty interest) and equal protection, respectively. Together these cases argued that laws prohibiting physicians from prescribing lethal doses of medication for their terminally ill patients violated the US Constitution.

In issuing opinions in the two cases the same day, the US Supreme Court majority opined that the historical state interest in preserving life coupled with the lack of an historical individual right did not support the challenge to the law in *Washington v Glucksberg* and, similarly, that the argument in *Vacco v Quill* failed to raise facts, giving rise to a finding that the New York law at issue in the case was unconstitutional. But writing for the Court, Justice Rehnquist in *Washington v Glucksberg* did acknowledge that a national debate was in process regarding PAS and that the debate should continue. In other words, although the Court found that the plaintiffs in the cases had no affirmative right that outweighed the state interest expressed in the Washington and New York laws, the laws permitting PAS as enacted by state legislative processes could also be constitutionally permissible. These 2 sentences paved the way for legislative efforts and ballot initiatives in a number of states permitting PAS. Oregon was the first state to enact and implement legislation, known as the Death With Dignity Act. Notwithstanding concerns about slippery slopes, overuse, and discriminatory application, over more than a decade of practice, the number of deaths under the Act remains small in terms of annual deaths in the state. In addition, a significant number of individuals who obtain prescriptions under the Act either delay using them or never use them, deciding instead to die of their underlying illness. Following Oregon, the states of Washington and Vermont have also passed laws permitting PAS. Montana has case law permitting PAS but not a statute.

Bringing the law to bear on the case of MA, determining whether she has the legal ability to receive a prescription for a lethal dose of medication from her physician depends on where she lives. Even in a jurisdiction that recognizes PAS, as included within the lawful practice of medicine, MA's right to the lethal prescription is not absolute. As in the *Cruzan* case, the state may impose limitations on her right to ensure that it adequately safeguards its interest in preserving life. These safeguards could include various measures such as second opinions, registration of prescriptions, multiple documented requests, and waiting periods.

In the discussion of the legal reasoning supporting local (individual state) enactment of laws permitting PAS, we have not considered the position of the physician vis a vis the law. There is little question that the AMA's opposition to PAS, as expressed in its amicus brief to the court, was known by the US Supreme Court in its consideration of the PAS companion cases; moreover, the fact that the largest organization of US physicians opposed PAS could only have weighed against the plaintiffs' claim that they had a protected right to the practice. On the other hand, now that a small number of states allow the practice and allow physicians in those states to participate in PAS, individual physicians are faced with whether and under what circumstances they will or will not grant their patients' requests for PAS. It is worth noting that not all physicians belong to the AMA and those who do not are not constrained by the ethics opinions of the AMA. Individual physicians themselves may feel that patient autonomy interests and humanity broadly justify PAS in the setting of terminal illness. Others may feel that the practice is sometimes warranted but that requests for PAS require additional careful consideration, safeguards, or both.

Returning to the case of MA helps illustrate this point. Suppose that MA does live in a jurisdiction that permits PAS and that MA's PCP believes that it would be ethically permissible to write a lethal prescription for MA given that she is terminally ill; this is only true if the PCP is convinced that this is *really* what MA wants, that is, that the decision reflects autonomy as guarded by an assessment of MA's ability to provide informed consent for the practice. In this scenario, MA's PCP may undertake additional questioning of MA or evaluate her for potential causes of altered decision-making. For example, is MA depressed? MA has stopped participating in activities she used to have interest in. Knowing that patients with cancer may become depressed and are then prone to making more restrictive decisions about their care and the future, MA's PCP may request a psychiatric consultation. The PCP might also ask that MA come to meet with her with a family member of loved one to have a more robust discussion of the decision to ensure that the PCP is comfortable that participating in PAS is ethically justified.

In summary, the case of MA serves as an illustration of the complex issues that arise in medical practice because medicine is practiced in a societal context. Moreover, clinical responsibilities, duties, and ethics—as in the case of a terminally ill patient like MA requesting to die—may come in conflict with legal principles and established law. Although it is critical for physicians to be aware of the law governing medical practice in the jurisdiction(s) in which they practice and the resources available to assist in navigating legal considerations, it is similarly imperative that physicians understand that their primary responsibility is to the ethical and competent care of their patients. Where the law appears to dictate that a physician act in a clinically counterintuitive manner, the physician must not act without careful consideration, employing available consultative resources, of alternative courses of action that meet legal requirements while also satisfying clinical and ethical obligations. Finally, when a law is permissive rather than prescriptive, such as PAS laws that permit but do not require physicians to issue prescriptions in the practice of PAS, physicians who have individual ethical objections to the practice need not compromise their morals but rather can help the patient, for example, by providing referrals to other providers.

COMPREHENSION QUESTIONS

3.1 Which of the following is illegal in all US jurisdictions?

A. PAS

B. Palliative sedation

C. Escalating doses of narcotics for analgesia when respiratory depression and death result

D. Euthanasia

E. Withdrawal of life support in a patient with a nonterminal illness

3.2 Ethical principles about decisions on end-of-life care include all of the following *except*:

A. *Primum non nocere*

B. Autonomy

C. Futility

D. Nonmaleficence

E. Due process

3.3 At the time of publication, in which of the following jurisdictions is PAS prohibited?

A. Massachusetts

B. Montana

C. Oregon

D. Vermont

E. Washington

ANSWERS

3.1 **D**. Euthanasia, also called active mercy killing, is illegal in every US jurisdiction. It is permissible in The Netherlands. Euthanasia is distinguished from PAS as follows. In euthanasia, the physician directly causes the patient's death; in cases of PAS, the physician provides a prescription to the patient to obtain a lethal dose of medication that the patient self-administers. Competent patients have the right to refuse all care, including life-sustaining care, even if such refusal will cause certain death and even if the illness is reversible. Finally, the principle of secondary effect refers to the permissible use of medications, such as morphine, in sufficient doses to treat suffering, even if those doses may secondarily hasten death.

3.2 **E**. All of the answers refer to ethical considerations with the exception of due process, which is a concept in constitutional law.

3.3 **A**. At the time of publication, Oregon, Washington, and Vermont all have legalized PAS by statute. Montana has case law allowing the practice. These are the only 4 states authorizing the practice in any way as of the time of publication. New Mexico has a case law that allows the practice, though it is currently being appealed.

KEY POINTS

▶ Patients have broadly recognized autonomy to refuse life sustaining or prolonging interventions, but access to legally permissible PAS is limited in the most US jurisdictions.

▶ The AMA opposes the practice of PAS.

▶ PAS is an issue that highlights the potential for conflict between ethics as articulated by organized medicine and legally permissible conduct.

▶ Physicians are never obligated to participate in PAS, even in jurisdictions in which the practice is legally permissible.

▶ Euthanasia, or active mercy killing, is illegal in all US jurisdictions. However, euthanasia must be distinguished from other interventions that are permissible and may secondarily cause death such as palliation and withdrawal of life-prolonging/sustaining care in cases of futility or competent patient choice.

REFERENCES

American Medical Association (AMA). Opinions 2.035 (1994), 2.20, 2.21, 2.211 (1996) and 2.201 (2008). In: AMA. AMA Code of Medical Ethics. Chicago, IL: AMA; 2008. http://www.ama-assn.org/ama /pub/physician-resources/medical-ethics/code-medical-ethics.page? Accessed June 7, 2014.

Black's Law Dictionary. 6th ed. St. Paul, MN: West Publishing Company; 1990.

Brendel RW, Epstein L, Cassem NH. Care at the end of life. In: Stern TA, Rosenbaum JF, Fava M, Biederman J, Rauch SL, eds. *Massachusetts General Hospital Comprehensive Clinical Psychiatry*. Philadelphia, PA: Mosby/ Elsevier; 2008:821-827.

Brendel RW, Schouten R, Levenson JL. Legal issues. In: Levenson JL, ed. *American Psychiatric Publishing Textbook of Psychosomatic Medicine: Psychiatric Care of the Medically Ill*. 2nd ed. Washington, DC: American Psychiatric Publishing; 2011:19-32.

Hall K, ed. *The Oxford Companion to the Supreme Court of the United States*. 2nd ed. Oxford: Oxford University Press; 2005.

Quill TE, Lo B, Brock DW. Palliative options of last resort—a comparison of voluntarily stopping eating and drinking, terminal sedation, physician-assisted suicide, and voluntary active euthanasia. JAMA. 1997;278:2099-2104.

A 24-year-old, third-year medical student married for 1 year comes into the student health clinic for a routine physical examination, including a pelvic examination and Pap smear. During the course of the examination, the nurse practitioner performing the examination obtains the Pap smear and also obtains cervical DNA assays for *Chlamydia trachomatis* (chlamydia) and *Niesseria gonorrhoeae* (gonorrhea). Other than contraceptive counseling and lifestyle counseling, the visit is unremarkable. Two weeks later, the patient receives a call from the clinic nurse indicating that the Pap smear was normal and human papillomavirus was negative. However, the cervical assay for chlamydia was positive. She is instructed to come in for treatment and to notify her sexual partners so they can also be treated. The nurse explains that "public health authorities" have been notified of her infection according to state regulations. The patient is very concerned that her husband will be contacted.

▶ Did the patient have a right to be informed prior to the examination that the chlamydia assay was going to be collected?
▶ Can the patient refuse to allow the student health clinic to release the results to the public health department?

ANSWERS TO CASE 4:

Public Health Ethics

Summary: A 24-year-old married student came into a student health clinic for a routine pelvic examination and pap smear. An assay for gonorrhea and chlamydia was performed. The patient was told that the public health authority has been notified and the patient is advised of need for treatment and her responsibility to notify her sexual partners so that they may also be treated.

- **Patient's right to be informed:** As with other testing, screening of sexually transmitted infections (STIs) should be voluntary and undertaken only with the patient's understanding of what testing is planned. The patient should be informed that she will be tested unless she declines; be provided with oral or written information about the infections she is being tested for and the meanings and courses of action for positive and negative results; and be given an opportunity to ask questions and to opt out of screening if she chooses. Consent for screening and diagnostic tests are generally incorporated in the patient's informed consent for medical care documentation and a separate consent for STI screening is typically not needed.

- **Can the patient prevent notification of the public health department?** The patient cannot prevent the student health center from notifying the public health authority of her positive result. Health information otherwise protected under the Health Insurance Portability and Accountability Act may be disclosed without patient authorization to public health authorities for the purpose of preventing or controlling disease, injury, or disability. Syphilis, gonorrhea, chlamydia, chancroid, HIV infection, and AIDS are currently reportable in each state. HIV and STI reports are kept strictly confidential.

ANALYSIS

Objectives

1. Describe the core functions of public health and the 10 essential services of public health.

2. Differentiate the principles of public health ethics and biomedical ethical values.

3. Understand the patient's right to privacy and confidentiality of information and exceptions when high likelihood of significant harm may develop.

4. Apply select principles of the ethical practice of public health to clinical scenarios.

Considerations

The patient in the scenario is a 24-year-old student who has a legitimate concern about the privacy of her personal relationships and the impact of a disclosure of her protected health information on her primary relationship. The patient's concerns should be handled with sensitivity and the clinician's approach should encourage the patient's full participation in a treatment plan from an informed point of view. The student health center's clinical staff members have a duty to provide the patient with prompt and effective treatment. However, clinicians should also provide emotional care in handling the apparent conflict the discovery of her infection presents. The USPSTF recommendations for screening for chlamydia and gonorrhea from 2014 recommend referral to "high-intensity behavioral counseling for patients with current or recent STIs" (www.uspreventiveservicestaskforce.org/uspstf/uspsstds.htm) and highlight the importance of post-test counseling as an opportunity to educate about risk-reduction strategies even among patients who test negative for an STI.

Clinical staff can be instrumental in putting the infection in perspective by explaining the prevalence of chlamydia in the patient's age cohort, the ease of transmission with sexual contact, and the likelihood that partners can be infected without showing signs or symptoms. Providing the facts about infection, treatment, and the importance of regular screening for sexually active adults should be brief, as patients receiving a diagnosis of an STI may not be receptive to retaining information because of the complex emotional factors in play. A better use of the limited time with the patient may include providing her with culturally and linguistically relevant resources she can consult at her leisure, such as websites, mobile phone applications, or pamphlets, as would informing her of numbers she can call to follow-up with questions.

Clinical staff can also assist the patient in preparing for the disclosure of the infection to her partner(s) by preparing through role play, scripting, or planning. Partners may be notified of potential exposure and treated through a variety of means, including:

- **Traditional patient referral:** The patient informs the partner(s) of infection and the partner must seek access to treatment.

- **Bring your own partner referral:** The patient informs the partner(s) of infection and brings them to the clinic for treatment.

- **Provider-assisted referral:** The provider or staff contacts the partner(s) for treatment and encourages the partner(s) to come in for treatment and also to disclose other potentially exposed individuals who may need to be notified. Confidentiality is maintained during this process.

- **Disease intervention specialist (DIS) referral:** A specially trained health worker (DIS) interviews the patient with the STI, performs a confidential contact investigation of the patient's identified partner(s), investigates partner(s) additional contacts, and provides prevention counseling and confidential treatment referral for all identified contacts to interrupt the chain of transmission. DIS referral for chlamydia infection is not available in all jurisdictions.

- **Expedited partner therapy:** Either the patient or a public health worker delivers the medications or a prescription from the clinic to the partner. Note that expedited partner therapy is not allowable in all states. Clinicians should check the laws and regulations in their public health jurisdiction.

It is vital that clinical staff assess the situation for possibility of aggression toward the patient upon disclosure and assist the patient in seeking services for

intimate partner violence if this is a possibility. Clinical staff can ease concerns about the involvement of external parties by collaboratively working with the patient to identify all her contacts and refer them to care. Follow-up on cases is vital, and clinical staff must be vigilant to ensure that all contacts are referred for care. Those not contacted may need to be referred to the public health authority for follow-up according to that jurisdiction's surveillance regulations.

APPROACH TO:
Public Health Ethics

DEFINITIONS

ASSESSMENT: A core public health function, assessment is the regular collection, analysis, and sharing of information about health conditions, risks, and resources in a community.

ASSURANCE: The third core public health function, assurance focuses on the availability of necessary health services through the community. It includes maintaining the ability of both public health agencies and private providers to manage day-to-day operations and the capacity to respond to critical situations and emergencies.

INTERDEPENDENCE: Interdependence is the belief that individuals have optimal health by living in community with other people; the health of an individual cannot be viewed as distinct from the health of the community.

POLICY DEVELOPMENT: The second core function of public health, policy development uses information gathered during assessment to develop local and state health policies and to direct resources toward those policies.

CLINICAL APPROACH

Core Functions of Public Health

According to the Centers of Disease Control and Prevention (CDC) Foundation, "Public health is the science of protecting and improving the health of families and communities through promotion of healthy lifestyles, research for disease and injury prevention and detection and control of infectious diseases. Overall, public health is concerned with protecting the health of entire populations." There are 3 core functions of public health: assessment, policy development, and assurance. Within the 3 core functions are 10 essential services, outlined by the Core Public Health Functions Steering Committee in 1994. The 10 essential services describe public health activities all communities should have in place to ensure the health of the public (Table 4–1).

Research, the 10th essential service, is a component of each of the public health functions. It is a necessary step in conducting an assessment to determine whether the findings are consistent with other similar situations or whether there is an existing solution. Research informs policy development by providing objective evidence for proposed actions, informing the public with tested best practices, and assisting communities to mobilize with strong evidence to back their plan.

<table>
<tr><th colspan="2">Table 4–1 • CORE PUBLIC HEALTH FUNCTIONS AND ESSENTIAL PUBLIC HEALTH SERVICES</th></tr>
<tr><td>I. Assessment allows public health practitioners to see the landscape in which they are operating, much as a clinician caring for an individual patient will first conduct a health history and perform a physical assessment of the patient's signs and symptoms. Assessment is a means of gathering information to make an informed plan of action. Within assessment there are 2 essential services:
1. Monitor the health status of populations.
2. Diagnose and investigate health hazards, disease, and infection.</td><td rowspan="3">Research for new insights and innovative solutions to health problems (encompasses all areas 1-9).</td></tr>
<tr><td>II. Policy development is the second core public health function and builds on the assessment function. Policy development takes the information gained through assessment and takes into consideration the findings within the context of the community's values and input to develop recommendations for action at a systems level. Within policy development there are 3 essential services:
3. Inform, educate, and empower people about health issues.
4. Mobilize community partnerships to address identified needs.
5. Develop policies that support systems-level change.</td></tr>
<tr><td>III. Assurance builds on assessment and policy development by translating identified need and policy support into the provision of quality services. Assurance includes 4 essential services:
6. Enforce laws or policies to protect the health of the public and ensure safety.
7. Link people to needed services and ensure care is available.
8. Ensure a competent workforce to support the public's health.
9. Evaluate the effectiveness, accessibility, and quality of health services.</td></tr>
</table>

Research contributes to the core function of assurance by feeding the evidence base for public health policies, demonstrating effective methods of service provision and contributing to a knowledgeable and competent workforce. System management is a thread woven throughout the core functions, because it is vital that these functions and essential services are complementary and not duplicative. It cannot stand as an essential service by itself, but instead is an element that must be incorporated in the context of the other services.

Public Health Values Versus Biomedical Ethical Principles

The most widely referenced medical ethics framework is that described by Beauchamp and Childress in *Principles of Biomedical Ethics*. This framework includes 4 principles meant to guide clinicians in their work with individual patients. In brief, the principles are as follows:

- *Autonomy* is the right for an individual to self-govern by rational principles and to make his or her own choices free from coercion.
- *Nonmaleficence* reflects the maxim stated in the Hippocratic Oath to "first, do no harm."
- *Beneficence* is the principle of seeking the best interests of an individual through careful weighing of risks and benefits.
- *Justice* describes the duty to act fairly and equitably when balancing competing claims, including for distribution of scarce resources, respect for individuals' rights, and respect for morally defensible laws.

The public health perspective has features that distinguish it from the biomedical perspective, and thus public health practice calls for a different ethical framework that is sometimes in tension with biomedical ethical principles. Medicine is practiced in a relationship between a clinician and an individual, and its ethical framework is designed to regulate potential abuses between the person in the relationship who holds the greatest power and influence (the clinician) and a person who is vulnerable (the patient). By contrast, public health practice occurs between primarily governmental institutions and populations or communities. Although power dynamics must still be regulated, principles must provide guidance for decision making about how whole communities operate including relationships between each person and other community members and between community members and institutions.

The Public Health Leadership Society outlines 11 values and beliefs inherent to the public health perspective, which underlie public health ethical principles. Among others, these include the values of *interdependence, participation*, and *scientific evidence*. The value of *interdependence* recognizes that each person's right to autonomy is not limitless but is interrelated with the boundaries of the rights of others. Said another way, no action is without impact to the greater community and, for the common good; each person's autonomy must be limited by consideration of how the person's choices impact others.

The value of *participation* is congruent with the concept of consent for public health. Public health institutions, which are themselves made up of individuals, function as "moral actors" for the populations they serve. To ensure that decisions are best designed to reduce harm, to benefit society, and to fairly and equitably balance public resources, individual and population rights, and implementation of laws, the value of *participation* asserts that individuals who are impacted by public health decisions must be provided with access and opportunity to provide input to the decision-making process.

The value of *scientific evidence* highlights the duty to look beyond impassioned opinion or hunches, by using of the full range of scientific tools in public health decision-making so that risks and benefits are weighed with a heavy reliance on integration of the scientific method and the highest-quality evidence available. **Research itself as a core public health function should be informed by the experience of those it involves, so that it accurately reflects the experience of the population being studied.** Best practice in research of communities now calls for community-based participatory research models, in which research about the communities is conducted by community members and research is subsequently shared with community members. This type of research results in greater buy-in among communities, resulting in more accurate data and a greater likelihood that the resulting recommendations will be accepted and implemented by the community.

Right to Individual Privacy Versus Protection of the Common Good

The provision of medical care to the individual human body is a complex interplay of moving organic parts, laden with ethical dilemmas. Even more complex is the ethical assurance of health for families, communities, and populations made up of these complex individuals. In the case study presented at the beginning of this chapter, the clinician is challenged to balance the duty to provide care that benefits the individual patient and preserves autonomy with the duty to protect the public's health, including assurance that her and her partner(s)' partners are notified and treated for suspected chlamydial infection. The aim of identification and treatment of all who were potentially exposed is to protect the public's health by preventing further spread of an infection known to cause significant morbidities, including pelvic inflammatory disease, infertility, and vertical transmission to infants. Partner treatment also prevents a vicious cycle of reinfection for the initial patient. **Thus, the biomedical ethics principle of autonomy is in tension with the public health value of interdependence.** Every effort should be made to preserve the right to privacy while also ensuring the health and safety of others in the community through contact tracking and reporting. Confidential partner notification—whereby partners are notified of possible exposure but not of the source of the exposure— serves to preserve individual privacy as much as possible while also protecting the common good.

Another example of the primacy of interdependence over the value of autonomy is public health's concern with the rights and needs of vulnerable populations, including those who may be disenfranchised or unable to advocate effectively for themselves. These populations include people with disabilities, minority populations, undocumented immigrants, incarcerated populations, individuals with low socioeconomic status, or low literacy among others. It is the responsibility of the public health system to ensure the health and well being of these groups within the context of the greater population. These groups are often left out of the traditional health care and social services systems due to lack of coordination of services to allow the system to be readily navigable or outright denial of services. Provision of care to vulnerable populations helps to ensure the health of the public by preventing introduction of disease, reducing disproportionate burden of illness among smaller groups, and thereby reducing the burden on the health care system.

The Ethical Practice of Public Health

An ethical framework must guide the core functions of public health and the implementation of the 10 essential services. Without guiding principles and moral standards that are population-focused rather than individual-focused, the core functions of assessment, policy development and assurance would not be achievable. These functions prioritize interdependence, participation, the scientific method, and other values that support the health, well-being, and dignity of individuals within a community. They also prize prevention of illness and disease over the cure, which is a priority in medicine.

In 2002, the Public Health Leadership Society under the auspices of the American Public Health Association (APHA) published the *Principles of the Ethical Practice of Public Health* that outlines 12 ethical principles underlying the practice. This document could be compared to the American Medical Association *Code of Medical Ethics* for physicians or the American Nurses Association's *Code of Ethics for Nurses*. The code is not meant to be a comprehensive ethical guide, since the practitioners of public health are often professionals from other fields with their own code of ethics. Rather, this code complements existing ethical standards by taking a population-based view and promoting the interdependence of people and the important role that living in community plays in the health of individuals.

Table 4–2 outlines the 12 principles and how each relates to the 10 essential services of public health to assist public health practitioners in managing ethical dilemmas and ensuring ethical practice.

Table 4–2 • TWELVE ETHICAL PRINCIPLES AND CORRESPONDING PUBLIC HEALTH SERVICE		
Ethical Principle	Core Functions and corresponding Essential Public Health Services	Example of Ethical Dilemma
1. Public health should address fundamental causes of disease and requirements for health, aiming to prevent adverse health outcomes.	**Assessment**: *Diagnose and investigate* causes of disease. **Policy Development**: *Inform, educate, and empower* communities on prevention. *Develop policies* to prevent adverse health outcomes.	Alcoholism leads to many chronic conditions. Should a public health practitioner focus on a patient's alcoholism before addressing his or her symptoms of chronic hepatitis?
2. Public health should achieve community health while respecting the rights of individuals in the community.	**Assessment**: *Monitor health* of communities to identify threats. *Diagnose and investigate* those threats with attention to the human rights of those involved. **Policy development**: *Develop policies* that move the community toward health considering both the rights of the individual and the protection of the community. **Assurance**: *Enforce laws* on protection of confidentiality and individual rights as well as laws that protect the health of communities.	Community leaders are concerned with the influx of fast-food restaurants in their town. Fast-food restaurants are drawn to the town because of the number of college students who eat fast food, enjoy it, and say they require it to accommodate their lifestyle. What is the responsibility of the community and what are their options?
3. Public health policies, programs, and priorities should be developed and evaluated through processes that ensure an opportunity for input from community members.	**Policy development**: *Mobilize community partnerships* so action is based on mutual understanding of the aims and impact of the change. *Develop policies* with input from those impacted by the policy. **Assurance**: *Evaluate* the impact of policies, programs, and priorities on the intended outcome as well as unintended consequences.	Research on a pressing health issue in an urban community is being conducted by the local hospital. A participatory model for the study has been proposed but will take more time and resources. Does the need for a fast turnaround on data to benefit the community outweigh the importance of community engagement in the process?
4. Public health should advocate and work for the empowerment of disenfranchised community members.	**Policy development**: *Inform, educate, and empower* disenfranchised communities so they have increased locus of control to make change happen. *Mobilize community partnerships* to enhance the linkages to service of vulnerable populations.	Do inmates being released from incarceration require transitional services from a public health perspective? What is the threat to the community if this group is not empowered?

(Continued)

Table 4–2 • TWELVE ETHICAL PRINCIPLES AND CORRESPONDING PUBLIC HEALTH SERVICE (*CONTINUED*)

Ethical Principle	Core Functions and corresponding Essential Public Health Services	Example of Ethical Dilemma
5. Public health should seek the information needed to implement effective policies and programs that protect and promote health.	**Assessment**: *Monitor health* to determine if existing policies are effectively supporting the health of the population or need revision. **Policy development**: *Develop policies* that address current trends in public health, changes in demographics, and population needs. **Assurance**: *Evaluate* existing policies and programs for return on investment, impact on health, and effectiveness. *Research* proposed changes to policy by determining if improved services or programs exist and would be appropriate in the community.	An urban health department receives a gift from a wealthy donor, which must be used to implement a community gardening project; the donor is a gardening enthusiast and just moved to the city. The health department is dubious that the community gardening project will work without significant investment of personnel and oversight, but does not wish to lose the funds. How should the health department proceed?
6. Public health institutions should provide communities with the information needed for decision-making and obtain the community's consent for their implementation.	**Policy development**: *Inform, educate, and empower* communities to participate in decision-making about research, policy, environmental changes, and other factors that may impact their health.	A highway may be built in a rural part of the state to allow residents quicker access to major cities and also allow trucks to travel more efficiently in their delivery routes. There is opposition from residents who say they did not ask for the road and are being used as an excuse to increase highway toll revenue from the trucks. How could this have been handled differently? How does this impact public health?
7. Public health institutions should act in a timely manner on the information they have within the resources and mandate given to them by the public.	**Assessment**: *Monitor health* to identify health threats in an efficient and respond in an organized manner.	A pertussis outbreak is suspected in a densely populated part of the state; the governor does not wish to create a panic by broadcasting the suspected cases publicly. What is the responsibility of the health authority?
8. Public health programs and policies should incorporate a variety of approaches that anticipate and respect diverse values, beliefs, and cultures in the community.	**Assurance**: *Link to/provide care* in a culturally competent manner so that both access to care and quality of care provided are assured.	A new population of Iraqi refugees has been resettled in a Midwest town hit hard by the 2008 recession. Public health leaders are concerned about potential tensions between the residents and the new arrivals that are both in need of jobs, public assistance, and medical care. How is this a public health issue?

(Continued)

Table 4–2 • TWELVE ETHICAL PRINCIPLES AND CORRESPONDING PUBLIC HEALTH SERVICE (CONTINUED)

Ethical Principle	Core Functions and corresponding Essential Public Health Services	Example of Ethical Dilemma
9. Public health programs and policies should be implemented in a manner that most enhances the physical and social environment.	**Policy development:** *Develop policies* to protect the cohesion and collective strength of communities. **Assurance:** *Enforce laws* to protect the community physically (environment) and socially (wellbeing of the community).	A neighborhood revitalization program promises mixed income housing in an area with a history of crime, but with an entrenched neighborhood association and residents who have lived there since the 1980s. What are the potential consequences of this program (positive and negative) to the physical and social environment?
10. Public health institutions should protect the confidentiality of information that can bring harm to an individual or community if made public. Justify exceptions on the basis of the high likelihood of significant harm to the individual or others.	**Assessment:** *Diagnose and investigate* with the privacy of the individual and protection of the community in mind. **Policy development:** *Develop policies* to protect the community when a high likelihood of harm exists. **Assurance:** *Enforce laws* to ensure the rights of the individual to autonomy do not impact the health of the community.	A young man comes to the clinic for sexually transmitted infection testing. He tests positive for syphilis and shares that he makes his income as a commercial sex worker. What are the potential ramifications of conducting a contact tracing to him, his relationship partner, and his clients? What type of behavioral interventions should take place with this client?
11. Public health institutions should ensure the professional competence of public health employees.	**Assurance:** *Ensure competent workforce* to protect the safety of those being cared for and ensure the evolution of the practice.	A prestigious physician with many years of experience working as a hospital clinician takes over as medical director of a public health department "to finish out his time" before retirement. What are the possible ramifications of this appointment?
12. Public health institutions and their employees should engage in collaborations and affiliations that build the public's trust in public health entities and the institution's effectiveness.	**Policy Development:** *Mobilize community partnerships* that link communities to public health entities such as health departments or advocacy organizations to promote understanding and collaboration.	A public health patient advocacy organization applies for and receives funding from a pharmaceutical company to implement a program they have wanted to do for years. The funder stipulates that any materials produced must be cobranded with their logo and partnering physicians must agree to visits from pharmaceutical representatives. What are the ethical implications of this sponsorship?

COMPREHENSION QUESTIONS

4.1 A family doctor has cared for a couple in his practice since they were first married, and the couple is now in their 50s. The wife presents to the doctor with an unusual rash on her palms that is faint and painless, and shares that she had "a bump" on the outside of her labia a few weeks ago that has since healed. Learning that she has had no new sexual partners, the physician sends her for a blood test. Testing confirms presence of syphilis. The provider feels compelled to handle the situation discretely because of his history with the family. Which of the following is the appropriate course of action for the physician?

A. Tell the wife she contracted an infection from the soil while gardening and that she and her husband should be treated. Conduct follow-up testing to ensure treatment success per clinical protocols.

B. Provide the wife with a full clinical picture of syphilis and how she was likely infected, and recommend treatment for her and her husband. Ask the wife to bring her husband in for treatment without contacting health authorities.

C. Invite both patients to receive the wife's test results together and develop a plan of action for treatment and contact tracing with their consent. Discuss the need for follow-up assays to determine treatment success and refer the patients to couples counseling.

D. Treat each patient as an individual case and as though they do not know one another. Based on the wife's results, contact her husband to come in for testing, explaining that he may be at risk for syphilis based on the results of the test of one of his sex partners. Offer treatment, contact tracing, follow up, and notify public health authorities.

4.2 Which of the following is an example of a clinician using patient-centered rather than public-health–centered clinical decision-making?

A. A patient has the right to make decisions about his or her cancer treatment plan based on a full picture of the risks and benefits it may incur.

B. A patient who lives in a dangerous neighborhood is at greater risk for obesity because of not having a safe environment in which to exercise and increased stress in his living situation.

C. A patient has tuberculosis and is participating in directly observed therapy. The patient is asked to determine the time and place for treatment to ensure compliance.

D. A patient is told the impact that his smoking has on the health of those she lives with, particularly as a risk factor for sudden infant death syndrome (SIDS) to her infant granddaughter.

4.3 Public health includes 3 core functions. Which of the following best describes the components of the core function of assessment?

   A. Researching pathways to care and barriers to service among newly arrived immigrants.

   B. Developing data profiles of special groups to depict the higher incidence of alcoholism among one group based on surveillance data.

   C. Conducting town hall meetings in the community to develop better community cohesion and a unified purpose.

   D. Supporting early entry into prenatal care through a nurse–social worker case management program.

ANSWERS

4.1 **D.** Although this is a difficult situation, it is paramount that the married couple be handled as though they do not know each other, confidentially, privately, and thoroughly. Reporting to the public health authorities is also important.

4.2 **A.** This is an example of beneficence and involves the patient's reviewing the cancer treatment risks and benefits on the individual patient. The other examples deal with public health issues.

4.3 **B.** Assessment means developing data profiles of special groups to depict the higher incidence of a disease or condition in a group. In this example, this refers to alcoholism in a specific group.

KEY POINTS

▶ Public health is the assessment of communities, the development of policy to address the needs and assets of communities, and the assurance of health of the individuals in those communities.

▶ Public health ethics differs from bioethics in its valuation of interdependence over autonomy and its recognition of the connection between the wellness of people and the wellness of their communities.

▶ Disease investigation and interruption of the chain of transmission are public health essential services. Individuals participate in public health through screening for STIs.

▶ The public is protected from infections and their sequelae by the interruption of infection through mandatory public reporting and public health partner testing and treatment infrastructure.

▶ Clinicians and laboratories should familiarize themselves with applicable reporting requirements within their public health jurisdiction. Contact state and local public health officials to clarify any questions about reporting requirements as well as to discuss regulations related to contact tracking (eg, partner notification) and expedited partner therapy.

REFERENCES

Bayer R. Ethics and infectious disease control: STDs, HIV and TB. In: Jennings B, Kahn J, Mastroianna A, Parker LS, eds. *Ethics and Public Health: Model Curriculum.* Published July 2003. http://www.asph .org/UserFiles/Introduction.pdf. Accessed May 5, 2014.

Beauchamp TL, Childress JF. *Principles of Biomedical Ethics.* 6th ed. New York, NY: Oxford University Press; 2009.

CDC Foundation. What is public health? Updated 2014. http://www.cdcfoundation.org/content/what-public-health. Accessed May 12, 2014.

Centers for Disease Control and Prevention. The public health system and the 10 essential public health services. Updated July 3, 2013. http://www.cdc.gov/nphpsp/essentialServices.html. Accessed May 12, 2014.

Conley E, Dahl J. *Public Health Nursing Within Core Public Health Functions: A Progress Report From Public Health Nursing Directors of Washington.* Olympia, WA: Washington State Department of Health; 1993.

Gostin L. Health care information and the protection of personal privacy: ethical and legal considerations. *Ann Intern Med.* 1997;127(suppl 2):683-690.

Lurie N, Fremont A. Building bridges between medical care and public health. *JAMA.* 2009;302:84-86.

Public Health Leadership Society. Principles of the ethical practice of public health. Version 2.2. Published 2002. http://www.apha.org/NR/rdonlyres/1CED3CEA-287E-4185-9CBD-BD405FC60856/0 /ethicsbrochure.pdf. Accessed May 5, 2014.

Thacker SB; Centers for Disease Control and Prevention. Early release: HIPAA privacy rule and public health: guidance from CDC and the U.S. Department of Health and Human Services. *MMWR.* 2003;52:1-12. http://www.cdc.gov/mmwr/preview/mmwrhtml/m2e411a1.htm. Accessed April 5, 2014.

Thomas JC. *Distinguishing Public Health Ethics From Medical Ethics.* Chapel Hill, NC: North Carolina Institute for Public Health. http://oce.sph.unc.edu/phethics/modules.htm. Accessed May 12, 2014.

A 32-year-old man with an artificial aortic valve is admitted into the hospital with acute shortness of breath. He is found to have aortic valve insufficiency and a large vegetation of the aortic valve. Physical examination reveals fresh track marks on his arms, and urinalysis shows opiates. The patient admits to using intravenous (IV) heroin. The patient is treated with IV antibiotics and is medically stabilized; however, the extent of the aortic valve damage is such that surgical replacement of the aortic valve is indicated. The cardiovascular surgical team is refusing to take the patient to surgery due to continued IV drug use and cites resource allocation and medical futility as reasons to deny surgery.

▶ What are the ethical issues involved with this patient?
▶ Does the cardiovascular surgical team have ethical standing to refuse surgery?

ANSWERS TO CASE 5:

Resource Allocation

Summary: A 32-year-old man with an artificial aortic valve is complaining of shortness of breath. He is found to have aortic valve insufficiency and a large vegetation of the aortic valve and needs surgical valve replacement. The patient admits to using IV heroin. The cardiovascular surgical team is refusing to take the patient to surgery due to continued IV drug use.

- **Ethical issues:** Resource allocation, medical futility, physician advocacy.

- **Grounds to refuse surgery:** The patient will likely continue IV drug use that will result in future complications and failure of the new artificial aortic valve. The artificial aortic valve and surgeon's time could be utilized for other patients who do not participate in behaviors known to negatively affect the outcomes of the procedure.

ANALYSIS

Objectives

1. Describe the ethical principles in health care resource allocation.

2. Describe the role of the physician in advocating for the individual patient's well-being and receiving treatment.

3. List the criteria used in deciding the equitable and appropriate allocation of resources that are limited in nature.

Considerations

The patient is experiencing shortness of breath due to aortic valve insufficiency likely due to his continued IV drug use; this drug use is a well-known cause for endocarditis. The patient has received an artificial aortic valve replacement in the past, and the patient has been evaluated for yet another artificial aortic valve replacement. The surgery team do not want to perform the surgery because they are frustrated that the patient has not taken care of his current artificial aortic valve and are concerned that the same thing will happen with the new one. They feel that the new artificial aortic valve and the team's time and resources would be wasted if the patient continues to use IV drugs and, instead, the valve and time to perform the surgery could be used for other patients. However, the surgery would be in the patient's best interest, and the patient's need for social and other support to avoid another failed surgery has not been addressed.

APPROACH TO:
Resource Allocation

DEFINITIONS

MEDICAL FUTILITY: A judgment that further medical treatment of a patient would not have useful or successful results.

RESOURCE ALLOCATION: The constellation of decisions and actions that prioritize health care needs.

CLINICAL APPROACH

Health care resources are regarded as limited in terms of both physical materials and human labor. There is a limit to the number of health care facilities, hospital beds, instruments manufactured, and organs, among other things. There is also a limit to operating room time and the number of tests that can be performed in a given day. In addition, the number of people who can become a health care professional and deliver care is limited. Whether health care is delivered in a private or public setting, the demand will always and necessarily exceed the supply. So who determines who receives these limited resources?

According to *The Principles of Medical Ethics* of the American Medical Association (AMA), "A physician shall be dedicated to providing competent medical service with compassion and respect for human dignity." A physician also has a duty to do all he or she can for the benefit of the individual patient as well as a societal duty to speak on behalf of patients regarding the allocation of health care resources.

Decisions regarding the allocation of limited medical resources among patients should be based on appropriate criteria relating to medical need. The criteria outlined by the AMA's Council on Ethical and Judicial Affairs include (1) likelihood of benefit, (2) urgency of need, (3) change in quality of life, (4) duration of benefit, and (5) the amount of resources required for successful treatment.

Likelihood of Benefit

These criteria prioritize patients who are assessed to have a greater likelihood of benefitting from treatment. The purpose of this resource allocation system is to maximize the use of limited resources to provide maximum benefit to society. Organ transplantation is an example of resource allocation based on these criteria. In the present case, the surgery team is using these criteria to argue that another patient who does not use IV drugs would benefit more from the time and money spent on an artificial aortic valve replacement by being able to utilize it for more years.

These criteria are used to allocate resources among patients and to determine whether treatment should be provided in situations where the likelihood of benefit is minimal. A treatment is defined as medically futile if it will not have useful or successful results. The surgery team believes another artificial aortic valve replacement in this patient is "futile" because he will continue to use IV drugs and will get another infection that will require another valve in the future.

The problem lies in predicting and defining outcomes. Placing a value on the potential benefit to an individual patient is also difficult. The patient in this case will likely benefit from a new artificial aortic valve even if it is for a shorter period of time than a patient who does not use IV drugs. There are also other nonmedical factors that contribute to a patient's likelihood of benefit, such as compliance, financial resources, and transportation. However, many of these factors are not permanent and can be overcome. Only those nonmedical factors or behaviors that directly affect the patient's likelihood of benefit should be considered.

Change in Quality of Life

Building on the likelihood of benefit criteria, limited resources would ideally be distributed to those who will likely have the greatest improvement in quality of life. As suggested earlier, defining quality of life and quantifying improvement are difficult tasks. The AMA defines quality of life in terms of functional status. Although functional status can be objectively assessed by physicians, the attitude toward a certain functional level is patient dependent. A disability may make life not worth living for some patients, whereas others may view it as acceptable. In this case, the patient's functional status, and thus quality of life, will likely be greatly improved with the new artificial valve replacement.

Duration of Benefit

These criteria are also an extension of the likelihood of benefit criteria. Those who benefit from treatment for a longer length of time should be given priority of scarce resources. For example, when all else is equal, patients who will survive for many years if treated in the intensive care unit (ICU) will benefit more from an ICU bed than patients who are expected to live only a few days or weeks. Again, there is a lack of certainty when determining duration of benefit. Many factors contribute to a patient's expected life span. Moreover, the degree to which a longer duration of benefit actually benefits the patient depends on the patient's subjective experience and values. In the present case, the surgery team is using this criteria to argue that an artificial valve in a patient who does not use IV drugs would last longer and be of more benefit. At the same time, not knowing the patient's comorbidities, this patient's expected life span may be longer than other patients with his condition, and this surgery is very likely to prolong it.

Urgency of Need

This criteria applies when the scarcity of the resources changes. When resources are especially scarce, priority should be given to the sickest patients until the scarcity situation improves. For example, kidney transplantations should be allocated to the most urgent cases first, whereas less urgent cases can be medically sustained until additional kidneys become available. These criteria can be applied to the present case when analyzing the surgery team's operating room time and staff. The patient appears to be stable and can be medically sustained for a period of time. However, these criteria should not be used to deny current patients treatment because others with more urgent need *may* present themselves. The question in this case refers to whether the patient should receive the treatment at all; it is not addressing the timing of the treatment.

Amount of Resources Required

In situations in which resources are exceptionally scarce, resources may be allocated to those who will require less of the resource, thereby maximizing the number of patients who could benefit from the resource. These criteria do not apply to this particular case.

The AMA has also outlined inappropriate and unethical criteria to allocate resources, including (1) ability to pay, (2) contribution of the patient to society, (3) perceived obstacles to treatment, (4) contribution of the patient to his or her own medical condition, and (5) past use of resources.

The surgery's team underlying bias toward the patient using IV drugs may play an important role in its decision-making process. However, the perceptions about those who use IV drugs and their contribution to society should not affect the team's decision-making. The team is also using the patient's previous use of the same resource and citing his continued IV drug as contributing to his own medical condition. In addition, efforts to address the patient's obstacles to successful treatment (eg, a drug rehabilitation program) have not been approached.

Based on the appropriate medical criteria, this patient should undergo the artificial aortic valve replacement surgery. The surgery should not be denied to the patient based on his past, current, or future IV drug use. Instead, the team should help the patient stop his drug use to prevent future infections and complications.

COMPREHENSION QUESTIONS

5.1 A physician director is trying to determine the best methodology in providing the last mechanical ventilator to 1 of 2 patients: one patient with HIV-infected pneumocystis pneumonia who has been unwilling to take his HIV medication, and another patient with influenza pneumonia. Which of the following is the most appropriate point to consider with regard to resource allocation?

   A. Likelihood of benefit

   B. Concern about political ramifications from HIV activists

   C. Current comparative quality of life

   D. Compliance with therapy

5.2 A 34-year-old man who abuses alcohol comes into the hospital with his third upper gastrointestinal bleed. He has been counseled to discontinue alcohol, but he has refused. Which of the following is the most appropriate reason to offer treatment to this man despite his noncompliance with therapy and contributory behavior to his medical condition?

A. Principle of nondiscrimination

B. Principle of autonomy

C. Principle of justice

D. Principle of altruism

ANSWERS

5.1 **A.** Likelihood of benefit should be considered for resource allocation. Concern about the possible political ramifications or prior compliance to therapy should not be an issue. The change in quality of life is important and, thus is more important than current quality of life.

5.2 **C.** The ethical principle of justice means that people are given treatment in a fair and equitable manner, and not based on characteristics such as ability to pay or perceived standing in society.

KEY POINTS

▶ Physicians have a duty to advocate for and prioritize the needs of their patients. They are also often faced with a societal duty to allocate limited health care resources.

▶ Resource allocation decisions should be made based on the following criteria: (1) likelihood of benefit, (2) urgency of need, (3) change in quality of life, (4) duration of benefit, and (5) the amount of resources required for successful treatment.

▶ Resource allocation decisions should not be based on the following criteria: (1) ability to pay, (2) contribution of the patient to society, (3) perceived obstacles to treatment, (4) contribution of the patient to his or her own medical condition, and (5) past use of resources.

REFERENCES

American Medical Association (AMA). Opinion 2.03. Allocation of limited medical resources. In: AMA. AMA Code of Medical Ethics. Chicago, IL: AMA; 1994.

Clarke OW, Glasson J, Epps CH, et al. Ethical considerations in the allocation of organs and other scarce medical resources among patients. Arch Intern Med. 1995;155:29-40.

A 25-year-old surgical resident sees a recruitment advertisement for a research study. The research team is looking for healthy volunteers to participate in a study comparing one magnetic resonance imaging (MRI) technique with another. Study participants will be compensated as much as $250 for their time. The resident calls the research coordinator to set up an appointment. Upon meeting the coordinator, the resident is given a consent form to read, which says that participants will be notified if significant abnormalities are found on the scan, and a referral to a neurologist will be provided. She signs the consent form and fills out a questionnaire to indicate that she had no educational or developmental problems, takes no medications, and has no diagnosed medical conditions. She has a head MRI scan one week later. The next day, she receives a phone call from a radiologist working with the research team who tells her that a neuronal migrational abnormality was found on her MRI scan and an appointment has been booked with a neurologist.

▸ What are incidental findings in research?
▸ Do researchers have to report incidental findings back to participants?
▸ What are the ethical implications of reporting incidental findings back to participants?

ANSWERS TO CASE 6:

Research Ethics

Summary: A 25-year-old surgical resident answers an advertisement for a research project comparing two MRI techniques. The consent indicates that participants will be notified if significant abnormalities are found on the scan, and a referral to a neurologist will be provided. One day after she has an MRI of the brain, she receives a phone call from a radiologist working with the research team who tells her that the MRI shows a neuronal migrational abnormality and an appointment has been booked with a neurologist.

- **Incidental findings in research:** Observations of potential clinical significance made during the course of research. Put another way, an incidental finding is any finding that has implications for the subject's personal or reproductive health, but which is beyond the scope of the research itself.

- **Required to report incidental findings to participants:** There are no national or international guidelines requiring the reporting of incidental findings to participants. However, one should consider the implications of incidental findings during the design of a research study.

- **Ethical implications of reporting incidental findings back to participants:** There may be risks of additional harm to participants if the findings are not accurate, if participants are not given proper information about the implication of the findings, or if additional expenses accrue to seek further medical care. However, there may be additional benefit to participants if the incidental finding results in earlier treatment than would otherwise have occurred.

ANALYSIS

Objectives

1. Define the term *incidental findings*.
2. Identify three sources of potential harm that could accrue to research participants from reporting of incidental findings.
3. Identify three strategies to help manage incidental findings.

Considerations

In this case, a 25-year-old healthy resident physician signs up for a research study on MRI techniques. The consent form specifies that any incidental finding would be communicated to the patient, and referral to a neurologist would be made. The resident has an MRI of the brain. The next day, she receives a telephone call regarding a neuronal migrational abnormality, and is told that an appointment has been booked with a neurologist. In consideration of the issue of incidental findings in research, it is important to consider the implications of incidental findings and to create a plan for addressing them as part of study design. The significance or veracity of these findings may be difficult to assess, and disclosure may result in benefit to the participant if it results in earlier, perhaps more effective treatment, or harm if results are inaccurate, are of unknown significance, or results in additional expense to the participant.

APPROACH TO:
Research Ethics

DEFINITION

INCIDENTAL FINDINGS: Observations of potential clinical significance made during the course of research. Put another way, an incidental finding is any finding that has implications for the subject's personal or reproductive health, but which is beyond the scope of the research itself.

CLINICAL APPROACH

The occurrence of incidental findings is thought to be 2% to 8% in brain imaging overall and may be as high as 50% in participants aged more than 65 years. The types of findings can include meningiomas, arteriovenous malformations, intracranial aneurysms, and malignant neoplasms, among others. The nature of the clinical significance may be immediate, future, or potential. For example, the presence of a brain tumor, even if the patient is asymptomatic, is of immediate significance as the likelihood of cure is much higher if the tumor can be treated before neurologic symptoms occur. The presence of an asymptomatic intracranial aneurysm is associated with a known likelihood of rupture that increases annually; as such, this represents a risk of future harm to the participant and, by initiating treatment early, one may reduce or eliminate the risk of harm.

The third category of incidental findings, those that may or may not be associated with a future clinical finding, is harder to consider. Neuronal migrational disorders represent an example of an incidental finding for which clinicians are unable to predict whether the participant will ever become clinically symptomatic. However, as some of the migrational disorders have a genetic component, there may be a risk of transmitting the abnormality to one's future offspring. As such, the risk of revealing such a finding to the participant must be balanced against the potential benefit, which cannot yet be quantified.

There are no universal or national guidelines from any country for what to do with incidental findings in research. There are several reasons for this. Some research techniques may not provide the same level of accuracy as the clinically accepted standard. For example, in neuroimaging, if the imaging modality does not provide the same level of resolution, or if a trained radiologist does not review the scans, the so-called incidental findings may not be accurate findings. There would be no benefit to individuals to be told that they had brain abnormalities when they did not; indeed, the potential for unnecessary worry, grief, and/or anxiety would be very high.

In other situations, the potential clinical significance of an incidental finding would require greater expertise to determine than that provided by the research team. One might need to take a more detailed history, or to perform a detailed physical examination to identify a possible clinical correlate for an incidental finding. In this scenario, an institutional review board (IRB) might require that the research team have a plan to send reports of incidental findings back to the participant's own physician, so that that individual could do a more complete assessment of clinical relevance before passing the findings along to the participant.

By accepting the responsibility of notifying participants of their incidental findings, the research team may further be constrained by a certain expected turnaround time between scan and feedback to the participant. However, many research studies involving imaging choose to use a single reviewer to avoid problems related to inter-reviewer reliability, and the research teams may, therefore, batch studies for review. The need to provide a quicker response may cause research teams to expand to accommodate the greater workflow. For example, if a researcher needs to hire a trained radiologist to interpret scans in real-time, then the overall cost of doing research will escalate.

There are additional ramifications of reporting incidental findings back to study participants. There may be an additional financial cost associated with required appointments with primary care providers, additional specialists, or additional imaging to clarify the nature of the incidental finding. In some circumstances, the patient's future insurability may be affected by the presence of a clinically asymptomatic finding. Bypassing the participant and going straight to the participant's primary care provider with incidental findings may increase the financial burden for participants if the finding gets into his or her medical chart before an assessment of the clinical significance of the finding is made. This latter situation may also be a violation of the participant's right to confidentiality with respect to research participation.

Most research studies make no intrinsic provision for these outcomes, and there is no standard IRB requirement for the informed consent process for research to include a statement informing potential research participants about the possibility of incidental findings being discovered.

Although these concerns apply to the research participant himself or herself, some incidental findings may be associated with a genetic tendency to pass along a propensity to certain lesions which may, ultimately, cause neurologic dysfunction. The potential for clinical consequences could, thus, apply to the participant, and also for the participant's future children, thus increasing the cost of health care delivery for future generations and increasing the potential for pain and suffering for the participant's children.

An interesting further consideration with respect to incidental findings is apparent when we consider autonomy as it pertains to study participation. Whereas participants have the right to consider study participation, because researchers do not routinely provide information about the potential for incidental findings, potential participants are not actually consenting to be screened for incidental findings.

In clinical care, there is an expectation that findings on imaging studies will be disclosed to patients for the purposes of improved health care delivery, even if those findings do not necessarily lead to treatment. However, in research, there may or may not be a potential for benefit through participation in a study. The primary goal of medical research is to produce generalizable knowledge; because of this, decision-making is focused at fulfilling the research mission. However, this does not take into account the very real potential for human suffering that could be alleviated in some participants should their incidental findings be brought to medical attention.

Some ethicists argue that a new framework needs to be adopted to deal with this dichotomy between clinical care and clinical research. Rangel suggests use of the ancillary care model, which was first proposed by Richardson and Belsky. In this, ancillary care is defined as "the clinical care in the research setting which goes beyond the requirements of scientific validity, safety, keeping promises, or rectifying injuries." She argues that incidental findings fall into this definition of ancillary care, and that management should be guided by the principles of non-exploitation of research participants and partial entrustment. In the model she suggests, the principle of partial entrustment recognizes that participants entrust some aspects of health to the discretion of the researcher. She develops an algorithmic approach to decision-making that weighs the type of research imaging with the urgency of the artifact, meaning the potential clinical significance of the finding.

Notably, the legal and regulatory requirements that exist around the world to ensure that potential research participants are adequately informed about the risks of research do not include rigorous or even suggested guidelines for what to do with findings that are not being evaluated and/or managed as part of the research study. However, Rangel suggests that IRBs should require researchers to have a per protocol plan for managing the discovery of incidental findings. Furthermore, she believes that IRBs should require investigators to document the discovery and ultimate decision-making of incidental findings.

Finally, Rangel supports having potential research participants understand via the consent process that incidental findings may be discovered during the course of an individual's study participation. To allow for participants to properly understand what this means, she proposes having some examples of potential findings included in the consent form, along with the potential courses of action that might ensue. Other researchers agree that the consent form and consent process should include information about the risks of discovery of incidental findings, and the plan to be followed for disclosure and assessment.

Booth and colleagues from the United Kingdom studied existing guidance documents from Europe and the United States pertaining to incidental findings and reviewed existing studies containing the Medical Subject Headings (MeSH) term *incidental findings*. They proposed a "sliding scale model" for disclosing incidental findings that would involve matching the mode of communication to the risk and severity of the finding, further suggesting that the optimal person to give participants the information about their incidental findings would be a clinician, whether the participant's own physician or a research physician. They also point out that potential participants should be informed if incidental findings may be incorporated as part of the participant's personal (ie, nonresearch) medical record, and if an enrolled participant chooses not to have information about incidental findings disclosed to himself or herself, then that wish must also be respected. The exception to this latter rule would be if the potential clinical risk to the participant would or could affect others; in that case, disclosure would be mandatory.

ANALYSIS AND DISCUSSION

Having considered the ethical implications of incidental findings, we turn to our case study and consider the implication for our surgical resident of having had an incidental finding of neuronal migrational abnormality identified on MRI. The neuronal migrational abnormality category encompasses a variety of disorders that all have, at their basis, a disturbance of neuronal genesis, migration, and/or organization. Some of the disorders are known to have genetic causes, but many are as yet not well understood. Furthermore, many of the ensuing lesions, while present at birth, are clinically silent for many years before causing patients to have seizures or other neurologic deficits.

Although we are told that our surgical resident participant is a healthy volunteer, we do not as yet know about her birth and early developmental history. If she had learning problems or was slow to achieve developmental milestones, then these could be subtle manifestations of her cortical malformation. Alternatively, at this time, she presumably functions at a normal cognitive level, so the significance of early developmental delay may be negligible. Evaluation by a neurologist or detailed neurocognitive testing might identify other manifestations of her lesion, but it would be difficult to determine whether or not this would result in a change in clinical management.

Equally likely is the fact that she may never have had clinical findings referable to this incidental lesion. Having said that, and knowing that neuronal migrational abnormalities can have a quiescent phase before becoming clinically active, we cannot predict whether this incidental finding will have implications for her. For example, some neuronal migrational abnormalities can result in seizures, and some of the seizure disorders can be refractory to medication therapy. In those cases, surgical excision of the causative lesion may be considered, with variable success.

Thus, we are unable to determine either the medical significance or urgency of this lesion for the participant herself.

However, we do know that this disturbance can be genetic for some people; therefore, there may be implications for the resident later in life. If she decides to bear children, some of them could inherit this condition from her. Without knowing exactly what genetic process has caused her disorder, she may not be able to obtain prenatal diagnostic testing. In that situation, having a clinical genetics assessment might be extremely valuable for the resident, and for her unborn children. A recent change in health care legislation in the United States means that people can no longer be denied health care coverage due to a pre-existing condition, but this will not necessarily prevent discrimination based on genetic findings. Thus, the resident will need to consider whether the potential risk associated with having a clinical genetics evaluation would be warranted. Optimally, consideration of the ramifications of discovery of an incidental finding should have been discussed with the resident before she consented to participate in this study.

COMPREHENSION QUESTIONS

6.1 A 45-year-old research participant undergoes positron emission tomography of the chest, and the results reveal an enhancing right lung mass as an unexpected finding. Which of the following is most accurate regarding incidental findings in research?

    A. Health care costs related to the incidental finding are generally covered by the research protocol.

    B. There are generally no clinical manifestations related to progression of an incidental finding.

    C. There are agreed-upon national and international guidelines regarding dealing with incidental findings.

    D. Research participants generally experience a significant amount of anxiety when they have an incidental finding.

6.2 Which of the following countries has mandatory guidance related to the management of incidental findings in research?

    A. United States

    B. United Kingdom

    C. United States and United Kingdom

    D. Neither the United States nor the United Kingdom

6.3 Which of the following factors may be used to determine whether or not incidental findings should be reported back to the participant?

    A. The potential for harm to the participant's unborn children.

    B. The potential for the research team to be sued.

    C. The lack of a specific statement in the informed consent form stating that incidental findings will be reported to the participant's personal physician.

    D. The lack of funding in the research budget for clinical care for participants.

ANSWERS

6.1 **D.** The potential for harm from progression of the lesion or from anxiety, either related to a true or false diagnosis, can accrue to any participant with an incidental finding. Research studies do not generally cover expenses related to the diagnosis and management of incidental findings; in these circumstances, the participant may be responsible for any costs related to receiving the necessary clinical assessment. There is no consensus on how to deal with incidental findings.

6.2 **D.** At this time, no country has mandatory legislation requiring a uniform approach to the discovery of incidental findings in clinical research.

6.3 **A.** The potential for harm to the participant and to his or her unborn children should be considered when assessing the significance of an incidental finding. It is more likely that a participant could sue a researcher for not disclosing an incidental finding than that she would for disclosing an incidental finding. The lack of a specific statement stating that incidental findings will be reported back to participants does not prevent the researcher from doing so. There is no legislative requirement for research teams to cover the cost of clinical care of an incidental finding.

KEY POINTS

▶ Research participants should be warned about the possible discovery of incidental findings as part of the consent process and should be given specific information about the clinical, emotional, and financial ramifications of such a discovery.

▶ Optimally, researchers should consider the possibility of identifying incidental findings before beginning a study and should develop a method of addressing them.

▶ At this time, there is no specific legislation and no generally accepted guidance about how to approach the evaluation and management of incidental findings in research.

REFERENCES

Booth TC, Jackson A, Wardlaw JM, Taylor A, Waldman AD. Incidental findings found in 'healthy' volunteers during imaging performed for research: current legal and ethical implications. *Br J Radiol.* 2010;83:456-465.

Illes J, Kirschen MP, Edwards E, et al. Practical approaches to incidental findings in brain imaging research. *Neurology.* 2008;70:384-390.

Illes J, Rosen AC, Huang L, et al. Ethical consideration of incidental findings on adult brain MRI in research. *Neurology.* 2004;62:888-890.

Rangel EK. The management of incidental findings in neuro-imaging research: framework and recommendations. *J Law Med Ethics.* 2010;38(1):117-126.

Richardson HS, Belsky L. The ancillary-care responsibilities of medical researchers. An ethical framework for thinking about the clinical care that researchers owe their subjects. *Hastings Cent Rep.* 2004;34:25-33.

Spalice A, Parisi P, Nicita F, Pizzardi G, Del Balzo F, Iannetti P. Neuronal migrational disorders: clinical, neuroradiologic and genetics aspects. *Acta Paediatrica.* 2009;98:421-433.

CJ, a 42-year-old woman with a history of breast cancer with pulmonary, hepatic, and central nervous system metastasis, presented in the emergency department (ED) complaining of shortness of breath, general weakness, and fever. She had just returned from visiting her boyfriend in California, where she had been hospitalized for sepsis, but left against medical advice (AMA) to return home. Her boyfriend, who did not know she had left, reported that she had become confused and exhibited unusual behavior while she was with him over the past month; he also admitted that she has been missing for 2 days. In the ED now, CJ presented with temperature of 39.2°C. She was alert but confused, exhibiting paranoid behavior and acute mania. She was hypotensive and hypoxic, with an SaO2 of 89% on room air. Chest radiography showed left lower lobe consolidation and fluid with a possible underlying mass. Her last chemotherapy session was 2 months ago, and additional chemotherapy was planned in 1 month. Several years ago CJ named her father as her health care proxy agent, with no alternate identified. Since that time, he had declined and was now living in a nursing home with slowly worsening dementia, unable to make informed decisions for himself or for his daughter. Her mother died of breast cancer 8 years ago. She was not married and had no adult children. Her sister and brother lived in the area, but they did not speak to each other very often. An ethics consultation was requested by the team to help determine how to approach the issue of informed consent.

► What is the purpose and role of ethics committees in health care institutions?
► What is the role of ethics consultation in addressing questions of ethics that arise in the clinical setting?
► How do we determine who speaks for the patient who lacks decisional capacity?

ANSWERS TO CASE 7:

Ethics Committees and Consultation

Summary: A 42-year-old woman with a history of end-stage metastatic breast cancer presented in the ED complaining of shortness of breath and fever with sepsis, including hypotension and hypoxia. She is confused. Her father has been named her primary proxy agent, with no alternate identified, but now he has dementia, and he is unable to make informed decisions for himself or for his daughter. The patient's mother died 8 years ago, and she was not married and had no adult children. Her sister and brother lived in the area, but they did not speak to each other very often. An ethics consultation was requested by the team to help determine how to approach the issue of informed consent.

- **Purpose and role of ethics committees:** The ethics committee provides consultation, education, and policy development to the institution, clinicians, patients, and their families.

- **Role of ethics consultation in the clinical setting:** Ethics consultation provides a forum for discourse and conflict resolution for ethical issues that arise in providing care to patients. It is accomplished through "ethics facilitation," a process which brings all the stakeholders to the table to discuss the facts of the case, identify the ethical questions, discuss the range of ethically defensible options to address the question, and facilitate consensus to move forward on one or more of the options identified.

- **Alternatives for determining who represents and gives informed consent for the patient who lacks decisional capacity:** Ideally, the patient has identified and legally appointed a health care proxy agent and instructed them on their wishes. There may also be a court-appointed guardian to represent the decisionally incapacitated patient. The family may also be a source of information and representation of the patient who cannot represent himself or herself.

ANALYSIS

Objectives

1. To identify the ethical components of patient care.

2. To understand the role and function of ethics consultation.

3. To appreciate the importance of identifying a spokesperson for the decisionally incapable patient.

Considerations

Modern health care requires the inclusion of the patient in decision-making. When the patient cannot speak for himself or herself, then his or her perspective is represented by legally appointed health care proxy agents, guardians, or family members. In complex and technologically advanced health care systems and a morally diverse society, difference of opinion on what is right or good (the essential questions of ethics) is the norm. To address these differences and conflicts, ethics committees have been established to provide education, policy development, and consultation on ethical issues that arise in clinical care. The physicians caring for the patient in this scenario must make an assessment of her decisional capacity. Having established with the help of psychiatric consultation that she lacked the ability to communicate a choice, understand relevant information, assess the consequences, and reason about choices for intervention, the physician had to identify who would speak for her. Although she had appointed a health care proxy agent, he was no longer able to function in this capacity for her. Because she had family members who knew her but had not stepped forward to speak for her, the team requested ethics consultation to assist in determining this. In concert with members of the team, the ethics consultants convened a meeting in which the team and family members could discuss the patient's condition, the current clinical questions, hear about past history that informs her likely choice, and decide together next steps in her care.

APPROACH TO:

Ethics Consultation

DEFINITIONS

DECISIONAL CAPACITY: The ability of a patient to communicate choice, understand relevant information, appreciate consequences, and reason about choices for intervention.

ETHICS COMMITTEE: An interdisciplinary group whose primary goals are to provide ethics education, policy development, and ethics consultation for a health care institution.

ETHICS CONSULTATION: A service provided by an individual, small team, or committee aims to facilitate discussion and negotiate conflict resolution of ethical issues that arise in patient care.

PRINCIPLES OF BIOMEDICAL ETHICS: The 4 primary values that together reflect aims of good health care: autonomy, beneficence, nonmaleficence, and justice.

CLINICAL APPROACH

In this case, the physician assessment of lack of decisional capacity and the need for clinical decision-making requiring informed consent led to the request for ethics consultation. In the consultation, the ethics consultant gathered information from the physicians, nurses, social worker, and chart that led to the need to facilitate a discussion with the patient's 2 primary family members and the team to sort out the wishes of the patient and their agreement on who would speak for her.

ANALYSIS AND DISCUSSION

Decisions about what is good or what is right—the essential questions of ethics—in patient care are guided by 4 fundamental principles that we strive to promote in providing care to patients: respect for autonomy, beneficence, nonmaleficence, and justice (Beaucamp and Childress, 2012). *Respect for autonomy* reflects the value of self-determination, which is both morally prized and legally reinforced. As health care technology has advanced, questions about what intervention a patient would want—or would not want—have become increasingly important. Medical interventions can sustain life even despite advanced physical or mental illness. Therefore, it is important for the patient living with severe debility or impairment to be able to express their preferences, choices, and experience, even if that means having a surrogate speak for her. *Beneficence* reflects the value of doing good and attempting to improve the condition of life for the patient. *Nonmaleficence* reflects an age-old expectation for physicians (and by extension all health care professionals) to "do no harm." There is now a strong expectation that the patient living with the treatment or disease will be the one to determine what constitutes "harm." Finally, the principle of *justice* reflects the value of treating patients fairly and attempting to distribute scarce resources in an equitable way.

These principles are sometimes in conflict, and a forum for discourse on ethical issues is necessary in a morally diverse society such as ours. This is increasingly true as health care technology interventions advance in scope, complexity and interdependence. In most health care institutions, this need is met by the ethics committee of the institution. Encouraged by law, regulation, and accreditation requirements, ethics committees serve 3 common functions: to provide education on ethical issues, to write institutional policies that provide guidance for practice, and to offer ethics consultation in specific cases. They are a common feature in large acute care facilities, with one survey showing that all hospitals with more than 400 beds had an ethics committee (Fox et al. 2007). Although practices vary, some features of health care institution ethics committee are shared: they tend to be multidisciplinary with wide representation from across the organization—physicians, nurses, social workers, chaplains, allied health services, and administrators. They include legal representatives from the organization as well as community members and/or former patients. The committees report to the leadership of the organization, often through the medical staff executive committee, chief executive officer (CEO), or the board of directors. Their authority derives from influence, inquiry, and moral suasion. They share interest in ethical issues with the organization's compliance office, the professional practice committee, the patient advocacy office, and the institution review board (IRB) for ethical concerns in research, but have a unique responsibility to help caregivers—including health care professionals, patients, and their friends and families—with clinical ethics questions that arise in the care of a specific patient.

Ethics consultation can be performed by an individual, small team, or full ethics committee. Its aim is to:

1. Promote an ethical resolution of the case at hand.

2. Establish comfortable and respectful communication among the parties involved.

3. Help those involved learn to work through ethical uncertainties and disagreements on their own.

4. Help the hospital ethics committee recognize patterns within the hospital and consider reviewing hospital procedures or policies (Andre, 1997).

These aims are accomplished by learning the facts sufficient to identify the ethical question or questions that are troubling any of the moral stakeholders. Stakeholders include those who have moral authority or responsibility for the patient, and then bringing the stakeholders together to discuss the facts and uncertainties of the situation, the range of ethically defensible options for addressing the ethical question, and finally helping the stakeholders reach a consensus agreement about which of the options will be chosen or pursued, even if only for a limited time and then re-considered (often referred to as a "time trial"). This approach, to addressing clinical ethical problems, described as ethics facilitation, relies on skills, knowledge, and process, identified in the *Core Competencies for Healthcare Ethics Consultants* (2011) from the American Society for Bioethics and Humanities (Table 7–1).

A critical element of ethically defensible clinical care is consistency with the wishes and values of the patient (reflecting respect for the principle of autonomy). However, the enactment of autonomy relies on the capacity to voice one's values and make decisions among possible choices that are consistent with those values. The exercise of autonomy requires cognitive and communicative abilities. For competent adults who can exercise autonomy, we allow a wide range of choices, even choices we disagree with—one is "allowed" to make "bad" decisions. When doing good (beneficence) and patient choice (autonomy) conflict, as they sometimes do (eg, allowing patient with emphysema to continue to smoke), we rely on an evaluation of cognitive and communicative ability, which is also called decisional capacity. Decisional capacity is also sometimes called competence, although competence and its related term *incompetence* are, strictly speaking, legal terms. Adults are legally

Table 7–1 • CORE COMPETENCIES FOR A HEALTH CARE ETHICS CONSULTATION	
Core Skills	**Core Knowledge**
Ethical assessment and analysis skills	Moral reasoning and ethical theory
Process skills	Common biologic issues and concepts
Facilitating formal meetings	Health care systems
Evaluative and quality-improvement skills	Clinical context
Interpersonal skills	Local health care institution Institutional policy Beliefs and perspectives of local patients Relevant codes of ethics and professional conduct and guidelines of accrediting organizations Relevant health law

assumed to be competent, until determined by a judge to be incompetent, when they are assigned a guardian. In health care, we make clinical judgments all the time on the ability of patients to make decisions for themselves, or, if lacking decisional capacity, to have their values and preferences expressed by someone they have chosen (a health care proxy agent or durable power of attorney for health care) or, more informally, a family member who knows their values and preferences.

With so much riding on decisional capacity, how is it determined? There are 4 criteria for assessing decisional capacity with regard to medical decision-making (Applebaum, 2007), which are based on legal standards of criterion. They include the following:

- Ability to communicate a choice
- Ability to understand relevant information
- Ability to appreciate the consequences of situation
- Ability to reason about choices for intervention

Physicians generally make informal assessments of decisional capacity; however, in complex cases it is often helpful to have psychiatrists, skilled at both interviewing and assessing the functional, organic, and psychoemotional impediments to reasoning and communication, involved in complex cases.

CJ was interviewed by a psychiatrist on 2 occasions and was assessed to lack decisional capacity. She showed only a superficial understanding of her metastatic disease (despite its having been explained to her on several occasions) and no understanding of the consequences of choices for intervention that were also explained to her. She did say she "came back to Boston because she wanted to live and be with her family." Because CJ lacked the capacity to make her own decisions, her "choice" or "voice" needed to be represented by others. Although she had appointed her father her health care proxy agent—her choice for her "voice"—he was no longer able to fulfill that role and her other family members needed to provide her perspective on health care choices and decision making—they needed to be her voice and reflect the choices they understood she would want. Because she had no specific advance care directive, such as a living will or other documents of her intentions and they would have to rely on conversations and statements she made to them before she became incapacitated. Ethically, this preserves the autonomy of the patient even when they themselves lose the capacity to do this.

On receiving the ethics consultation request from the resident on the team, the ethics consultant read through the patient's chart and talked to her nurse and to the social worker involved in the case. They corroborated the facts of the situation. The nurse added that the patient frequently asked about her sister, Joyce, and inquired about whether Joyce knew she was in the hospital, and also asked about why her father had not been in to see her, despite being reminded of his nursing home residence and disability. She also said that she heard from other nurses who had cared for her that Joyce and her brother did not get along and rarely spoke to one another, based on residual disagreement about the end-of-life care of their mother. The social worker added that, on a prior hospitalization, CJ had been encouraged to complete another health care proxy form, because her father was not longer able to speak for her, and while she spoke about both her sister and brother, she did not follow through on completing the form that would have accomplished that change. The social worker also told the ethics consultant that although she had encouraged both Joyce and her brother, James, to meet, come in, and to talk with the team about CJ's situation, they had visited but not committed to meet with the team.

The ethics consultant recommended that they hold a formal ethics consultation meeting—2 ethics consultation service members, with the clinical team and the family. The goals of the meeting were to discuss CJ's current clinical situation, the expected clinical needs she would have, the goals of care recommended by the team, and to hear Joyce's and James' understanding of what CJ would want for her treatment. An additional goal was to see if the siblings would agree to have one of them act as spokesperson in communicating with the team. This was done within the next 2 days, and at that meeting, the initial tension that was sensed between Joyce and James subsided somewhat as they talked about how loyal to their mother CJ had been through her illness, especially toward the end of her life when CJ moved in with her mother and father to help care for her at the end of her life. Although she died in the intensive care unit, the decision was based on their mother's request that "everything possible be done" for her, despite some disagreement within the family (Joyce disagreed, trying to convince her mother to accept comfort-oriented care and hospice, while James encouraged her to "fight on"). CJ had been clear that she, too, would want aggressive care if she were to develop breast cancer like her mother. The ethics consultants reinforced the responsibility of those speaking for the patient to voice and defend the values and choices of the patient, not their own perspective and choice. This point helped CJ's siblings reach agreement that James be spokesperson for CJ, keeping Joyce informed of her clinical condition and the team's recommendations for treatment.

Almost immediately, the team needed permission from someone speaking for CJ to place an inferior vena cava (IVC) filter to prevent pulmonary emboli, which they both agreed CJ would want. The ethics consultants also encouraged the team and family to remain vigilant for a time when CJ might regain decision-making and could complete another health care proxy document. The ethics consultants summarized the discussion and recommendations in a note in the patient's chart and continued to follow the case, checking in weekly with the treatment team.

COMPREHENSION QUESTIONS

7.1 What is the single most important ethical principle to consider in deciding clinical issues?

A. Autonomy.

B. Justice.

C. Nonmaleficence and beneficence considered together.

D. There is no single most important ethical principle. The 4 principles are weighed against one another as they apply to the particulars of a clinical situation.

7.2 What is the primary reason health care institutions have developed ethics committees?

A. The US federal government requires ethics committees as a way to insure consumer input.

B. In a morally diverse culture such as ours, ethics committees have promoted discourse on ethical issues in clinical care, ensuring discussion about ethical issues in health care from all the stakeholders involved.

C. Licensing regulations for hospitals require ethics committees.

D. Ethics committees grew out of the focus on patient's rights and are an attempt to equalize the imbalance of power that clinicians hold over patients.

7.3 The purpose of ethics consultation in clinical care is to do which of the following?

A. Provide a "court of last resort" in controversies and conflicts that arise in care of patients.

B. Create forum for venting the frustrations and difficulties of complex acute patient care.

C. Promote an ethical resolution of the problem presented in a particular case by establishing respectful communication among all the parties involved.

D. Clarifying the legal limits and rights to all the parties involved in a case conflict.

ANSWERS

7.1 **D.** It is tempting, especially in an individualistic culture, to choose the principle of respect for autonomy as the "single most important principle." However, it is not true that respect for autonomy trumps the other principles. The 4 principles are intended to provide a frame or template of the primary values, which must be considered in determining morally defensible action in health care. Their application to the particular case under consideration provides an opportunity to weigh their relative importance against one another, all things considered.

7.2 **B.** Health care ethics committees were borne out of the need for a forum for discourse between the various stakeholders in medical decisions, when technology development created situations in which determining the "right" thing to do or the "good" choice was not clear. Encouraged by legal requirements and accrediting bodies, they were developed to meet the need for moral deliberation in a diverse society with regard to the applications and opportunities of newly developing technology in health care delivery.

7.3 **C.** Health care ethics consultation aims to create the space and conditions for respectful dialogue among all the moral stakeholders involved in the care of a patient, including the voice of the patient and family members. In modern health care, it is no longer defendable that the good of the patient is determined solely by the attending physician. Although differences in power and authority continue to challenge our claim of "patient- and family-centered care" and well-functioning and egalitarian "health care delivery teams," our aim is to attempt to preserve the voice and perspective of the patient (autonomy), the intent and obligations of clinicians (beneficence and nonmaleficence), and, to do this fairly (justice), our human imperfections require the space and encouragement as well as a format for managing our conflicts and uncertainties as we work together for the well-being of the patient.

KEY POINTS

▶ In a morally diverse society such as ours, a forum is needed to facilitate discourse in situations of moral uncertainty or conflict. The forum that has developed in health care institutions is the ethics committee.

▶ There has been an explosion of ethical questions in health care due to the development of technology coupled with strong respect in society for self-determination and individual rights.

▶ Four ethical principles in health care—autonomy, beneficence, nonmaleficence, and justice—reflect the important fundamental values in health care. No single principle can be identified as "superior" or more important than the others in all cases.

▶ The principle of autonomy relies on the capacity to communicate and reason about choices. When a patient lacks decisional capacity, his or her autonomy is preserved through surrogate decision-makers speaking for the patient.

▶ Ethics consultation is a function of health care ethics committees. Its aim is to provide a forum for ethical questions in a particular patient's care to be raised, all viewpoints to be heard, options considered, and a consensus reached in determining next steps.

REFERENCES

American Society for Bioethics and Humanities. *Core Competencies for Healthcare Ethics Consultation.* 2nd ed. Glenview, IL: American Society for Bioethics and Humanities; 2011.

Andre J. Goals of ethics consultation: toward clarity, utility, and fidelity. *J Clin Ethics.* 1997;8:193-198.

Applebaum PS. Assessment of patients' competent to consent to treatment. *N Engl J Med.* 2007;357: 1834-1840.

Beauchamp T, Childress J. *Principles of Biomedical Ethics.* 7th ed. Oxford: Oxford University Press; 2012.

Fox E, Myers S, Pearlman RA. Ethics consultation in United States hospitals: a national survey. *Am J Clin Ethics.* 2007;7:13-25.

A 70-year-old woman is seen in your office for an annual visit. She has a history of atrial fibrillation for which she takes oral Coumadin. Over the last year, her International Normalized Ratio (INR) has ranged between 2.0 to 3.0. She has no other medical problems and takes no other medications. Her only new complaint is "forgetfulness." Recently, she has had what she calls more "senior moments." She occasionally forgets words and misplaces her keys. The forgetfulness does not interfere with her daily activities, and she continues to work part time in the volunteer office of a nearby hospital. She denies urinary incontinence, difficulty with walking or balance, changes in mood or appetite, weight changes, and problems with her vision. She does not drink alcohol. There are no significant findings on her physical and neurologic examinations. A depression screen is negative. All laboratory studies are within normal limits, including B12, folate, rapid plasma reagin (RPR), and thyroid stimulating hormone (TSH). She asks about gingko biloba, which a friend recommended taking to improve her memory.

► What is your response to gingko biloba?
► What is the best approach in discussing complementary or alternative medications with your patient?

ANSWERS TO CASE 8:

Complementary, Alternative, and Integrative Medicine

Summary: A 70-year-old woman is seen in your office for an annual visit. She has a history of atrial fibrillation and has been therapeutic on Coumadin over the previous year. Her only complaint is new forgetfulness. The workup is negative and her memory problems are likely a normal symptom of aging. She asks about taking gingko biloba.

- **Response to gingko biloba:** Advise her not to take gingko biloba, because of its possible interaction with warfarin. It is an herbal supplement sold over-the-counter. Many believe it can help with memory and cognition, but more research must be done, and there may be risks associated with its use. Gingko biloba may be associated with an increased risk of bleeding, especially in patients who are taking other anticoagulants such as warfarin.

- **How to discuss complementary and alternative medicine (CAM):** Ask all patients if they use CAM during the comprehensive history in an open-minded manner. It is important to be open and nonjudgmental and understand the different reasons patients may use CAM.

ANALYSIS

Objectives

1. Define complementary, alternative, and integrative medicines.

2. Describe effective ways to discuss and work with patients who wish to pursue nontraditional therapies.

3. Describe resources to find out scientific evidence and safety of various nontraditional therapies.

Considerations

This 70-year-old woman with a history of atrial fibrillation for which she takes Coumadin asks about the use of gingko biloba to improve her memory. The most important first step is a comprehensive history, physical examination, and laboratory work-up to rule out reversible causes of dementia, such as hypothyroidism, B12 deficiency, and syphilis. Polypharmacy, depression, and normal pressure hydrocephalus can also cause similar symptoms in elderly patients. It can be difficult to distinguish memory loss that is a normal symptom of aging from non-reversible causes dementia, such as Alzheimer disease; however, if memory loss does not interfere with day-to-day functioning, as in this case, then it is more likely to be benign.

Once you determine that her memory problems are likely a common symptom of aging and not pathologic, it is important to provide reassurance and appear open and non-judgmental when answering her question about gingko biloba. Although many believe that gingko biloba may improve cognition and memory, there is still more research that needs to be done, particularly to determine the dose and length of treatment. Case studies have reported that gingko biloba may be associated with an increased risk of bleeding, particularly in patients taking other anticoagulants, such as warfarin. Therefore, in this case, the patient should be advised not to take gingko biloba, as the risks may outweigh the benefits.

APPROACH TO:

Complementary, Alternative, and Integrative Medicine

DEFINITIONS

ALTERNATIVE MEDICINE: Use of a nonmainstream approach in place of conventional medicine.

COMPLEMENTARY MEDICINE: Use of a nonmainstream approach together with conventional medicine.

INTEGRATIVE MEDICINE: The practice of medicine that reaffirms the importance of the relationship between practitioner and patient, focuses on the whole person, is informed by evidence, and makes use of all appropriate therapeutic approaches, health care professionals, and disciplines to achieve optimal health and healing.

CLINICAL APPROACH

Complementary medicine is defined as the use of a nonmainstream approach together with conventional medicine. Alternative medicine is different in that it is the use of a nonmainstream approach in place of conventional medicine. In the United States, alternative medicine is less common than complementary medicine. Integrative medicine focuses on the whole person, not just the disease, emphasizes the relationship between patient and physician, is informed by evidence, and makes use of all possible therapeutic approaches, practitioners, and disciplines to achieve optimal health and healing.

In a National Health Interview Survey from 2002, 75% of American adults reported having used CAM at some time. Patients more likely to use CAM were women, those with a higher education, and those who had been hospitalized within the last year. The reasons for using CAM varied, but more than one-half of the adult patients who used CAM believed that CAM combined with conventional medical treatments would help. Less than one-third believed conventional therapies would not help them. Thirteen percent felt conventional medicine was too expensive.

ANALYSIS AND DISCUSSION

What Are the Most Common Complementary Health Approaches?

The National Center for Complementary and Alternative Medicine divides the therapies into 2 subgroups, that is, mind and body practices and natural products. The most commonly used mind and body practices among adults are deep breathing, meditation, chiropractic and osteopathic, massage, yoga, progressive relaxation, and guided imagery. Other practices include movement therapies, Tai chi and qi gong, healing touch, and hypnotherapy. Natural products include herbs, vitamins, minerals, and probiotics, which are sold over the counter as dietary supplements. According to the 2007 National Health Interview Survey, the most common natural product used by adults was fish oil/omega 3. Although 17.7% of American adults had used a nonvitamin/nonmineral natural product in the previous year, research to prove they are safe and effective is still ongoing. It is especially important to consider potential interactions, as some patients fail to report use of natural products to their physicians.

Ginkgo biloba

Gingko biloba is a medicinal herb sold over-the-counter in the United States. Many believe it can improve memory and cognition. Although more studies must be performed to identify the diseases and symptoms for which it is most useful, as well as the ideal dose and duration of treatment, it is thought to be beneficial in age-associated dementia, Alzheimer disease, and vascular dementia. Possible mechanisms of action include improving cerebral blood flow, reducing reperfusion injury, inhibiting platelets, and various neuroprotective processes such as antioxidation and antiinflammation. Although gingko biloba is sold over-the-counter, its use is not without risks. Case studies report unusual bleeding in patients taking gingko biloba. The risk of bleeding seems to be higher in patients taking other antiplatelet drugs, such as non-steroidal anti-inflammatory drugs (NSAIDs), aspirin, and anticoagulants, possibly secondary to the inhibition of platelet-activating factor due to gingko use.

Notably, gingko biloba is not the only herbal supplement thought to have potential interactions with warfarin. Many recommend that patients taking warfarin avoid gingko biloba, garlic, ginger, and ginseng.

Communicating With Patients

Speaking with patients about CAM can be difficult for physicians, as CAM includes medical interventions not typically covered in the curriculum of many US medical schools. Before initiating a discussion about CAM, physicians should consider why patients utilize these therapies. Reasons may include a desire for more control over their medical care, to enhance quality of life, and to boost the immune system. Other patients turn to CAM because they are dissatisfied with attitudes of physicians and feel conventional therapies have failed. Interestingly, patients who use CAM commend CAM providers on the time spent with patients, the way they explain illnesses, the continuity in care, and the personalization of care. Patient satisfaction with CAM may not correspond with improvements in symptoms, which means that patients respond to more than just the treatment itself.

There are multiple reasons patients may not initiate a conversation with their physician about CAM. Patients may be afraid of being judged or not want their physician to think they are ungrateful for the care they have received. Other patients may not understand that CAM can interact with biomedical treatments or that withholding information about its use from their physician can be dangerous.

Physicians have their own reasons for not initiating discussions about CAM. For some physicians, it is a lack of knowledge on the subject and a fear of appearing uniformed. Others may not believe that CAM can help their patients.

One way that physicians may talk to their patients about the use of CAM is to make it part of the comprehensive history, along with asking about the use of drugs and alcohol. Asking patients what medications they use at home is not sufficient, as many patients do not consider CAM as medication. One way to approach the topic is to ask, "Are you taking anything else, such as vitamins, herbs, or homeopathic remedies? Have you tried any other practices, such as acupuncture or yoga?" It is important for physicians to appear nonjudgmental and supportive. In addition to facilitating a discussion about CAM, providers should review issues of safety and efficacy and follow-up with patients to review the response to therapy and monitor for adverse effects. It is also important to document these interactions. This strategy helps both patients and physicians integrate CAM into their conventional medical therapy, which may help avoid potential and serious interactions.

Resources
The Internet has a wealth of information on CAM for both patients and physicians. When reviewing a website before recommending it to a patient, check who runs the website, if they are selling a product, and if the information is evidence based and up to date. Some examples include:

- National Center for Comprehensive and Alternative medicine (www.nccam .nih.gov)

- Evidence Report Summaries from the Agency for Healthcare Research and Quality (www.AHRQ.gov)

- Hospital websites, for example, Memorial Sloan Kettering Cancer Center (www.mskcc.org)

COMPREHENSION QUESTIONS

8.1 A 46-year-old man is taking warfarin anticoagulation. You ask about CAM medications. Which of the following may lead to interaction with the warfarin and bleeding complications?

A. Garlic

B. Grape seed abstract

C. Green tea

D. Goldenseal

8.2 As you are considering how to incorporate CAM therapy in your practice, which of the following findings have been noted in studies?

A. Physicians who recommend CAM are typically viewed by patients as subpar or quacks.

B. Typically, physicians who recommend CAM are positively viewed by patients because of the time they spend with their patients.

C. Physicians who recommend CAM are generally not board certified.

D. Physicians who recommend CAM generally have a higher job satisfaction.

ANSWERS

8.1 **A.** Many experts advise patients on warfarin to avoid gingko biloba, garlic, ginger, and ginseng.

8.2 **B.** Physicians who incorporate CAM or have discussions of CAM in their practice are generally viewed by patients as spending more time and are viewed positively by patients. There is no evidence of differences in board certification rates or job satisfaction.

KEY POINTS

▶ Complementary medicine is the use of a nonmainstream approach together with conventional medicine, while alternative medicine is the use of a nonmainstream approach in place of conventional medicine.

▶ Ask all patients about the use of herbal supplements, homeopathic remedies, and other practices such as acupuncture or yoga.

▶ Although herbal supplements and vitamins are sold over the counter, their use is not without risks, and many can interact with conventional medical therapies.

▶ All physicians and patients should be aware of the potential interaction and increased risk of bleeding with the gingko biloba, garlic, ginger, and ginseng in patients taking anticoagulants (eg, warfarin).

REFERENCES

Barnes PM, Powell-Griner E, McFann K, Nahin RL. Complementary and alternative medicine use among adults: United States, 2002. *Advance Data.* 2004;343:1-20.

Barnes PM, Bloom B, Nahin RL. Complementary and alternative medicine use among adults and children: United States, 2007. *CDC Natl Health Stat Rep.* 2008;12:12-16.

Diamon BJ, Bailey MR. Ginkgo biloba: indications, mechanisms, and safety. *Psychiatr Clin N Am.* 2013;36:73-83.

National Center for Complementary and Alternative Medicine. Complementary, alternative, or integrative health: what's in a name? Published May 2013. http://nccam.nih.gov/health/whatiscam. Accessed May 1, 2014.

Pappas S, Perlman A. Complementary and alternative medicine: the importance of doctor-patient communication. *Med Clin N Am.* 2002;86:1-10.

Royal Australian College of General Practitioners. Integrative medicine. Published 2011. http://curriculum.racgp.org.au/statements/integrative-medicine. Accessed May 1, 2014.

Vaes LP, Chyka PA. Interactions of warfarin with garlic, ginger, gingko, or ginseng: nature of the evidence. *Ann Pharmacotherapy.* 2000;34:1478-1482.

Zollman C, Vicker A. Complementary medicine and the patient. *BMJ.* 1999;319:1486-1489.

The week after graduating from medical school, you fly home to a family wedding. Your oldest family friend approaches you and offers her congratulations. You thank her, but then are caught off guard when she asks your opinion about the risk of vaccination for pediatric patients. She is currently raising her 3 grandchildren but none has been vaccinated for routine diseases due to the grandmother's fears about possible adverse events. She tells you that she does not trust her pediatrician, but she has known you your whole life. So, if you think that she should vaccinate the children, she says she will do it. You know the associations between autism and vaccinations have been disproved, and you are a strong proponent of vaccination for individual and herd immunity, so you answer her questions and advise her to have all 3 grandchildren vaccinated as soon as possible.

▶ Was a physician–patient relationship formed?
▶ If one of the children has an adverse reaction to a vaccination you recommended, are you potentially liable?

ANSWERS TO CASE 9:

Physician–Patient Relationship

Summary: As a newly graduated medical doctor, you are approached at a social event and asked to provide medical advice regarding the risks and benefits of childhood vaccines; specifically, you are asked to make a recommendation for providing routine immunizations for the 3 grandchildren of a family friend. You advise the grandmother to have the grandchildren immediately vaccinated.

- **Was a physician–patient relationship formed?** Yes, after giving a recommendation on medical matters, a physician–patient relationship was formed.

- **Liability should one of the children have an adverse event to a vaccination you recommended:** Yes, you would have liability because a physician–patient relationship has been formed.

ANALYSIS

Objectives

1. Understand the most common circumstances under which a physician–patient relationship is formed.

2. Describe the ethical concept of fiduciary duty and describe how it applies to the physician–patient relationship.

Considerations

Most physicians are all too familiar with the scenario described above in which a friend or family member asks for an opinion or advice on a medical matter during a social gathering. Once the helpful opinion or advice is proffered, a formal physician–patient relationship with all its attendant obligations is formed, including any ethical and legal obligations. Sometimes it is difficult to determine when the physician–patient relationship is formed; however, once such a relationship is created, the physician has a fiduciary duty to the patient and may incur legal liability if a breach of that duty occurs. For example, supplying medical advice about a specific circumstance may be viewed as practicing medicine, rather than simply stating the consensus of a professional medical organization. Nevertheless, giving advice on medical issues—no matter the venue or the relationship—may certainly be viewed as the beginning of a physician–patient relationship.

APPROACH TO:

Physician–Patient Relationship

DEFINITION

PHYSICIAN–PATIENT RELATIONSHIP: A relationship that carries obligations for both the physician and the patient. Once formed, the physician owes the patient a fiduciary duty—that is, a duty to act in the best interests of the patient when formulating treatment plans and applying the ethical principles of beneficence, nonmaleficence, autonomy, and justice. In addition to the ethical obligations that accompany the physician–patient relationship, legal ramifications may also exist. The relationship has justifiable limits, and the physician may discontinue the relationship under certain circumstances; however, steps must be taken to avoid the physician abandoning the patient.

CLINICAL APPROACH

The establishment and maintenance of a mutually beneficial physician–patient relationship is fundamental to the ability of a physician to provide appropriate care and treatment to patients. The physician–patient relationship is based on the concept of medicine as a profession, thus creating a fiduciary duty that extends from the physician to the patient. The underlying tenets of the physician–patient relationship are the ethical principles of beneficence, nonmaleficence, autonomy, and justice. Recognizing the importance of such a relationship underscores the need for clarity as to precisely when such a relationship is formed, thereby placing the physician in a fiduciary relationship with the patient. Once a physician-patient relationship is formed and a fiduciary duty is established, the physician has an obligation to act in the best interests of the patient.

ANALYSIS AND DISCUSSION

Ethical Considerations

The ethical concept of being a patient was introduced into medical ethics in the 18th century by Scottish physician-ethicist John Gregory (1724–1773). Gregory wrote the first text in English on professional medical ethics. In the centuries between the Hippocratic texts (fifth and fourth centuries BCE) to the early 18th century, the relationship between a physician and a sick person (*aegrotus* in the Latin texts on medical ethics) was contractual and based on mutually negotiated self-interest. Physicians had no duties other than those agreed to with the sick individual contracting for services. Physicians were also mainly guided by prudence, the virtue that schools one in the discipline of identifying then acting to protect one's self-interests. This resulted in physicians routinely stopping treatment of the desperately ill and leaving them to their own devices, so that the disease, not the physician, was blamed for the ensuing death—no small consideration in a highly competitive market for the services and coin of the well-to-do who could afford the fees of the physicians.

Gregory changed this model with his invention of the ethical concept of medicine as a profession, which requires 3 sustained commitments: (1) the physician commits to becoming and remaining scientifically and clinically competent, (2) the physician makes the protection and promotion of the patient's health-related interests, the physician's primary concern and motivation, and keeps individual self-interest systematically secondary, and (3) the physician keeps the interests of physicians as a group, or guild interests (which had dominated the practice of medicine for centuries), systematically secondary. These commitments transformed physicians into professional physicians and the sick into patients. Gregory was the first to use the word "patient" to mean an individual protected by the professional commitments of physicians.

In Gregory's account, the ethical concept of becoming a patient is straightforward: (a) an individual is presented to a physician (or other health care professional), and (b) there exist forms of clinical management that are reliably expected to result in net clinical benefit for that individual. Note that the concept is based on beneficence. An individual does not need to originate his or her moral status and an individual does not need to have rights to be a patient, which is a requirement for making contracts.

The individual can be presented to a physician in the usual way, physical presentation, face-to-face; however, other ways exist in which a patient may present to a physician. In Gregory's day, the great doctors received letters from individuals with their medical stories and a request for help and responded to them with a diagnosis and treatment plan. These individuals became patients. In contemporary communications, media, including telemedicine, phone conversations, e-mail, and social media, provide alternative forums in which individuals may present to physicians and become patients. On rounds in an academic setting, the great doctors have long been those who could work up a differential diagnosis for an individual based on the report of the learners on the team alone without seeing or examining the patient. We have a concept for this in medical education: the students and residents presented the patient to the attending physician.

In the case that opened this chapter, the physician's family friend presented her 3 grandchildren and the physician offered forms of medical care—giving advice about vaccinations—that are reliably expected to result in net clinical benefit. Ethically speaking, these 3 grandchildren became the physician's patients, to which the physician owed and provided the standard of care for medical advice in the preventive care of children.

Legal Considerations

The physician–patient relationship is the legal framework upon which the concept of medical malpractice lies. In the absence of a physician–patient relationship, a physician owes no specific duty to an individual; without a duty to the patient, no breach of duty exists and, thus, no professional liability. The legal definition of when a physician–patient relationship is formed will vary based on state laws and appropriate governing statues; however, some general guiding principles can be employed (see Table 9–1).

The earliest case that raised the question of the existence of a physician–patient relationship was that of *Hurley versus Eddingfield*, a case decided by the Indiana Supreme Court in 1901. Dr Eddingfield was a general practitioner in Indiana and had previously served as the family physician to Charlotte Burk. Ms Burk experienced complications during childbirth, and Mr Burk sent word to Dr Eddignfield requesting his presence to assist in the delivery of the neonate; Mr Burk tendered payment in advance. Dr Eddingfield refused to attend to Ms Burk for unknown reasons and the infant was stillborn. The Indiana Supreme Court held that a physician is free to determine whom he or she will treat and under what circumstances. In this case, Dr Eddingfield did not owe a duty to Ms Burk and could not be held legally liable.

Table 9–1 • CREATION OF A PHYSICIAN–PATIENT RELATIONSHIP	
Actions That May Create a Physician–Patient Relationship	**Actions Not Likely to Create a Physician–Patient Relationship**
Providing advice to friends or relatives	"Curbside consultations"/informal advice to a colleague
Supervising midlevel practitioners providing care and treatment	Evaluation/treatment of a patient for a third party (ie, insurance, workers' compensation, pre-employment physical examinations)
Writing prescriptions	
Engaging in phone, social media, or e-mail correspondence	
Accepting walk-in patients	
Diagnosing and/or treating a patient	
Performing online consultations	
Interpreting data (ie, test results, radiographs)	

The Indiana Supreme Court went further and established that no duty exists on the part of the physician to render aid in an emergency; this concept is also known as the duty to rescue. This is a key area in which medical ethics and the law do not agree—ethically speaking, once a physician comes upon the site of an emergency to render aid, the injured party is considered to have presented themselves for treatment, thus establishing a physician–patient relationship. The physician should stop and help by stabilizing the patient to the extent possible, seeing to it that 911 is called, and turning over management of the patient's condition and problems to emergency medical services as soon as possible.

Legally, though physicians are not required to do so, physicians are protected in their willingness to render aid by so-called "Good Samaritan" laws. In fact, physicians have an ethical obligation to render aid in emergencies, as shown above. Good Samaritan laws should be supported in all jurisdictions to encourage physicians to fulfill their professional responsibilities while concurrently protecting them from liability. This is true so much so that the American Medical Association (AMA) states that physicians have the right to choose their patients except in an emergency situation. The AMA *Code of Medical Ethics* is not legally binding, but it does set out guidelines physicians should follow and often leads the way for new legislation in controversial areas.

What if instead of a family friend requiring this information at a social gathering, a fellow pediatrician asked whether or not you would recommend a certain vaccination for one of his patients? In general, states are reluctant to find existence of a physician–patient relationship when the physician provides informal consultation to a colleague in the form of a "curbside consultation." Similarly, examinations performed at the request of a third party such as an insurance company or employer will not typically result in the formation of a physician–patient relationship because the intent of the care provided to the patient is to provide information to the third party, not to provide care and treatment of the patient.

COMPREHENSION QUESTIONS

9.1 You are a gastroenterologist working for a large health care system with an impressive website that offers online resources to the public. Based on this online content, a woman you have never met or treated decides that her bloating symptoms are due to a gastrointestinal cause that she treats with over-the-counter medication. Six months later, she is diagnosed with stage 3 ovarian cancer. You are informed by a patient of yours who is friends with the woman that she intends to sue you for delay in diagnosis of her cancer based on your physician–patient relationship. Was a physician–patient relationship formed and do you have potential liability?

A. A physician–patient relationship was formed and you have potential legal liability to the patient for delayed diagnosis.

B. No physician–patient relationship exists and you have no legal liability to the patient for delayed diagnosis.

C. A physician–patient relationship exits, but you have no legal liability to the patient for delayed diagnosis since you had nothing to do with the decision of the health care system to post the online resources.

9.2 You are a resident in general surgery and decide to start a blog. On your official blog site, readers have the opportunity to post comments and feedback. A man posted information about his recent laparoscopic cholecystectomy and mentioned that he was experiencing excruciating shoulder pain the day following surgery. You replied to his post indicating that shoulder pain was very common following laparoscopic procedures due to retained carbon monoxide gas and may cause irritation. Based on your post, he did not seek medical care and subsequently died due to undiagnosed bleeding. Was a physician–patient relationship formed and do you have potential liability?

A. No physician–patient relationship exists and you have no legal liability to the patient's estate for wrongful death.

B. A physician–patient relationship was formed and you have potential legal liability to the patient's estate for wrongful death.

C. A physician–patient relationship exits, but you have no legal liability to the patient for delayed diagnosis because you had a statement on your blog that all questions about personal medical conditions should be referred to the individual's physician.

ANSWERS

9.1 **A.** In the era of electronic communication, many ways exist in which a physician–patient relationship can be formed even in the absence of a face-to-face consultation. In the case of online resources, it is important that patients understand that the medical tools being provided do not take the place of a visit and examination by a qualified medical professional. To this end, those providing online medical resources will protect themselves from legal claims by providing wording on their website indicating that providing the information online does not create a physician–patient relationship.

9.2 **B.** When the man posted personal medical data on your blog, he was officially presented for treatment and a physician–patient relationship was created. The presence of a disclaimer on the blog informing all readers to consult their own physician will likely be viewed as insufficient to protect the person who owns the blog and prevent the finding of a physician–patient relationship. The fact that the person hosting the blog decided to provide advice to the patient is further evidence that the relationship was created. Thus, the physician responding to the man's posting has potential liability for his wrongful death.

KEY POINTS

▶ The formation of the physician–patient relationship may more readily occur from the ethical perspective as compared with the binding requirements of the law.

▶ Once a physician–patient relationship is established, the physician owes the patient a fiduciary duty to act in the patient's best interests.

▶ There are 2 notable exceptions to the formation of the physician–patient relationship: (1) "curbside consultations," and (2) examinations and treatment performed at the behest of a third party.

REFERENCES

American Medical Association (AMA). Opinion 10.01. Fundamental elements of the patient-physician relationship. In: AMA. *AMA Code of Medical Ethics.* Chicago: AMA; 2008.

American Medical Association (AMA). Opinion 10.015. The patient-physician relationship. In: AMA. *AMA Code of Medical Ethics.* Chicago: AMA; 2008.

Fromme EK. Ethics case: request for care from family members. *Virtual Mentor.* 2012;14:368-372.

Folkl A. The patient-physician relationship: classic questions and new directions. *Virtual Mentor.* 2012;14:365-367.

Hurley v Eddingfield, 156 Ind 416, 59 NE 1058 (Ind 1901).

Parsi K. Duty to treat: conscience and pluralism. *Virtual Mentor.* 2007;9:362-364.

Simon RI, Shuman DW. The doctor-patient relationship. *Clinical Manual of Psychiatry and Law.* 2007; 17-36. http://focus.psychiatryonline.org/article.aspx?articleid=52460. Accessed May 1, 2014.

A patient of yours, a 57-year-old man, presents to the emergency department with exacerbation of chronic obstructive pulmonary disease (COPD). The emergency medicine physician on duty conducts an evaluation, initiates treatment, and plans to admit the patient when he fails to show significant improvement after 2 hours. You receive a phone call at home informing you that the patient is being admitted and that you need to come in to the hospital to further assess and treat the patient. You state that you have no obligation to come into the hospital and explain that because the patient will not comply with your treatment recommendations, you had planned on terminating your physician–patient relationship.

▶ Are you ethically or legally obligated to come in and admit the patient?
▶ What are the consequences of your failure to admit the patient?

ANSWERS TO CASE 10:

Patient Abandonment

Summary: A 57-year-old man with exacerbation of COPD requires admission to the hospital, but you do not wish to provide any further care and treatment for this patient. You would like to terminate your physician–patient relationship due to the patient's continued noncompliance with your medical recommendations.

- **Are you ethically or legally obligated to come in and admit the patient:** Yes, you are obligated because you have not formally terminated the physician–patient relationship and you still have a duty to the patient.

- **Consequences of failing to admit patient:** You will have abandoned the patient.

ANALYSIS

Objectives

1. Understand when a physician–patient relationship is formed.

2. Describe a process for termination of the physician–patient relationship.

3. Define patient abandonment and describe a clinical situation in which a physician has abandoned a patient.

Considerations

Failure of a patient to comply with recommended medical treatment can be grounds for discontinuation of the physician–patient relationship; however, processes must be followed to ensure that the discontinuation of the relationship does not result in patient abandonment. In the scenario described, the physician has not taken the necessary steps to formally discontinue the physician–patient relationship; thus, he or she still has a duty to provide care for the patient. Failure to fulfill those obligations is equivalent to patient abandonment, which has negative legal, hospital, and state medical board consequences.

APPROACH TO:

Discontinuation of the Physician–Patient Relationship

DEFINITION

PATIENT ABANDONMENT: Failure to provide appropriate care and treatment for a patient prior to the proper termination of the physician–patient relationship.

CLINICAL APPROACH

Ethical Considerations

In professional medical ethics, the relationship between a physician and patient is asymmetrical. The physician has more demanding obligations to the patient than the patient has to the physician. In addition, although patients should be prudent and implement agreed-upon plans for self-care, some patients will be imprudent. This behavior may be voluntary or involuntary, a clinical distinction that can often be challenging to make.

The ethical asymmetry of the professional physician–patient relationship means that the physician bears the burden of proof to end the relationship without the patient's agreement. In this respect the professional relationship with a patient is not contractual; the distinction is important, because failure of one party to keep one's agreement is grounds for voiding a contract. The physician continues to have obligations despite the patient's behavior.

The most fundamental ethical obligation of a physician is to see to it that his or her patients receive appropriate, timely, and effective clinical management of their conditions, diseases, or injuries. The physician either attends to this care himself or herself or via referral when the skill level required to meet the patient's clinical needs exceed those of the physician. This ethical obligation requires that the ending of the professional relationship without the agreement of the patient does not disrupt the patient's care and thus violate the physician's obligation to protect the patient's health-related interests. These ethical requirements shape the law of abandonment.

Legal Considerations

Once a physician–patient relationship is established, the physician is obligated to continue treatment of the patient until such a time as the relationship is terminated. Some common reasons a physician may terminate the relationship with a patient include failure to pay for services rendered, failure to comply with prescribed treatment, difficult/demanding patients, and repeated failure to appear for appointments.

In general, a physician–patient relationship may be terminated in 1 of 3 ways: (1) agreement of the patient and the physician to terminate the relationship (eg, the patient is moving out of state and the treating physician helps the patient locate a new doctor), (2) a unilateral act by the patient without involvement of the physician (eg, requesting medical records for transfer to another practice), or (3) a unilateral act by the physician (eg, sending the patient a termination letter). To avoid the accusation of patient abandonment, it is necessary to follow a series of steps to formally terminate the physician–patient relationship, even though it might seem as if the patient unilaterally terminated the relationship by engaging in certain behaviors such as refusing to pay their medical bill. The amount of time a patient is given to find alternative care must be reasonable based on factors such as availability of providers and the severity of the patient's condition.

Table 10–1 • RECOMMENDED APPROACH TO TERMINATION OF THE PHYSICIAN–PATIENT RELATIONSHIP
1. Inform the patient of your intention to terminate the relationship.

2. Prepare a letter of termination that includes the following information:
  a. Recount the salient points from the termination discussion.
  b. Provide the reason for termination.
  c. Indicate a termination date.
  d. Explain physician availability for emergencies until the termination date.
  e. Inform the patient that names of other potential treating physicians can be provided.
  f. State that medical records will be available to the patient or to the new physician.
  g. Discuss need for additional treatment, if necessary.

3. Send the letter via certified mail with return receipt requested.
4. Allow the patient ample time to locate a new physician (ie, 30–90 days).
5. Provide the patient's medical records to the new physician when authorized by patient.
6. Provide list of other medical professionals on patient request.
7. Inform the patient of the potential consequences for failing to seek further treatment.

Reprinted with permission from Clinical Manual of Psychiatry and the Law, (Copyright ©2007). American Psychiatric Association. All Rights Reserved.

One approach to termination of the physician–patient relationship is presented in Table 10–1.

Even after notification, the physician must be available to the patient for emergencies or urgent conditions until the "transition time." Certain medical conditions are viewed as emergent conditions and terminating the physician–patient relationship is not generally allowed such as pregnancy in the third trimester. This is because a pregnant woman in the third trimester of pregnancy may have complications or impending delivery.

COMPREHENSION QUESTIONS

10.1 You are an on-call obstetrician/gynecologist when a new patient presents to your practice; she has her first appointment scheduled 4 days from now. However, she is complaining of chest pain and would like to know what to do. You inform the woman that because she has not been seen in the practice as yet, you will not be providing her any advice or recommendations by phone and that she needs to present for her appointment to receive care from your group. You further explain that, if she is really worried about her condition, then she can report to the emergency department to receive care. What is the proper description of this exchange?

A. No physician–patient relationship exists, so no patient abandonment occurred.

B. A physician–patient relationship exists; however, because you are the only on-call partner, patient abandonment did not take place.

C. A physician-patient relationship exists, so patient abandonment occurred.

10.2 The patient in question 10.1 died approximately 12 hours after speaking to you by phone due to a massive myocardial infarction. One week later, you receive notice of a lawsuit filed by the patient's spouse for wrongful death. Assuming a physician–patient relationship did exist, what best describes your ethical and legal position vis-à-vis the patient?

A. A fiduciary duty did exist, but you did not breech your duty to this patient because you recommended that she visit the emergency department.

B. A fiduciary duty was present, and you breached that duty when you failed to speak to the patient about her symptoms and failed to facilitate immediate treatment.

C. No fiduciary duty existed because you are an obstetrician/gynecologist with no expertise in acute myocardial infarction; thus, the patient would have been better treated in the emergency department.

D. A fiduciary duty did exist, but you did not breach that duty because you referred the patient to the emergency department.

ANSWERS

10.1 **C.** This patient called and was scheduled for an appointment in the office. Ethically, a physician–patient relationship was created because this patient presented to the health care facility for care and treatment through the scheduling of an office visit. Furthermore, from a legal perspective, providing a new patient with an appointment is generally considered the creation of the physician–patient relationship, absent an explicit statement to the contrary.

10.2 **B.** Because a fiduciary duty was present based on the appointment, you breached that duty when you failed to speak to the patient about her symptoms and failed to facilitate immediate treatment.

KEY POINTS

▶ Once a physician–patient relationship is formed, it may be discontinued by either party.

▶ When unilaterally terminating the physician–patient relationship, the physician must abide by both ethical imperatives and legal requirements to avoid patient abandonment.

REFERENCES

American Medical Association (AMA). Opinion 10.015. The patient-physician relationship. In: AMA. *AMA Code of Medical Ethics*. Chicago: AMA; 2008.

American Medical Association (AMA). Opinion 8.115. Termination of the physician-patient relationship. In: AMA. *AMA Code of Medical Ethics*. Chicago: AMA; 2008.

Auckley D. When the patient-physician relationship is broken. *Virtual Mentor*. 2008;10:548-552.

Levin M. The abandoned patient. *Insurance Law Journal*. 1965; 165 Ins. L.J. 275.

Simon RI, Shuman DW. The doctor-patient relationship. *Clin Man Psychiatr Law*. 2007;17-36.

You admit a 78-year-old man to your service for acute pneumonia. His condition rapidly deteriorates, and he spends 2 weeks in the intensive care unit before his condition improves. He is discharged home after 6 weeks in the hospital and is home in time to celebrate the New Year holiday. You rounded on the patient each day during his hospitalization, including during your holiday vacation. The patient's wife is so appreciative of your dedication and support during the hospitalization that she brings you a designer briefcase as a thank you gift. You find the briefcase via an Internet retailer and discover the bag costs $2000.

▶ Can you accept the briefcase?
▶ What if the gift had instead been a $20 bottle of wine?

ANSWERS TO CASE 11:

Boundary Issues

Summary: After a prolonged hospitalization, the grateful wife of a patient attempts to give you a briefcase that costs $2000 for your dedication and for the excellent care her husband received.

- **Can you accept the briefcase?** You cannot accept the briefcase based on its value.

- **Could you accept a bottle of wine?** You may be able to accept a gift of lesser or nominal value based on individual institutional policies.

ANALYSIS

Objectives

1. Identify types of boundaries encountered as a physician.

2. Identify circumstances in which professional boundary issues may be violated.

3. Describe concerns that stem from physicians accepting gifts from patients.

4. Describe concerns about connecting with your patients on social media websites.

Considerations

While some boundary violations are clear, such as entering into a sexual relationship with a patient, others are not as clear as in the case of gifts. Although it may be flattering to receive gifts from patients expressing their gratitude for the care you provide, receiving particularly lavish or expensive gifts is problematic. In this case, the patient's family offered a briefcase of significant value, which should not be accepted.

APPROACH TO:

Boundary Issues

DEFINITION

PROFESSIONAL BOUNDARIES: A set of conditions that describe the *limits* of a fiduciary relationship—in other words, a relationship in which a person (the patient) entrusts his or her welfare to another person (the physician) who receives a fee for performing a service.

CLINICAL APPROACH

Types of Boundaries

There will always be an inherit power differential between a patient and a physician. Despite our best efforts as providers, laypersons may not fully understand their medical conditions, possible complications, or treatment options. Patients trust and depend upon us as their providers to take care of them to the best of our ability. It is this dependency, and its subsequent power differential, that can lead to potential boundary issues between provider and patient.

It is important to distinguish between boundary crossing and boundary violations. Minor boundary crossings are not exploitative and may be helpful in some instances. Imagine the soothing effects of rubbing a patient's hand during a painful lumbar puncture, a behavior that counters the usual recommendations about touching outside the physical examination. Boundary crossings can be distinguished from damaging boundary violations, which are universally unethical. The most extreme form of a boundary violation is any sexual contact between a current patient and physician. Many instances of physician–patient sexual relationships are preceded by nonsexual boundary crossings that may lead to a boundary violation. Other possible boundary problems that may arise and must be considered include gifts, misuse of the physical examination, and dual relationships.

Sexual Boundary Violations

The most easily recognized boundary violations in medicine are sexual in nature. Physician–patient sexual relations of any type are considered to be inappropriate and unethical regardless of who initiated the relationship. A sexual encounter with a patient constitutes a breach of trust that is fundamental in the physician–patient relationship. A person seeking care is often at his or her most emotionally or physically vulnerable, making mutual consent to a sexual encounter or relationship impossible. Sexual relationships between former patients and physicians is less absolute, but they should be approached with extreme caution.

Gift Giving

Patients may wish to show caregivers appreciation by bringing gifts to their provider. Although small gifts as cookies or alcohol during the holidays may represent benign boundary crossings rather than serious violations, more expensive gifts have been cited as problematic from 2 standpoints. First, gift giving may be a conscious or unconscious bribe by the patient, designed to keep aggression, negative feelings or unpleasant subjects out of the doctor–patient relationship. For example, the patient may bring the doctor and the staff lunch to keep them from getting upset about frequently missing scheduled appointments. Second, there is often a secret or even explicit expectation of some reward or acknowledgment involved in performing services or bestowing a gift, whether that be better care or the expectation of improved outcomes. There are no definitive rules or fixed values to determine when a physician should or should not accept a gift. The American Medical Association (AMA) suggests that, when deciding to accept a gift, the physician should evaluate if he or she would be comfortable if their colleagues, or the public, knew about acceptance of the gift.

Physical Examination

Patients are often anxious and uncomfortable during a physical examination but often will go along with what the physician believes is necessary. For example, during his annual examination, a male patient who abuses alcohol may submit to a breast or testicular examination even though he does not question you, nor does he understand that you are evaluating for gynecomastia or testicular atrophy associated with his chronic disease. At best this can lead to failure to keep future appointments or transferring to another doctor; at worst, it could lead to a sexual harassment lawsuit. The physician should always explain all parts of the physical examination, but particular care needs to be undertaken to explain to a patient why examining the genitals, breasts, or other sensitive areas is necessary. If the patient hesitates, then the physician should encourage questions or expressions of concern that can then be clarified. Because the physician cannot know how a certain patient is likely to respond to various aspects of touching in the physical examination, clear communication is of paramount importance. A chaperone should always be considered, particularly when performing an examination on a patient of the opposite sex.

Dual Relationships

An essential element of the physician's role is the fiduciary duty that is owed specifically that what is best for the patient must be the physician's first priority. Dual relationship refers to any relationship that coexist simultaneously beyond that of physician–patient relationship, for example, dual relationships may exist with family members, friends, sexual partners, employees, or business associates. These dual relationships have the potential to undermine the physician's ability to focus primarily on the patients' well-being, and can affect the physician's judgment. This concept is central to why physicians should not treat family members. It may be difficult to see the harm in caring for your aunt if you imagine just providing annual well women examinations. However, imagine this same aunt who you know to be struggling for years with infertility, but you now are managing because of profuse bleeding whom you know requires emergency hysterectomy to save her life. Would you be able to perform it? Would you be able to eat holiday dinner with her if you eliminated her ability to carry a child by performing the hysterectomy? Relationships outside the physician–patient relationship can affect the physician's judgment and can compromise his or her objectivity.

The ability to separate oneself from dual relationships becomes more difficult for providers in rural settings where they may be the only physician in a town or are returning to small towns where they grew up. It has been suggested that boundary guidelines must be applied flexibly in rural areas where a provider may be the only provider for hundreds of miles; however, the same principles of boundaries should still be recognized and maintained.

Boundaries and Social Media

The Internet has positively impacted the ability for the medical profession to exchange and relay information to the public in a way never experienced before.

However, in social media, a provider's personal presence on social networking sites must still respect physician–patient boundaries. In 2011, the AMA issued guidelines on professionalism in the use of social media. The AMA recommends that physicians consider separating personal and professional content online, and there should be no differences in the online and in-person physician–patient relationship. It argues that online friendships with patients may open the door to boundary violations whether online, in person, or possibly romantic. A request from a patient to connect with a physician via a social networking website should be declined, and the patient should be referred to the physician's professional page.

COMPREHENSION QUESTIONS

11.1 A patient comes to your office for treatment of depression. Over the course of several months her condition dramatically improves and the patient is extremely grateful for all of your help. The patient is an executive chef at a restaurant in your city, and she invites you for a complimentary meal with her at her restaurant. You are unsure of her intentions, but you do find her attractive and would not be opposed. What should you do?

    A. Accept the dinner invitation.

    B. Decline the dinner invitation.

    C. Refer the patient to another provider and go to dinner.

    D. Refer the patient to another provider and decline the dinner invitation.

11.2 A 29-year-old man presents to your office for an annual examination. While obtaining the patient's history, he begins to make suggestive comments and then asks if you are married. Your next step in managing this patient's condition is which of the following?

    A. Ignore the question and continue your examination.

    B. Reprimand the patient and continue your examination.

    C. Answer his question and continue your examination.

    D. Inform him that you do not answer personal questions and continue with a chaperone.

    E. Refer the patient to another physician.

ANSWERS

11.1 **B.** It is never acceptable to have a romantic relationship with your patients. No matter what the patient's intentions, it is possible that accepting the dinner invitation could lead to a boundary violation, the most serious of which would be a sexual relationship. A relationship with a former patient is less well defined, but relationships between a psychiatrist and a patient are never acceptable even after the physician–patient relationship has ended. Referral to another provider and then accepting the dinner invitation is generally frowned upon despite the termination of the physician–patient relationship.

11.2 **D.** Patients may not be aware of the correct boundaries of a therapeutic relationship, so it is important that you clearly delineate the locations of those boundaries. Simply inquiring into your personal life prior to establish physician–patient boundaries is not enough to warrant referring the patient to another provider. Reprimanding or ignoring the question also does not aid in advancing your professional relationship, and, instead, may interfere with your ability to care for him in the future. While answering the question may help to establish rapport in some instances, in this case, the patient may have been attempting to engage in a social or sexual relationship, which would be a violation of professional boundaries.

KEY POINTS

▶ Boundary crossings do not necessarily cause damage to the physician–patient relationship.

▶ Boundary violations are universally unethical and damage the physician–patient relationship.

▶ Physician–patient sexual relations of any type are inappropriate and unethical regardless of who initiates the relationship.

▶ The physician should always explain all parts of the physical examination, especially during examination of the genitals or breasts. Always consider a chaperone.

▶ Small gifts from grateful patients may not be boundary violations, but always be cautious.

▶ Maintain separate personal and professional social media presences and do not connect with your patients on your personal social media page. Always maintain the same boundaries online as you do in your office.

REFERENCES

American Medical Association; Council on Ethical and Judicial Affairs. Sexual misconduct in the practice of medicine. *JAMA.* 1991;266:2741-2745.

Nadelson C, Notman MT. Boundaries in the doctor-patient relationship. *Theor Med Bioeth.* 2002;23:191-201.

Simon RI, Williams IC. Maintaining treatment boundaries in small communities and rural areas. *Psychiatr Serv.* 1999;50:1440-1446.

Spence SA. Patients bearing gifts: are there strings attached? *BMJ.* 2005;331:1527-1529.

A second-year internal medicine resident is asked by a close friend, MW, to refill some blood pressure medication. This friend is a 32-year-old man who works at the local diner, and he has not seen his doctor for several years. Recently, while shopping at the grocery store, he had an automated blood pressure reading of 150/92 mm Hg. MW has taken lisinopril in the past. He has the name and phone number of the pharmacy where he had filled the prior prescription.

▶ How should the second-year resident respond?
▶ What is the next step that the resident should undertake?

ANSWERS TO CASE 12:
Prescribing for Friends and Family Members

Summary: A 32-year-old man with a history of hypertension has not been seen by his primary care physician recently and is now without his prescribed medication. His current blood pressure is 150/92 mm Hg. He approaches his close friend who is an internal medicine resident and asks him to refill his medication.

- **How should the resident respond?** The resident should not prescribe the medication. The resident is beyond his authority to prescribe medications to his friend who is not a patient of his institution. In addition, his physician–patient relationship is not being supervised by a licensed physician, and MW's blood pressure is only mildly elevated. Unless an emergency situation has occurred, a physician should not prescribe to family members, friends, colleagues, employees, or themselves.

- **Next Step:** The resident should provide support and alternatives for his close friend. The resident can provide possible referrals, educate his friend on his condition, and support his friend in helping to navigate the health care system.

ANALYSIS

Objectives

1. Describe the requirements for medical care of friends or family members.

2. List the potential consequences of rendering medical care without a proper history, physical examination findings, and medical records.

3. Describe the particular issues of a resident in training providing medical care outside of his or her clinical assignments.

Considerations

Family members and friends commonly see their relationships with physicians as an opportunity to obtain a better handle on their own medical care. Many times friends or family may utilize this relationship as a method of understanding their condition, getting an unofficial second opinion, or, as in this case, as a manner of convenience to obtain a refill following a lapse in care. This is a dilemma that all physicians will face, likely on a regular basis, and will begin when the physician is undergoing training as a resident. In this case, the resident is asked by a friend to prescribe a medication that the patient was previously taking. It may seem harmless, but the act of prescribing (practicing) without the requisite history and examination, documentation in the medical record, and acting under the hospital authorized setting (a physician-in-training permit) are all reasons that this action would be inappropriate. Moreover, if the resident does prescribe (though innocently), the action may be grounds for termination from his residency.

APPROACH TO:
Prescribing for Friends and Family

DEFINITIONS

SELF-PRESCRIBING: Prescribing medications for oneself, usually without a formal evaluation.

TREATMENT OF FRIENDS AND FAMILY: Rendering medical care for close friends, family members, or both, usually without formal evaluation and documentation in the medical record.

CLINICAL APPROACH

It is important to recognize how potentially treating friends, family members, or both may change the established relationship. It is often difficult for friends and family members to share all aspects of their health condition with a physician whom they already have a personal relationship with. It is also difficult for physicians to properly obtain a complete history or perform a physical examination on friends and family members. This can result in suboptimal care that may even fall outside of the physician's area of expertise.

ANALYSIS AND DISCUSSION

Each state, hospital, and residency program may have their own nuances when it comes to prescribing for friends or family members; therefore, it is imperative for all physicians to be familiar with the recommendations, policies, and laws associated with the prescriptive authority. Typically, it is ethically permissible to prescribe medications in (1) emergency situations, (2) when not prescribing could cause significant distress, and (3) when the prescription is for a controlled substance related to an immediate need. The most commonly prescribed medications in these circumstances are antibiotics, antihistamines, and oral contraceptive agents. In addition, once the physician engages in this care, it tends to continue, with the "patient" asking for more favors in the future.

Power of the Pen

Studies have shown that 65% to 83% of physicians write prescriptions for medications for themselves or family members. Although this appears to be a common occurrence, it is important for physicians to understand that the physician's professional objectivity is difficult to maintain when treating individuals that the physician interacts with socially. In its *Code of Ethics*, the American Medical Association (AMA) describes how "the physician's personal feelings may unduly influence his or her professional medical judgment, thereby interfering with the care being delivered." A large number of physicians also self-prescribe, which, likewise, presents hazards such as incomplete medical evaluation, a lack of objectivity, and potential for abuse. In fact, 12% of physicians who self-prescribe have been noted to prescribe anxiolytic or other habituating medications.

Most state medical boards discourage the treatment of friends, family members, or self. However, if there is an emergency, or if medical treatment is necessary and difficult to obtain, then a physician may prescribe medication. These patient interactions still require the same procedures and protocols for patients seen in a health care facility, including performing a history and physical examination on the patient, keeping a medical record, and, ultimately, accepting the responsibility for the medical liability associated with treatment outcomes. In addition, many third-party payers will not reimburse for care rendered by relatives of patients, even if performed in the appropriate office setting.

Mousmman and colleagues gives the following cautions for prescribing for friends or family members:

- Avoid unless an emergency

- Obtain a medical and drug history

- Perform an appropriate and thorough examination

- Create a medical record with reason for prescription

- Inform the individual of the risks, benefits, and adverse effects

- Initiate follow-up care

- Maintain confidentiality and compliance with Healthy Insurance Portability and Accountability Act (HIPAA)

- Before prescribing, check for any other alternatives

In its *Code of Ethics*, the AMA states that "physicians generally should not treat themselves or members of their immediate families. Professional objectivity may be compromised when an immediate family member or the physician is the patient; the physician's personal feelings may unduly influence his or her professional medical judgment, thereby interfering with the care being delivered."

The case previously illustrated showcases how a physician in training who is asked to refill a prescription for his friend can bring an additional level of complexity to this common occurrence. Residency is a period of time when the physician in training is practicing medicine under the direct supervision of a licensed physician. When a resident prescribes a medication to a patient who is not part of his or her health care system, including friends and family members, he or she is performing medical management without the direct supervision of a licensed physician. In the scenario, the issue was hypertension; however, sometimes a more intimate examination is called for such as a pelvic or breast examination. Because of the nature of these examinations, the physician and "patient" may not wish to undergo these examinations, further compromising the care of the patient.

Depending on the residency training program, the resident contract may or may not specifically forbid residents from independently writing prescriptions for patients outside of the program. Nonetheless, should the resident write the prescription, a physician–patient relationship has been established. Therefore, this relationship holds the same legal responsibilities found with an established office visit, opening the resident to all the liability associated with the outcomes. Furthermore, as the resident practicing medicine without the direct supervision of an attending physician, the resident is at risk for breach of contract with his or her home institution or even employment termination, depending on the policies outlined by the residency program.

Summary

It is in the best interest of the patient and the physician to decline the patient's request to refill the prescription. Although this may cause tension between the 2 friends, so can establishing a physician–patient relationship. Resident physicians should be discouraged to prescribe medication to individuals who are not patients of their home institutions. However, as a practicing physician, it is ethically permissible to prescribe medications in emergency situations. Once the emergency has passed, the physician should help connect the patient to the proper resources, including physician referrals, as soon as possible to establish appropriate ongoing medical care.

COMPREHENSION QUESTIONS

12.1 Dr Mandy Peterson, a first-year resident, is on a demanding medical rotation in an intensive care unit. Early one morning she realizes she is now out of her oral contraceptive pills. There are no refills left on her prescription. Knowing that she will be unable to take time away from her current rotation for a medical appointment, she asks a fellow obstetrics/gynecology resident if she will refill her prescription. The obstetrics/gynecology resident should do which of the following?

A. Prescribe the medication for 1 month and instruct the resident to follow-up as soon as possible with her primary obstetrician/gynecologist.

B. Give her fellow resident the medication from the sample closet at her resident clinic.

C. Inform the resident that most obstetricians/gynecologists will refill a prescription for a short period of time with the caveat that the patient will follow-up as soon as possible.

D. Instruct the resident to purchase condoms from the pharmacy.

12.2 Which of the following reasons does the AMA state is a reason not to prescribe or render medical care for immediate family members?

A. Lack of medical record documentation

B. Lack of objectivity

C. Lack of confidentiality

D. Lack of informed consent

ANSWERS

12.1 **C.** In most situations, the physician's office will authorize a short time refill of medication under the agreement that the patient will schedule an appointment at a reasonable time. Refilling the medication by the resident without proper examination and documentation and to a nonpatient is problematic.

12.2 **B.** The main reason the AMA gives for why physicians should not treat family members is lack of professional objectivity. The physician's personal feelings may unduly influence his or her professional medical judgment, thereby interfering with the care being delivered.

KEY POINTS

▶ Treatment of friends, family members, and self is common among physicians.

▶ The most commonly prescribed medications for family members are antibiotics, antihistamines, and oral contraceptive agents.

▶ In general, treating a friend or family member is not prudent due to difficulty to maintain professional objectivity.

▶ Residents in training must restrict their practice of medicine to their hospital-assigned roles.

▶ Treatment of friends of family members requires the same standard as that of any other patient, including history and physical examination, proper assessment, counseling of the patient, and documentation in the medical record.

▶ Self-prescribing is inappropriate.

REFERENCES

Aboff BM, Collier VU, Farber NJ, Ehrenthal DB. Residents prescription writing for nonpatients. *JAMA.* 2002;288-232.

American College of Physicians. *Ethics Manual.* American College of Physicians, Philadelphia, PA. http://www.acponline.org/ethics/ethicman.htm. Accessed, September 15, 2014.

American Medical Association (AMA) Section E-8.19. In: AMA. *AMA Code of Medical Ethics.* Chicago: AMA; 2008.

Moussman D, Farrell H, Gilday E. Should you prescribe medications for family and friends? *Curr Psychiatry.* 2011;10:10-14.

Puma JL, Stocking CB, LaVoie D, Darling CA. When physicians treat members of their own families. *N Engl J Med.* 1991;325:1290-1294.

You are a busy family physician, and one day your nurse hands you a phone message in the middle of your clinic duties. The wife of one of your patients has called to discuss concerns about the health of her husband, Sam. She informed the nurse that she thinks her husband is addicted to prescription pain medications and would like to know if you have observed any signs of addiction during your visits. You last saw Sam 2 weeks ago, and you did think he was behaving strangely. He seemed very preoccupied and disengaged. In addition, he seemed sad, and you inquired about his emotional health because he was very out of character. You were concerned about possible depression, although Sam denied it.

► What are the ramifications of discussing Sam's care with his wife?

ANSWER TO CASE 13:

Confidentiality

Summary: A patient's wife phones you to discuss concerns regarding her husband's possible addiction to pain medications.

- **Ramifications of discussion:** Discussing Sam's care with his wife violates patient confidentiality.

ANALYSIS

Objectives

1. Define confidentiality in terms of the physician–patient relationship.

2. Describe current US federal regulations with regard to patient confidentiality.

3. Understand the common exceptions to patient confidentiality.

Considerations

Patient confidentiality is an important principle in the physician–patient relationship. All reasonable and appropriate attempts to protect patient confidentiality must be made; however, there are certain circumstances where the health or well-being of the patient or others may supersede the need for patient confidentiality. In the case of Sam's wife, it would be a violation of Sam's expectation of privacy to discuss his private health information without his consent. His wife should be informed that you are unable to provide her with this information due to concerns over confidentiality.

APPROACH TO:

Confidentiality

DEFINITIONS

CONFIDENTIALITY: Similar to the idea of informational privacy, confidentiality is the duty to protect personal information from others who have no right to it.

PRIVACY: A term often used interchangeably with confidentiality, privacy is the freedom from exposure to, or intrusion by, others. It can refer to the privacy of your body, disclosure of your personal information, or your ability to independently make decisions.

ANALYSIS AND DISCUSSION

Ethical Considerations

Physicians are charged with the duty to protect patient's health information. During the famous oath attributed to Hippocrates, ancient Greek physicians pledged to respect confidentiality in these words: "What I may see or hear in the course of the treatment or even outside of the treatment in regard to the life of men, which on no account one must spread abroad, I will keep to myself, holding such things shameful to be spoken about." In 1803, Thomas Percival discussed confidentiality in his book, *Medical Ethics*, which is considered to be the first code of medical ethics. Patient confidentiality is centered on the ethical principles of respect for autonomy, beneficence, and nonmaleficence.

Under the principle of autonomy, patients have the right to control who has access to both their person and their personal health information. Any disclosure of that information without patient consent fails to respect autonomy. Furthermore, patients are more likely to share sensitive health information if there is no concern that the information will be publicly shared. This, in turn, allows the physician to better care for the patient, promoting the ethical principle of beneficence. Finally, disclosure of protected health information in violation of confidentiality may, in fact, cause harm to the patient. In this case, there is no guarantee that the patient's wife is interested in this information so that she may help or aid her spouse. They could potentially be in the middle of a contentious divorce, and this information may be used against Sam in court, allowing his wife to negotiate a more advantageous settlement at his expense.

Legal Considerations

The legal obligations of patient confidentiality are grounded in common law, state law, and US federal law. Current US federal regulations were established by the 2003 Health Insurance Portability and Accountability Act (HIPAA) to obtain standards for health care confidentiality. The Privacy Rule implemented new regulations that require providers to protect the confidentiality of "individually identifiable personal health information" in any form, whether that be electronic, written, or oral. Personal health information includes information that relates to a person's physical or mental health, the provision of health care, or the payment for health care. The regulations apply to all health care organizations, including hospitals and physicians.

Under the HIPAA regulations, patient's health information is protected with few exceptions. The health information can be disclosed without written permission if: (1) the patient makes the disclosure on his or her own, (2) the physician needs the information for his or her own care, in regard to payment or in regard to health care operations, (3) when the patient gives "informal" permission to discuss health information with family members, and (4) disclosure is related to national priority purposes (Table 13–1). For disclosures made in error, the HIPAA regulations assess monetary penalties per violation. The US Office of Civil Rights of the Department of Heath and Human Services is responsible for overseeing and enforcing the privacy rules.

Although patient confidentiality is essential, there are several exceptions to this obligation under law. Examples of the exceptions include the duty to warn, the duty to report certain conditions, and the duty to inform legal guardians about the care of minors. The duty to warn concerns a physician's obligation to break patient confidentiality to protect the safety of a nonpatient. In situations where there is clear evidence of danger to other person, the practitioner must determine

Table 13–1 • NATIONAL PRIORITY PURPOSES BASED ON THE 2003 HIPAA PRIVACY RULE
Health information can be disclosed when:
• Required by law
• For public health activities (eg, tracking disease, vital statistics)
• Reporting abuse, neglect, or domestic violence
• For health oversight (eg, health inspections)
• Needed for judicial or law enforcement proceedings
• Disclosures about deceased persons are needed (eg, to medical examiners)
• Organ and tissue donation
• Averting a serious health threat
• Completing certain types of health research
• Needed for specialized government functions (eg, military missions)
• Processing workers' compensation claims

the degree of seriousness of the threat and warn the victim, warn the police, or counsel a patient until the patient is no longer felt to be a threat. This principle was established in the Supreme Court case *Tarasoff v Regents of the University of California*. In this case, a California psychologist requested that campus police arrest a patient he believed was dangerous and had threatened to kill Ms Tarasoff. The patient was released following assurance to the police that he would stay away from the victim, and the victim was never notified. She was murdered by the patient 2 months later. Laws vary from state to state in regard to the degree of harm necessary to trigger the duty to warn. In some states, the requirements are less rigorous than others.

Physicians have long been held responsible of the duty of reporting certain conditions, such as tuberculosis and sexually transmitted infections, for the good of public health. Lists of reportable conditions are kept by the state health boards and can include bioterrorism agents (eg, anthrax) and epidemic diseases (eg, severe acute respiratory syndrome). In addition to these conditions, most states have laws requiring or allowing the report of patients who are unable to safely operate a motorized vehicle. Finally, any health care professional who has reason to suspect that a child has been abused or neglected must report this immediately to the local child protective services division. The reporting individual is protected from liability unless it is shown that the person making the report acted in bad faith or with malicious intent.

In order for legal guardians of minors to make educated decisions concerning the minor, the guardian must have full access to the minor's protected health information. However, The American Medical Association (AMA) states that physicians who care for minors have an ethical duty to include them in the medical decision-making process as a way to promote their autonomy. And while minors can request confidential services, it is recommended that the health care provider attempt to understand their concerns and encourage them to include their parents or guardians in the decision-making process. When an immature minor requests contraceptive services, pregnancy-related care, including pregnancy testing, prenatal and postnatal care, and delivery services, treatment for sexually transmitted infections, drug and alcohol abuse, or mental illness, physicians must recognize that requiring parental involvement may be counterproductive to the health of the patient. Physicians should encourage parental involvement in these situations; however, if the minor continues to object, his or her wishes ordinarily should be respected. In agreement with the AMA, many states have established laws allowing for confidential treatment of minors in the certain situations stated above. As state laws vary, it is important for all providers to be familiar with the common exceptions of patient confidentiality in their states.

COMPREHENSION QUESTIONS

13.1 A 16-year-old girl presents to your office without her parents. She reports that she had recently had unprotected sex with her boyfriend. She is concerned she may have gonorrhea. She does not want her parents to know that she is requesting sexually transmitted infection screening because "they will kick me out of the house if they knew." What is your obligation to her in most states in regard to patient confidentiality?

   A. You are unable to perform any testing without permission from her parents because she is a minor.

   B. You perform the sexually transmitted infection testing due to the duty to warn (as she may be spreading gonorrhea to other partners).

   C. You perform the sexually transmitted infection testing due to exceptions of the duty to inform legal guardians in the care of a minor.

13.2 You are a psychiatrist and one of your patients was recently fired from his job. At your last visit, you were concerned about his mental stability. During previous visits, you have established that your patient is an avid hunter and has easy access to a gun. In the mail today, you find a letter where he describes a detailed plan to kill his former boss along with himself. You believe the threat is credible and the former boss is at risk. What is your obligation in regard to patient confidentiality?

   A. You contact the authorities immediately as you believe the threat is credible, and the duty to warn supersedes patient confidentiality in this situation.

   B. You are upset but unable to contact the authorities because there is no situation that warrants breaking patient confidentiality.

   C. You call the patient to have him come in to discuss his current mental status.

13.3 A 38-year-old man presents to your clinic. He is a long-distance truck driver. He admits that he abuses alcohol and typically drinks at least 6 beers a day. He reports that he experiences withdrawal symptoms if he does not drink. You are concerned about his safety because he is frequently driving his truck while under the influence. What is you obligation in regard to patient confidentiality?

    A. You develop a plan to treat him for alcoholism and advise him that it is against the law to drive a motor vehicle under the influence.

    B. You develop a plan to treat him for alcoholism and advise him that it is against the law to drive a motor vehicle under the influence. You also contact the authorities to report that he is not able to safely operate a motorized vehicle in his current medical condition.

    C. You develop a plan to treat him for alcoholism and advise him that it is against the law to drive a motor vehicle under the influence. You also contact his wife to let her know that he is not able to safely operate a motorized vehicle in his current medical condition.

13.4 A 26-year-old woman presents to your office with complaints of hand pain that she attributes to an injury that occurred at her work while operating a machine. Radiographs are obtained, and a care plan is developed. A representative from her place of employment contacts your office a few days after the visit. Your patient has filed a workers' compensation claim due to the hand injury. The representative would like copies of your office visit and radiologic findings. What is your obligation to your patient in regard to patient confidentiality?

    A. You inform the representative from her place of employment that you are unable to give any copies of her medical record because doing so violates her confidentiality.

    B. You inform the representative that you are going to fax her entire medical record today.

    C. You inform the representative that you are going to fax only the portions of the medical record relevant to the hand injury.

ANSWERS

13.1 **C.** Most states allow for adolescents to be screened for sexually transmitted infections without the consent of their legal guardians. This exception is to encourage adolescents to be screened for sexually transmitted infections.

13.2 **A.** The duty to warn has been established in cases where there is a possibility of serious harm to a nonpatient. As long as you feel the threat to a nonpatient is credible, it is your duty to contact the authorities or the possible victim.

13.3 **B.** Most states have laws requiring or allowing the report of patients who are unable to safely operate a motorized vehicle. Until this patient's alcoholic dependence is adequately treated, he is not able to safely operate a motorized vehicle and the proper authorities should be notified.

13.4 **C.** Under the HIPAA Privacy Rule, medical records can be disclosed to process workers' compensation claims. To protect your patient's confidentiality, only medical records related to the claim should be disclosed.

KEY POINTS

▶ The physician–patient relationship must be protected by protecting patient confidentiality.

▶ The legal implications of patient confidentiality have been established by common law, state law, and federal law including under the HIPAA federal regulations.

▶ There are exceptions to patient confidentiality that include the duty to warn, the duty to report reportable conditions, and the duty to inform legal guardians of the care of minors.

REFERENCES

American Medical Association (AMA). Opinion 5.055. Confidential care for minors. In: AMA. *AMA Code of Medical Ethics*. Chicago: AMA; 2013. http://www.ama-assn.org/ama/pub/physician-resources/medical-ethics/code-medical-ethics/opinion5055.page. Accessed March 31, 2014.

Higgins GL. The history of confidentiality in medicine. *Can Fam Physician*. 1989;35:921-926.

Moskop JC, Marco CA, Larkin GL, et al. From Hippocrates to HIPAA: privacy and confidentiality in emergency medicine part I: conceptual, moral, and legal foundations. *Ann Emerg Med*. 2005;45.1:53-59.

Office of Civil Rights. Standards for privacy of individually identifiable health information; security standards for the protection of electronic protected health information; general administrative requirements including civil monetary penalties: procedures for investigations, imposition of penalties, and hearings. Regulation text. 45 CFR Parts 160 and 164. December 28, 2000, as amended: May 31, 2002, August 14, 2002, February 20, 2003, and April 17, 2003. http://www.hhs.gov/ocr/privacy/hipaa/news/2002/combinedregtext02.pdf. Accessed February 20, 2014.

Office for Civil Rights. Summary of the HIPAA privacy rule. http://www.hhs.gov/ocr/privacy/hipaa/understanding/summary/. Accessed February 20, 2014.

Riech WT. Oath of Hippocrates. In Post SG: *Encyclopedia of Bioethics*. Vol. 5. New York, NY: Macmillan Publishing Company; 1995: 2632.

Tarasoff v Regents of the University of California, 17 Cal 3d 425, 551 P.2d 334, 131 Cal. Rptr. 14. 1976.

MS is a 28-year-old woman who has had asthma ever since her early childhood. She arrives in the emergency department (ED) with a severe asthma attack, accompanied by her sister. The attending physician, Dr V, begins treatment with inhaled and intravenous medications, but believes MS is on the verge of respiratory arrest and tells her that she needs to be intubated and placed on a ventilator. MS refuses, indicating that she believes she will recover without intubation. She asks Dr V to call her father Dr S, a physician, which he does. Dr S reviews the situation with Dr V and suggests that Dr V should wait to see if MS makes a recovery, because his experience with his daughter's asthma leads him to believe she will recover without intubation or mechanical ventilation. After this conversation, Dr V reassesses MS. She has not worsened significantly since his last evaluation, but given that she is not clearly improving Dr V is convinced that she will experience respiratory arrest and quite possibly die as a result. Despite the continued objections of MS and her sister, he indicates that he is going to sedate and intubate her. When she resists, Dr V instructs ED staff to restrain her while he sedates and intubates her, placing her on a mechanical ventilator.

- ▶ What are the elements of informed consent or informed refusal?
- ▶ What are *emergency consent* and *implied consent*?
- ▶ Does MS have decision-making capacity?
- ▶ If MS lacks decision-making capacity, does Dr V need to seek consent for intubation from her family?

ANSWERS TO CASE 14:

Informed Consent

Summary: This is a case in which a physician overrode the refusal of a patient and her surrogates. He did so because he believed the patient would die if he did not, and he thought that this meant that he was not required to seek consent for intubation. This case is adapted from a real case that ended up in court, and, as the legal rulings and the discussion that follows showed, the physician was mistaken to believe that he was not required to seek informed consent for intubation, even if it were true that the patient would die without it.

- **What are the elements of informed consent or refusal?** To provide consent or refusal, the patient must be competent—meaning that she is cognitively capable of understanding the situation and the choices she is facing—and capable of expressing a choice. The physician must disclose the appropriate information about the situation and the risks and benefits of the treatment options. The patient must demonstrate understanding of the situation and the disclosed information. The patient must be able to make a decision voluntarily, free of coercive pressure from caregivers or others. Finally, the patient must consent to one of the treatment alternatives.

- **What is *emergency consent* or *implied consent*?** When a patient lacks decisional capacity and no surrogate is available, physicians are authorized to provide treatment without obtaining explicit consent to protect the patient from serious harm or death.

- **Does MS have decision-making capacity?** We do not have enough information to fully answer this question. The answer depends on her ability to understand her situation and make a reasoned choice between the alternative treatment options. As the discussion will show, however, whether MS was competent or not was not precisely relevant to the question of whether Dr V should have intubated her.

- **If MS lacked decision-making capacity, then did Dr V need to seek consent for intubation from her family?** In brief, yes. Because appropriate surrogates were available, and because enough time was available to fully inform them and seek their opinion, Dr V was obliged to seek consent for intubation or, if it was not forthcoming, to honor their informed refusal. This is true even if the patient is at risk of dying.

ANALYSIS

Objectives

1. Understand the elements of informed consent/refusal.

2. Understand the elements of decision-making capacity (competence).

3. Understand the role of surrogate decision-makers with respect to informed consent/refusal.

Considerations

When a patient has decision-making capacity, or when an appropriate surrogate is available to make decisions for him or her, and when time is available to seek informed consent, physicians are obliged to seek it. When an intervention is invasive, painful, or risky, physicians generally must explicitly seek at least verbal consent before proceeding. In some situations, such as surgery under general anesthesia or participation in research, the consent should be documented in writing, usually in documents designed for the purpose, which are then signed by the patient or his or her surrogates. The requirement for informed consent is so strong that physicians may not override a competent patient's voluntary and informed refusal even in order to save his or her life.

APPROACH TO:
Informed Consent

DEFINITIONS

BEST INTERESTS: Surrogates who do not know the patient (or surrogates for patients who have never been competent such as children or cognitively challenged patients) cannot exercise substituted judgment and must make decisions on the basis of a best-interests analysis (ie, all things considered, what is in the best interests of this patient?).

COMPETENCE: A patient who has decision-making capacity is said to be competent. Although *competence* has a specific legal meaning, the terms *capacity* and *competence* are usually used interchangeably in the clinical setting and in discussions of the ethics of consent.

INFORMED CONSENT: When a competent and informed patient (or his or her surrogate) voluntarily authorizes a medical intervention, he or she is said to have provided informed consent. In this case, when the term informed consent is used, it can be read as "informed consent or refusal."

SUBSTITUTED JUDGMENT: A surrogate who tries to make the decision that the patient would have made, using knowledge of the patient's (premorbid) values, beliefs, and interests, is said to be exercising substituted judgment.

SURROGATE: Any individual who is authorized to make decisions on behalf of an incompetent patient is a surrogate decision-maker. Only surrogates who know the patient can exercise substituted judgment.

CLINICAL APPROACH

Competent patients must be provided the opportunity to consent to or refuse medical interventions. Authorized surrogates can provide consent or refusal for the incapacitated patient. When a physician can obtain consent, she must. When consent cannot be obtained (because the patient is incompetent and no surrogate is available, and no time is available to seek a surrogate), then clinicians can invoke the doctrine of emergency consent (also known as presumed consent) on the assumption that the incapacitated patient would want medical therapy intended to improve quality or quantity of life.

ANALYSIS AND DISCUSSION

The doctrine of informed consent requires that competent patients have an opportunity to consent to or refuse any medical therapies. An authorized surrogate provides informed consent or refusal for incompetent patients. A number of criteria must be met for consent or refusal to be considered informed (Table 14–1). A signed informed consent document is not a substitute for ensuring that these criteria are met.

First, the patient or her surrogate must be competent—that is, capable of understanding his or her medical situation, the alternative treatments, and probability of benefits or harms from each alternative. The patient must also be able to communicate a choice. In the case described in this chapter, it seems likely that MS was competent, but even if she was not, she had her sister with her and her father was available by phone and we have no reason to question their competence.

Caregivers must disclose the information relevant to the decision. The amount of information that must be disclosed will vary depending on the gravity and urgency of the situation, but should meet the "reasonable person" standard. That is, caregivers should disclose the information that a reasonable person would want to know when faced with a decision such as the one being considered. This includes but is not limited to information about the current medical situation, the alternative treatment courses (including no treatment), and the probable or expected outcomes of the various alternatives. The reasonable person standard may not meet the needs of an individual patient because it might seem to demand more or less information than the particular patient would want. For this reason, clinicians should tailor the information disclosed to the needs of the individual patient. In other words, the reasonable person standard is only a starting point for determining what information needs to be disclosed.

In the case of MS, Dr V had the opportunity to disclose whatever information he felt was relevant to the situation, and he was motivated to do so because he wished to persuade MS that intubation was the course she should pursue. We can assume

Table 14–1 • ELEMENTS OF INFORMED CONSENT
Competence: The patient or surrogate is cognitively capable of understanding the situation and the choices he or she faces and of expressing a choice.
Disclosure: Clinicians have shared information about the current situation and the risks and benefits of various treatment alternatives.
Understanding: The patient or surrogate shows appreciation of the situation and the disclosed information.
Voluntariness: The medical decision is made free of coercive pressure from caregivers or others.
Consent: The patient or surrogate expresses a choice among alternatives.

that he disclosed the most obviously important facts: that he believed she would die without intubation, and that the risks of intubation were minimal.

The patient or surrogate should demonstrate understanding of the information that has been disclosed. Caregivers can usually adequately assess understanding through conversation and exchange of ideas. If the patient or surrogate asks appropriate questions and can weigh the benefits and burdens of treatment alternatives, then understanding is usually adequate. If the patient can provide comprehensible reasons for choosing one alternative over another, then understanding is likely to be adequate. The mere act of agreeing ("consenting") to a course of therapy does not necessarily reflect understanding. Exchange of ideas between patient and caregiver is usually required to ensure understanding.

In the case of MS, it seems clear that, even if MS had not fully understood Dr V's position, her sister and her physician father certainly would have.

A patient or surrogate's consent must be made voluntarily—that is, free of coercive pressure. Coercion occurs when a clinician employs incentives (usually negative) to pressure a patient to make a particular choice. Negative incentives can be explicit (eg, threatening to stop providing care) or subtle and implicit (eg, exaggerating the risks of a given course of action). Even making patients express their choice repeatedly, in the hopes that they will eventually change their decision to a preferred choice, can be coercive—this is known as badgering. Family and friends can also exert coercive pressure. The term *coercion* should usually be reserved for pressure applied by one person to another. Although severe illness can put patients under great pressure and can severely restrict the choices available to a person, the mere existence of illness should not be considered coercive.

Coercion does not seem to have been a feature of MS's case. Coercion would obviously have been an issue if Dr V had threatened MS somehow—perhaps by implying that if she refused intubation, he would refuse to provide any other medications or treatments for her asthma. More subtly, coercion would be an issue if he had exaggerated the risks or discomforts associated with treatment short of intubation. In theory, family and friends can also coerce patients, although it was not a feature of this case, because MS's sister and father supported her refusal.

Finally, the patient or surrogate must either implicitly or explicitly provide consent. Note that the act of consenting is only the final step in a process of providing informed consent, which is why a signed consent document is not a substitute for truly informed consent.

Implied (or Presumed or Emergency) Consent

In some situations, time or medical urgency does not permit a conversation about patient preferences or might preclude a search for an appropriate surrogate. In these circumstances, clinicians are permitted to proceed with lifesaving or medically necessary interventions, on the assumption that the patient would consent. This is called implied, presumed, or emergency consent. This form of consent is justified only in time sensitive or urgent situations. Once the emergency has passed, the usual methods of consent and decision-making apply.

Dr V in this case seems to have erroneously believed that the emergency consent doctrine allowed him to override MS's voluntary, competent, informed refusal.

Competence and Decision-Making Capacity

The terms *competence* and *capacity* both refer to a patient's ability to understand his or her circumstances, understand the choices he or she is faced with, and the ability to make a decision. Some argue that "competence" is a strictly legal term, to be used only when a court makes a ruling about a patient's decision-making capacity; however for most purposes the distinction can be ignored. Competence is not an all-or-nothing quantity, and many patients' competence is limited but not absent. Patients can generally be placed somewhere on a spectrum between fully competent for all decisions and utterly incompetent. Patients can be competent for one type of decision but not for another; therefore, competence must always be considered with respect to the type of decision the patient is facing.

Generally speaking, the more serious the consequences of the decision, the higher the threshold for determining competence. For example, there are many patients whom we would consider competent to make choices about what to have for lunch but whom we would not consider competent to make decisions about surgery or life-sustaining treatment. Determining competence does not necessarily require the expertise of a neurologist or psychiatrist; however, for difficult or marginal cases, or cases in which the medical or legal consequences are particularly weighty, these experts can be helpful.

In MS's case, it would be reasonable to set the bar quite high when assessing her competence, because Dr V believed that the decision she was making (refusing ventilation) was likely to result in her death. But importantly, even if Dr V wanted to claim that MS was not competent, he had no plausible reason to believe the same of her sister or father.

To make a competent choice between treatment alternatives, the patient must be able to (1) appreciate his or her current situation and expected consequences, (2) understand the treatment options and their expected outcomes, (3) reason about treatment options, and (4) communicate a choice.

The ability to appreciate, understand, and reason about treatment options can be difficult to assess at times. Many patients with psychiatric diseases have the cognitive ability to understand their situation and options, but they should not be considered competent to make important medical decisions for themselves. For example, a suicidally depressed patient is usually presumed to lack decision-making capacity because his disease may distort his reasoning and appreciation of the circumstances. Patients who have just recently experienced a debilitating injury may sometimes refuse life-sustaining treatment in the hours or days following their injury and meet the usual criteria for competence, but a compelling argument can be made that life-ending decisions should be delayed, if possible, to allow for some emotional recovery from the sudden disability, as well as for some time to elapse so that he or she can appreciate what life will be like with the new disability.

Summary

In the case of MS, there was an unfortunate result. Dr V intubated MS, and she recovered from the acute asthma attack. However, a couple of years later, when she suffered another asthma attack, she adamantly refused to go to the hospital out of fear of being intubated again, and she died. Her father sued Dr V for his care in the first asthma attack, claiming that Dr V was required to seek her consent for intubation (or respect her refusal), and that his failure to do so resulted in his daughter's overwhelming fear of going to the ED, which eventually resulted in her death. The case eventually was heard by the Massachusetts Supreme Judicial Court, which ruled that Dr V violated his duty to respect his patient's refusal.

COMPREHENSION QUESTIONS

14.1 Which of the following statements about informed consent is false?

    A. Competent and informed patients have the right to refuse any medical therapies, even if refusing them would result in their death.

    B. In a life-threatening emergency, even properly authorized surrogates cannot refuse life-sustaining treatment on behalf of someone else.

    C. To be considered competent to provide informed consent, a patient must be capable of communicating a choice.

    D. In the clinical setting, competence and decisional capacity are interchangeable terms.

14.2 A 23-year-old woman with a history of severe depression has just attempted suicide by hanging and is brought to the ED. She has tracheal swelling that within minutes threatens to obstruct her airway, and ED physicians believe she will die if she is not intubated. At this moment, however, she is alert and conversational, and appears to understand everything that is communicated to her. Which of the following represents the most appropriate care?

    A. Observing that the patient is capable of understanding her situation, the doctors honor her refusal of intubation.

    B. Believing that she is incompetent because she has just attempted suicide, doctors spend 15 minutes attempting to reach the patient's parents to ask whether it would be appropriate to intubate her.

    C. The physicians simply wait until the patient loses consciousness (and thus capacity), and then intubate her on the basis of the emergency consent doctrine.

    D. The physicians briefly attempt to persuade the patient to assent to intubation; however, when this fails, they override her refusal and intubate her despite her objections. They take care to avoid any additional harm while restraining her.

14.3   Which of the following is not an element of informed consent?

A.   Voluntariness: The medical decision is made free of coercive pressure from caregivers or others.

B.   Competence: The patient or surrogate is cognitively capable of understanding the situation and the choices he or she faces and of expressing a choice.

C.   Documentation: Informed consent must be documented in writing and the document must be signed by the patient or his or her surrogate.

D.   Disclosure: Clinicians have shared information about the current situation and the risks and benefits of various treatment alternatives.

ANSWERS

14.1   **B.** Properly authorized surrogates can make any decision that the patient could have made if she were capable. This includes decisions to refuse or forego even life-sustaining therapies. It is uncontroversial that competent patients have the right to refuse any and all medical therapies. Patients who are incapable of communicating a choice cannot be considered decisionally capable. Note that this does not include situations in which communication is merely *difficult*, because even patients who cannot speak can often communicate a choice.

14.2   **D.** An otherwise healthy patient who has just attempted suicide is considered incompetent by definition and cannot refuse life-sustaining therapies. In this case, a life-threatening emergency exists, and, in the absence of immediately available surrogates, the doctors can intubate this patient on the basis of the emergency (presumed) consent doctrine. Intubation should not be delayed while surrogates are sought. The strategy of waiting for the patient to lose consciousness has 2 major flaws: (1) The delay risks unnecessary harm because the loss of consciousness implies some degree of hypoxia, and (2) it assumes that the patient's initial refusal must be honored and then seeks a work-around to avoid the obligation to honor that refusal. If the refusal should have been honored in the first place, then it should be honored after she loses consciousness. It should be noted that if surrogates *had* refused intubation on this patient's behalf (not one of the answers), then there would be a strong case for overriding their refusal as well.

14.3   **C.** Documentation is not a necessary part of informed consent, although in special situations (eg, surgery, human subjects research), policies may require an informed consent document as proof that some minimal standard has been met. A signature on an informed consent document is not a substitute for truly informed consent in which a competent patient or her surrogate voluntarily consents to an intervention after understanding the relevant information disclosed by her clinician.

KEY POINTS

▶ Clinicians are required to obtain informed consent (or honor informed refusal) from a competent patient or his or her surrogates.

▶ When consent cannot be obtained because the patient is incompetent or has no available surrogate, clinicians are permitted to treat under the doctrine of presumed, or emergency, consent.

▶ Clinicians are obliged to disclose the information about treatments and alternative treatments that the patient would find salient. A useful starting point is to reflect on the "reasonable person" standard, that is, what would the average person want to know to make this decision? Further disclosure should then be tailored to the needs of the individual patient.

REFERENCES

Appelbaum S. Assessment of patients' competence to consent to treatment. *N Engl J Med*. 2007;357: 1834-1840.

Berg JW, Appelbaum PS, Lidz CW, Parker LS. *Informed Consent: Legal Theory and Clinical Practice*. 2nd ed. New York, NY: Oxford University Press; 2001.

Faden RR, Beauchamp TL. *A History and Theory of Informed Consent*. New York, NY: Oxford University Press; 1986.

A 29-year-old man with no known past medical history was brought to the emergency department (ED) via ambulance after a high-speed motor vehicle accident. As the ED physician on duty, you are asked to evaluate him. The patient complains of headache and constant right-sided chest pain that is worse with inspiration. Your examination and evaluation are significant for several broken ribs and a large right pneumothorax. You recommend chest tube placement and inpatient admission for continued management. He agrees to the plan of care, but after a few minutes, he suddenly becomes uncooperative and demands to be immediately discharged.

▶ How do you deal with the patient's wishes to discontinue care?
▶ Can the patient be restrained or sedated for placement of the chest tube?

ANSWERS TO THE CASE 15:
Medical Intervention Against Patient's Will

Summary: A 29-year-old patient with pneumothorax and multiple rib fractures wishes to be discharged from the ED against medical advice. You medical opinion is that he needs to be admitted for continued care.

- **Dealing with the patient's wishes to discontinue care:** Assess his decision-making capacity, and if the patient is deemed to have decision-making capacity, then the patient may refuse care. If the patient lacks decision-making capacity, then a surrogate decision-maker should be appointed.

- **Can the patient be restrained or sedated for placement of the chest tube?** This patient is likely to be lacking decision-making capacity and may be restrained and sedated for placement of the chest tube.

ANALYSIS
Objectives

1. Understand the concept of autonomy and how autonomy may be exercised.

2. Discuss the essential elements for determining medical decision-making capacity.

3. Understand the selection and role of surrogate decision-makers.

Considerations
Patients with appropriate decision-making capacity have the right to refuse care, even when the refusal is not in their best interest or may cause personal harm. It is essential for physicians to be able to determine decision-making capacity and understand the role of surrogate decision-makers when capacity does not exist. In this case, the patient has the right to refuse care in the ED. If care is forced upon him, then the physicians involved may be held criminally liable for battery. If there is any doubt as to the patient's decision-making capacity, then an evaluation should be conducted and a surrogate decision-maker appointed, if appropriate.

APPROACH TO:
Medical Intervention Against the Patient's Will

DEFINITIONS
ADVANCE DIRECTIVE: A written instruction or durable power of attorney for health care relating to the provision of medical care when the individual is incapacitated.

CAPACITY: The ability of a patient to understand, manipulate information, and communicate a rational health care decision.

DURABLE POWER OF ATTORNEY: A document designating an agent or proxy to make health care decisions when the patient is no longer able to do so.

INFORMED CONSENT: The willing acceptance of a medical intervention by a patient after the adequate disclosure of the nature, risks, benefits, and alternatives of that intervention.

LIVING WILL: A written legal document that conveys the health care wishes of a person in the event he or she becomes incapacitated. A living will may state specific care, treatment, or procedures that the patient desires or would refuse under specific circumstances, such as, cardiopulmonary resuscitation (CPR), intubation, or artificial nutrition. The document becomes effective when the attending physician certifies the patient has a terminal or irreversible condition and the patient is unable to communicate his or her wishes.

CLINICAL APPROACH

Ethical Considerations

Ethical dilemmas can be examined in the context of the 4 basic principles of medical ethics: autonomy, beneficence, nonmaleficence, and justice (Table 15–1).

Respect for the autonomy of competent patients is demonstrated by accepting their informed decisions, even when they refuse recommended treatments or act contrary to their best interests. The option of refusing treatment is fundamental to the concept of informed consent. If patients must consent to treatment, then, in turn, they have the right to decline treatment.

To give informed refusal (or consent), patients must have appropriate decision-making capacity, which must mean that they are able to understand the nature, risks, benefits, and alternatives of a course of treatment, including that of doing nothing, and the probable outcomes of both acceptance and refusal of the proposed treatment. The information relevant to the decision should be provided to the patient in an understandable manner. The ultimate decision must be made free of coercion.

The assessment of decision-making capacity focuses on whether a patient can understand and properly manipulate information regarding a specific treatment or

Table 15–1 • ETHICAL PRINCIPLES
Beneficence: The duty to promote good and act in the best interests of the patient and the health of society.
Nonmaleficence: The duty to do no harm to patients.
Autonomy: The duty to respect and foster a patient's choice free from coercion.
Justice: The equitable distribution of the life-enhancing opportunities afforded by health care.

Table 15–2 • ESSENTIAL ELEMENTS OF DECISION-MAKING CAPACITY
Ability to express a choice
Ability to understand relevant information
Ability to appreciate the situation and its consequences
Ability to reason with relevant information

course of action and communicate a rational decision (Table 15–2). It does not require that a patient be sober or free of mental illness.

Legal Considerations

Physicians have a duty to treat, and it is a duty that arises with the initiation of the physician–patient relationship and is implied when the patient presents for care, regardless of whether there was a pre-existing relationship. However, both law and ethics dictate that a patient has the right to refuse medical care, and forcing a patient to unwillingly undergo treatment constitutes battery. A properly executed against medical advice (AMA) discharge severs the physician–patient relationship and with it the physician's duty to treat. When a patient signs an AMA, he or she is exercising the right to refuse care and voluntarily assumes the risk of his or her injury.

An assessment of decision-making capacity focuses on a patient's ability to understand and communicate a rational decision. Occasionally, a person in need of medical care may not be able to make decisions on his or her own behalf. If a patient is not capable of making a decision, then a physician cannot ethically or legally allow a decision, such as leaving AMA, which is not in the patient's best interests. In such situations, the patient's decision-making power is taken away and given to a surrogate. The first step in this process is to determine if the patient has previously communicated specific wishes about medical treatments or decisions prior to becoming incapacitated. The next step is to determine who should serve as the surrogate decision-maker.

Advance planning encourages individuals to select a reasonable person to decide medical issues on their behalf and decide how he or she would wish to be treated if he or she become unable to participate in medical decisions. The wishes of the patient may be stated in legal documents, generally referred to as advanced directives and may include a durable power of attorney, a directive to physicians, and a living will. A durable power of attorney authorizes individuals to appoint another person to act as his or her agent to make health care decisions after he or she has become incapacitated, whereas directives to physicians and living wills document the forms of treatment that the patient wishes to have in the event of a serious illness. If the patient has not selected a surrogate decision-maker, then next of kin has traditionally been utilized in the United States.

COMPREHENSION QUESTIONS

15.1   A 21-year-old woman presents to the ED via ambulance unconscious and with severe abdominal trauma following a robbery. She is hypotensive, and your brief survey reveals a hemoperitoneum. In your best judgment, she needs to go to the operating room for emergent laparotomy. At this time, she cannot consent to surgery and her next of kin is not available. What should you do next?

A.   Perform conservative measures until the next of kin can be identified or the patient resumes consciousness.

B.   Proceed with emergency surgery as it can be assumed that the patient would opt for treatment in her best interest.

C.   Request a psychiatric consult to document the patient's absence of decision-making capacity.

D.   Attempt to get a court order to perform surgery.

15.2   A 32-year-old practicing Jehovah's Witness presents to the hospital with chest pain and shortness of breath and is found to be severely anemic with a hemoglobin level of 3.2 g/dL. She is accompanied by her husband and sister. You are consulted as the hospitalist, and you recommend that she be admitted for a blood transfusion; however, the patient declines due to religious reasons. You are certain that the patient and her family understand the risks and benefits of the procedure. What is your next best step?

A.   You respect the patient's wishes and admit her for observation alone.

B.   You should administer the transfusion under the premise that she has unclear mentation with such severe anemia.

C.   When the patient is alone, you again discuss your recommendation for blood transfusion.

D.   You discharge the patient because she is declining your recommended treatment and there is nothing else that you can do to mitigate her symptoms.

15.3   A 93-year-old man with terminal cancer and multiple medical comorbidities was admitted to your internal medicine service overnight. He is well known to you and recently verbally reconfirmed his previously stated decision not to undergo CPR or be put on a respirator while in the office. You are reviewing his chart and note that code status has not been addressed when a "code blue" is called to his room. When you arrive, CPR is in progress. What should you do?

A.   Continue CPR until the next of kin returns to the room and can be asked about the patient's wishes.

B.   Assume that the patient would want all resuscitative measures because code status was not documented in the chart.

C.   Halt CPR since this is in line with the patient's most likely wishes.

D.   Administer chest compressions but not intubation.

ANSWERS

15.1 **B.** Physicians should provide emergency care unless it is known that the patient or surrogate would refuse such care.

15.2 **C.** You must ensure that your patient's decision is free from coercion, including that of family and friends.

15.3 **C.** The patient has clearly and consistently expressed that he did not desire life-prolonging treatment and had specifically stated that he did not desire CPR in case of cardiac arrest. CPR should be halted.

KEY POINTS

▶ Patients with decision-making capacity have the right to refuse care.

▶ Informed refusal is the refusal of a medical intervention by a patient after adequate disclosure of the nature, risks, benefits, and alternatives of that intervention.

▶ Know the role of surrogate decision makers and how to proceed when decision-making capacity does not exist.

REFERENCES

Jonsen AR, Siegler M, Winslade WJ, Jonsen AR, Siegler M, Winslade WJ, eds. *Clinical Ethics: A Practical Approach to Ethical Decisions in Clinical Medicine*. 7th ed. New York, NY: McGraw-Hill; 2010.

Levy F, Mareiniss D, Iacovelli C. The importance of a proper against-medical-advice (AMA) discharge: how signing out AMA may create significant liability protection for providers. *J Emerg Med*. 2012;43:516-520.

Lo B. *Resolving Ethical Dilemmas: A Guide for Clinicians*. 4th ed. Philadelphia, PA: Lippincott Williams & Wilkins; 2009.

Nelson LJ, Milliken N. Compelled medical treatment of pregnant women: life, liberty, and law in conflict. *JAMA*. 1988;259:1060-1066.

West JM. Ethical issues in the care of Jehovah's witnesses. *Curr Opin Anesthesiol*. 2014;27:170-176.

A 64-year-old gravida 3 para 3 Latino woman comes to the gynecology clinic with a reluctant chief complaint that she sometimes soils her underpants. She speaks Spanish only and her history is obtained with the aid of her granddaughter because the clinic interpreter was busy with other patients. She states that her stools have become soft and she has had 2 to 3 bowel movements per day for the last year, with an accident every week or more, depending on how often she has diarrhea. If she has diarrhea she may have 2 or 3 accidents a week. Her medical history is remarkable for diabetes and chronic hypertension. She had a hysterectomy for pelvic organ prolapse 5 years prior. She also had a normal colonoscopy performed 3 months ago. Her review of systems is positive for hot flashes. Her medications listed in her electronic medical record are glyburide and captopril; however, she admits to take them irregularly. She admits that she does not trust the medications and prefers more natural remedies. In fact, she started taking herbal remedies and has been taking oral aloe vera every day for about 1 year to "clean" her body; she informs you that this is a common practice in her community in Guatemala where aloe vera is recommend by the village healer. Her more recent laboratory studies show glycated hemoglobin of 8.0 mg/dL. Her physical examination shows atrophic vaginitis, with a normal perineum and an adequate rectal sphincter tone. No evidence of pelvic organ prolapse was visualized.

▶ What is your approach to the patient's medications?
▶ How should you address the patient's natural medications?
▶ How do you address her problems without the aid of an interpreter?

ANSWERS TO CASE 16:
Cross-Cultural Issues

Summary: A 62-year-old woman with fecal incontinence–associated diarrhea presented to you. Her work up ruled out a rectal or colonic mass. Her symptoms started shortly after she decided to "clean" her body with aloe vera and some other home remedies. You reviewed the literature and found out that aloe vera can act as a potent laxative and can interfere with the absorption of oral hypoglycemic medications. You would like her to discontinue the aloe vera and home remedies that you believe are leading to diarrhea and fecal incontinence.

- **Approach to the patient's medications:** Attempting to force a patient to do anything will rarely achieve the expected results. The patient will do whatever she thinks is best, and, if you do not earn her trust, then she may not comply with your recommendations. Rather, you need to explore why she believes that she does not need to take the medications as prescribed. Is she afraid of the adverse events? Are the medications too expensive?

- **Approach to the natural medications:** It is always a good practice to be open to patient ideas during the encounter and to further explore their practices. In this particular case you learned that the patient relies on herbs for most of her maladies. You do not really know much about herbs; however, you consult the National Institutes of Health (NIH) Center for Complementary and Alternative Medicine website (http://nccam.nih.gov/health/herbsataglance.htm) and discover that, in large amounts, aloe vera can be a potent laxative and can interfere with the absorption of oral hypoglycemics. This is likely the trigger for her diarrhea and fecal incontinence. You offer this as an explanation of her chief complaint and explain that stopping the aloe vera may improve her symptoms, emphasizing the importance of her continuing to take glyburide and review with her the outcomes of poorly controlled diabetes.

- **Discussing problems without the aid of the interpreter:** You must wait for a qualified trained interpreter before discussing problems with the patient. Relatives are more susceptible to modify what the patient is saying or omit details they may view as embarrassing because they think they are trying to help. A professional interpreter is trained to relate a message without interjecting opinion. Relying on informal interpreters may mean that a provider or institution is violating Title VI of the Civil Rights Act of 1964. For institutions that receive federal funding, Title VI and its supporting regulations guarantee individuals with limited English proficiency any language assistance they need to guarantee "meaningful access" to health care and social services.

ANALYSIS

Objectives

1. Recognize models of adequate cross-cultural communication.

2. Review the importance of patient negotiation to improve treatment compliance.

3. Plan how to effectively work with medical interpreters.

4. Evaluate your own self-awareness to provide culturally competent care.

Considerations

Failure to elicit a cross-cultural competent history can jeopardize physician–patient interactions and obstruct patient care. A basic knowledge of cultural diversity and health care perceptions is necessary to earn a patient's trust and to ensure patient adherence to treatment plans. Some insight into our own biases and prejudices is important so as not to impact patient care. In this case, an officially recognized interpreter should be immediately engaged. Once the interpreter is in place, it is then possible to speak openly with the patient about her views on traditional medications. It is important to understand her point of view and to be open to her perspective to establish a therapeutic physician–patient relationship. Once the relationship is established, it is then possible to discuss with her the ways in which her current herbal medications may be contributing to her fecal incontinence.

APPROACH TO:

Cross-Cultural Competency

DEFINITIONS

CULTURE: Refers to integrated patterns of human behavior that include the language, thoughts, actions, customs, beliefs, and institutions of racial, ethnic, social or religious groups.

COMPETENCE: Implies having the capacity to effectively function as an individual or an organization with regard to autonomous decision-making within the context of cultural beliefs, practices, and needs by patients and their communities.

CULTURAL COMPETENCE: A set of congruent behaviors, knowledge, attitudes, and policies that come together in a system, organization, or among professionals that enables effective work in cross-cultural situations.

Table 16–1 • KLEINMAN'S QUESTIONS
What do you think has caused your problem?
Why do you think it started when it did?
What do you think your sickness does to you?
How severe is your sickness? Will it have a short or long course?
What kind of treatment do you think you should receive?
What are the most important results you hope to receive from this treatment?
What are the chief problems your sickness has caused for you?
What do you fear most about your sickness?

CLINICAL APPROACH

Providing health care in a culturally competent manner requires an understanding of different factors, both social and cultural, that may influence patient's response to various treatment plans. To be versed in cultural competence we must assess our knowledge, skills, and attitudes pertinent to the subject.

Knowledge

There are different models that help us understand the patient's explanatory models of his or her health (Tables 16–1 and 16–2). Becoming familiar with these types of questions is necessary to improve the communication with our patients, and to facilitate the negotiation of the treatment plan. Familiarity with different communication styles, including verbal, body language, and tone of voice, and personal distance would also help establish a good respectful relationship while you get to know your patient. In addition, the role of different family members as decision-makers can help inform the dynamics of the encounter with the patient. Some populations are more prone to seek the help of traditional healers as a first approach. Being aware of these relationships will assist in obtaining a more complete patient history. Health care professionals must show respect and tolerance for these practices to establish a mutually respectful relationship with the patient.

Skills

Quality history taking skills are essential to gain patient trust and truly understand the patient's beliefs as to why he or she is ill, suffering, or living with

Table 16–2 • THE ETHNIC MNEMONIC
Explanation (How do you explain your illness?)
Treatment (What treatments have you tried?)
Healers (Have you sought any advice from traditional healers?)
Negotiate (Mutually acceptable options)
Intervention (Agreed on)
Collaboration (With patient, family, and healers)

Table 16–3 • WORKING WITH INTERPRETERS
Do not depend on children, relatives, friends, or nonmedical staff to provide language interpretation.
Hold a brief preinterview with the interpreter.
Allow enough time for the interpreted sessions.
Use carefully chosen words to convey your meaning and limit the use of gestures.
Speak clearly in a normal voice and not too fast or too loudly.
Avoid jargon and technical terms.
Ask only one question at a time.
Expect the interpreter to interrupt when necessary for clarification.

chronic disease. This also translates into being able to engage the patient in the decision-making for the plan of care. This "negotiation" and patient participation is essential to ensure patient compliance with the treatment plan. Working with language interpreters is an essential skill for a provider in a multicultural community, and it adds another layer of complexity in patient care. There are unique aspects to consider and specific skills to develop when working with interpreters (Table 16–3).

Attitudes

It is important to perform routine self-assessments to ensure one's own personal biases and behaviors are not negatively impacting the therapeutic relationship. Experiences from the past influence the way in which health care professionals relate and react to patients. This influence can be conscious or unconscious and can lead to development of stereotypes of different patient populations in our minds. There is no one correct way to treat a particular ethnic group; each patient is an individual, and the knowledge and tools for intervention should be applied in a patient-centered approach (Table 16–4). In addition, there are intergenerational differences that make overgeneralization dangerous. At the end of the next cross-cultural patient encounter, reflect on the following questions: (1) What did you think about the encounter?, (2) Did you take into consideration the patient's perspective?, (3) What did you do to better understand the patient?, and (4) How would you manage this patient's condition differently during the next encounter?

Table 16–4 • IMPORTANT ATTITUDES FOR COMPETENT CROSS-CULTURAL CARE
Avoid stereotyping.
Consider all patients as individuals first, as members of minority status, and then as members of a specific ethnic group.
Never assume that a person's ethnic identity tells you anything about his or her cultural values or patterns of behavior.

COMPREHENSION QUESTIONS

16.1 You have been working in the emergency center for 10 months, and tonight have been assigned to all female patients that present with vaginal bleeding. You have noticed that almost all patients that present with a diagnosis of a miscarriage want no form of medical treatment, only to allow "God to do his will." Your first patient is a Spanish-speaking 16-year-old girl diagnosed with a miscarriage. Of the following choices which action would represent a lack of competent cross-cultural care?

A. Consult an interpreter to interview the patient because you do not speak Spanish

B. Arrange outpatient follow up after a full history and physical examination

C. Offer all forms of treatment for miscarriage, including observation, medical, and surgical management

D. Perform a complete history and examination and offer her a prayer to ease her pain

16.2 You are a surgical intern and working at a preoperative clinic. Your next patient presents with a long history of abdominal pain due to a ventral hernia that you can see on examination when she sits up. She is 32 years of age, speaks Spanish and English and is accompanied by her mother who only speaks Spanish. She would like surgical management and you are explaining the risks, benefits, and alternatives to the procedure. After each explanation and before she signs off on the consents, she discusses the details with her mother in Spanish. Her mother does not appear to want that her daughter has mesh implanted during the surgery; because of this, the patient is not going to consent to the surgery. You are getting frustrated. Which of the following cross-cultural approaches to care may help to elicit buy-in for what you consider the standard of care for hernia repair?

A. Request medical interpretation in order that her mother has the consents explained to her in Spanish.

B. Recognize that possibly in this patient's culture that her mother may be entrusted to make most of the family's medical decisions and include the mother in the process.

C. Have the patient sign off on the mesh procedure anyway; if she decides not to proceed with the case, then she can cancel prior to the surgical date.

D. Rationalize with the patient that the decision is hers and not that of her mother.

ANSWERS

16.1 **D.** Although it is tempting to offer prayer, without knowledge of this particular patient's religious or cultural beliefs, you are assuming that, perhaps like other patients you have taken care of with a similar condition, she wants "God to do His will." Without a specific statement by the patient ascribing to this belief, offering prayer or assuming the patient has a religious affiliation based on past experiences is stereotyping and not a competent attitude to employ in cross-cultural care.

16.2 **B.** Recognizing that the patient's mother, even though she is 32 years of age, may be responsible for ensuring her family's health is important; therefore, allowing them more time to think about the case planned and engaging her mother in the decision-making process will help build trust and may ultimately accomplish your goal, that is, providing her with the surgery that she needs and that you feel is the standard of care. Having her sign a consent form without her mother's permission or rationalizing that the decision is the patient's and not her mother's decision is likely to have the opposite effect.

KEY POINTS

► Cross-cultural competent care improves physician–patient interactions.

► Patient negotiation is a key strategy for improved patient compliance.

► Use of interpreters improves patient care and should be guaranteed in federally funded hospitals and clinics.

► Self-assessment of your own beliefs and experiences may help to limit stereotyping and provide better patient care.

REFERENCES

Kaczmarczyk JM, Hueppchen NA, Abbot JF, et al. The preceptor and cultural competence. Association of Professors of Gynecology and Obstetrics Effective preceptor series. https://www.apgo.org/binary/Preceptor9.pdf. Accessed September 22, 2014.

Kobylarz FA, Heath JM, Like RC. The ETHNIC(S) mnemonic: a clinical tool for ethnogeriatric education. *J Am Geriatr Soc.* 2002;50:1582-1589.

Management Sciences for Health. The Provider's Guide to Quality and Culture. Management Sciences for Health, Cambridge, MA. http://erc.msh.org/mainpage.cfm?file=1.0.htm&module=provider&language=English. Accessed September 22, 2014.

Miller NB. Social work services to Urban Indians. In: Green J, ed. *Cultural Awareness in the Human Services.* Prentice-Hall. Englewood Cliffs, NJ; 1982:182.

South-Paul J, Axtell S, Betancourt JR, et al. *Cultural Competency Education for Medical Students.* Association of American Medical Colleges. https://www.aamc.org/download/54338/data/culturalcomped.pdf. Accessed September 22, 2014.

You attend the cesarean delivery of a 27-year-old primigravida with a history of generalized anxiety disorder, dysthymia, pre-eclampsia, and concerns for a possible bleeding behind the placental (placental abruption). A 37-week, appropriate for gestational age, male infant is successfully delivered. After routine resuscitation by the neonatologist, the infant is well appearing as is the new mother. For teaching purposes and per policy, you have requested that the placenta be sent to pathology for evaluation of placental abruption. The infant and mother are discharged home routinely after 4 days. One week later, you receive the report from pathology, which confirms the presence of a small, retroplacental hemorrhage. However, the report goes on to describe increased syncytial knots, villous agglutination, distal villous hypoplasia, and intervillous fibrin, findings which are consistent with placental underperfusion. A literature search suggests that these findings may be associated with short- and long-term neurodevelopmental impairments in premature infants. At the mother's next follow-up visit, she shares her concerns that the serotonin-specific reuptake inhibitor (SSRI) she took throughout pregnancy, her pre-eclampsia, or perhaps the surgical anesthetics used during the delivery may negatively impact her son's development. She states that she began sharing these concerns with her son's pediatrician at the 2-week visit but stopped because the pediatrician seemed very busy. You are unsure whether to disclose the pathology results with the mother, specifically the findings consistent with underperfusion, because you are concerned about potentially contributing to her anxiety about her infant son or worsening her depressive symptoms.

▶ What is your ethical and/or legal obligation to disclose the pathology results to the patient?
▶ When, if ever, is it appropriate to withhold medical information from a patient?
▶ When, if ever, is it appropriate to deceive a patient?

ANSWERS TO CASE 17:

Deception to Patients

Summary: A 27-year-old primigravida mother with generalized anxiety disorder, dysthymia, and pre-eclampsia is worried that her full-term, healthy appearing newborn son may suffer negative neurodevelopmental consequences as a result of any one of numerous risk factors. The placental pathology report describes findings consistent with placental underperfusion, a condition that may be associated with neurodevelopmental impairments in premature infants. You are unsure whether to disclose these results with her due to concerns over her mental health.

- **Ethical and/or legal obligation to disclose the pathology results to the patient:** Ethically, the pathology results should be disclosed based on the ethical principle of respect for autonomy. Legally, the physician should disclose all clinically relevant information that a "reasonable person" would want in making a medical decision.

- **When, if ever, is it appropriate to withhold medical information from a patient?** Information may be withheld where the physician believes the information may harm the patient (therapeutic privilege).

- **When, if ever, is it appropriate to deceive a patient?** It is never permissible to deceive a patient.

ANALYSIS

Objectives

1. Understand the ethical principles that generate the obligation to veracity (truth telling).

2. Understand the ethical principles that may justify withholding information from the patient.

3. Identify criteria necessary to justify deception.

Considerations

This 27-year-old first-time mother has a generalized anxiety disorder for which she receives treatment in the form of an SSRI. Due to concerns for placental abruption, you ordered and have received the pathology report on the placenta. In addition to confirming a small abruption, the pathologist mentions findings consistent with placental underperfusion, which may be associated with adverse neurologic outcomes in premature infants. This finding is of questionable significance to your patient, because these results are not conclusive and relate specifically to premature newborns. Conversely, you suspect that no studies have been performed that look at this association in term newborns; it may be appropriate to say that the literature can neither prove nor disprove the association with neurodevelopmental impairments in term newborns. It is also possible that the findings of placental abruption and of underperfusion are related to your patient's pre-eclampsia. Your patient voices her concerns to you about her newborn son's long-term neurodevelopment, citing her medication use, the use of anesthetic medications during her cesarean delivery, and her pre-eclampsia as possible risk factors. She has tried to discuss her concerns with her son's pediatrician, but she remains unconvinced by the pediatrician's reassurances. Because you have observed that the infant appears healthy, it would be appropriate to investigate why she is concerned about her son, for example, has she observed anything about his behavior that led her to worry about his neurodevelopment?

In a patient with a known mood disorder in the setting of a major life stressor, it would be appropriate to screen her for depression using an appropriate screening tool. In accordance with the ethical principle of nonmaleficence, you wish to avoid full disclosure of the pathology results. You are concerned that disclosing this information to this anxious-appearing, first-time mother may increase her level of anxiety, leading to emotional or psychological issues, and potentially exposing her son to future medical procedures. You are also concerned that she may believe that her pre-eclampsia led to the findings described in the pathology report and that disclosure of this information will lead to her feeling guilty, triggering a worsening of her depressive symptoms that could potentially lead to a major depressive episode. However, you are afraid that not revealing this information constitutes a form of deception, violating your obligation to veracity, which is rooted in the principle of respect for patient autonomy. An ethically rigorous and empirically justified process by which to weigh these competing claims is necessary to make a morally justifiable choice and to act on it.

APPROACH TO:
Truth Telling and Withholding Information

DEFINITIONS

DECEIVE: To intentionally cause another person to believe what is false. Deception is the act of doing so.

LIE/LYING: To make a believed false statement to another person with the intention that he or she believes the statement to be true.

PATERNALISM: Intentionally overriding a person's known preferences or actions with the goal of benefitting or avoiding harm to the person whose preferences or actions are overridden.

THERAPEUTIC PRIVILEGE: A justification used to withhold information from patients with the belief that disclosing such information would cause the patient very grave harm.

VERACITY: The principle of truth telling and the duty to avoid deception in patient interactions.

CLINICAL APPROACH

Ethical and Legal Considerations

There are 4 principles that form the framework of medical ethics: beneficence, nonmaleficence, justice, and respect for autonomy (Table 17–1). No principle is superior to the others; rather, all 4 must be considered to evaluate the ethical appropriateness of an action. From the interplay of these four principles, secondary principles, standards, patient rights, rules, and codes of conduct are derived which help guide the practice of medicine.

In this case, the physician's obligation to veracity primarily stems from the principle of respect for autonomy. For a patient to act autonomously, he or she must be able to make meaningful decisions in regard to his or her present and future health. To do so, the patient must have relevant and accurate information. This creates an obligation on the part of the physician to provide that information. Furthermore, it can be argued that withholding information may negatively impact the patient if the withholding of information results in a negative consequence or prevents a positive outcome—a line of reasoning supported by the principles of nonmaleficence and beneficence, respectively.

The law reflects establishing the right to informed consent wherein the patient has a right to all relevant information needed to make an informed choice and should be free of any undue influence or coercion. Two different legal standards are commonly used to decide what information is "relevant" and, thus, must be disclosed. The first is the "reasonable person" standard, whereby a physician must disclose all medical information, which a "reasonable person" would be expected to want when making medical decisions. However, empiric ethics research reveals that physicians grossly underestimate the amount of information that their patients want, while patients assign a higher degree of relevance to their medical information. Patient preference for disclosure persists even after being counseled about the questionable clinical significance of the information. These empiric data obligate physicians to err on the side of greater disclosure or to have explicit discussions with their patients about the types of information they desire. Furthermore, when the physician fails to give the patient all relevant information regarding a procedure, the patient's ability to give informed consent is precluded.

Should the physician go on to perform a procedure without consent, this is an assault on the patient, which is considered to be another violation of the patient's

Table 17–1 • PRINCIPLES OF MEDICAL ETHICS	
Beneficence	The duty to promote good and to act in the best interests of the patient and the health of society.
Nonmaleficence	The duty to do no harm to patients.
Justice	The equitable distribution of the life-enhancing opportunities afforded by health care.
Respect for Autonomy	The duty to protect and foster a patient's choices free of coercion.

autonomy. To account for these shortcomings, a second "subjective" standard was developed, wherein the physician must disclose all information considered "material" or "significant" to the decision-making process of the particular person or patient. Although obstacles to a patient obtaining the desired information may remain, this standard puts the burden on the physician to assess his or her patient's desired level of disclosure.

The most common justification for nondisclosure is the concept of therapeutic privilege, which holds that a physician (or other medical practitioner) may at, his or her discretion, withhold medical information from a patient (as this information relates to the diagnosis, prognosis, treatment options, and risks associated with these options) if, in his or her opinion, the information would harm the patient or would then leave him or her unable to make rational decisions. The justification for this paternalistic act is derived primarily from the principle of nonmaleficence, the goal of which is to avoid harm to the patient. The inherent conflict of therapeutic privilege with the principle of respect necessitates that the physician who relies on it to justify nondisclosure of information to his or her patient and he or she must do so after a rigorous analysis of the moral appropriateness of the decision. A successful justification must rely on specific facets of the case, because this is necessary to counter the default obligation to full disclosure. Conversely, the justification must be limited to the specific case, so as to not provide a "blanket justification" to be used to justify nondisclosure in seemingly similar but critically different scenarios. To do so, the physician must take into account the patient's psychological state. It would be extremely difficult, if not impossible, to argue that a patient without a psychiatric disturbance (either chronic or acute) would be exposed to sufficient harm from full disclosure so as to outweigh the violation of their autonomy and the potential benefits of full knowledge of his or her disease and the potential treatment options. Five potential reasons have been suggested by Richard and colleagues for when to resort to the use of therapeutic privilege. These are as follows:

1. To allow the patient to come to terms with events, both factually and emotionally.

2. To prevent decision-making at a time of relative incapacity precipitated by overwhelming anxiety or stress.

3. To prevent physical or psychological harm (eg, prevent severe psychological stress).

4. To preserve hope.

5. To maintain the patient's long-term autonomy.

These reasons must still be weighed against violating the patient's short-term autonomy and the potential consequences thereof in order to weigh the moral appropriateness of a decision to violate the patient's autonomy (Figure 17–1). The algorithm in Figure 17–1 has been slightly modified for purposes of simplicity; it is also worth acknowledging that the algorithm involves subjective reasoning and, thus, may result in reaching a faulty conclusion.

The Council on Ethical and Judicial Affairs of the American Medical Association (AMA) states that information should never be permanently withheld from

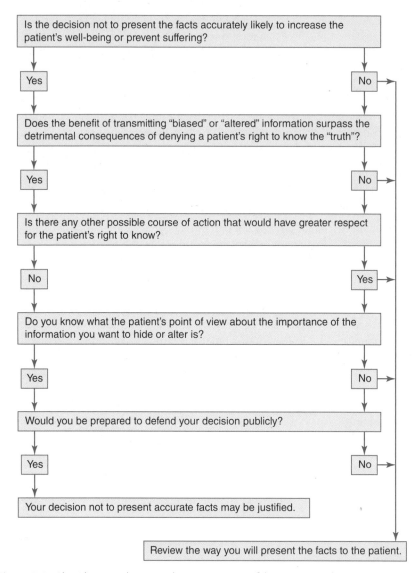

Figure 17–1. Algorithm to evaluate moral appropriateness of therapeutic privilege.

patients, because doing so violates the patient's trust in the physician. Rather, the AMA advocates that beneficence may allow a physician in select circumstances to postpone full disclosure of information to patients whose capacity to make competent medical decisions may be compromised or when disclosure is otherwise medically contraindicated. Delayed disclosure is not justified when a physician merely intends to prevent a patient's refusal of medically necessary treatments or to instill hope for the future. It is important to note the conflict between the position taken on preserving hope by Richard and colleagues (of

French-Canadian nationalities) and the AMA. This difference likely reflects the heightened importance put on respecting patient autonomy in the United States, an importance reflected in the cultural views on rights and in the law. As a result, a practitioner in the United States may choose to be more forthcoming if he or she is considering the preservation of hope as the reason to withhold information from the patient.

In the case described above, the obstetrician should pay close attention to the mother's emotional and psychological state. Evidence of worsening of her anxiety disorder or the development of depression (eg, postpartum depression) warrants evaluation and treatment. If her psychological symptoms are severe enough at this initial visit, then the obstetrician may consider temporarily delaying a full discussion of the results of the pathology report until her symptoms have improved. At that time, the physician may choose to discuss with the patient how much detail she desires, thus making it possible to discuss the results of the pathology report to the level of detail the patient desires.

COMPREHENSION QUESTIONS

17.1 What ethical principle does the physician's obligation to veracity (truth telling) *primarily* derive from?

A. Principle of beneficence

B. Principle of nonmaleficence

C. Principle of respect for autonomy

D. Principle of double effect

E. Principle of justice

17.2 Invoking therapeutic privilege to justify withholding information from a patient depends *most* on which ethical principle?

A. Principle of beneficence

B. Principle of nonmaleficence

C. Principle of respect for autonomy

D. Principle of double effect

E. Principle of justice

17.3 Decisions to withhold information from patients can best be described as which of the following?

A. Virtuous

B. Compassionate

C. Paternalistic

D. Utilitarian

E. Autonomous

17.4 What should the physician evaluate to appropriately invoke therapeutic privilege to justify nondisclosure?

   A. How much the patient desires the information?

   B. The patient's emotional/psychological state.

   C. The consequences of pursuing either full disclosure or nondisclosure.

   D. If the desire to withhold information is due to a desire to prevent the patient from refusing medical treatment.

   E. All of the above.

ANSWERS

17.1 **C.** The principle of respect for autonomy obligates the physician to provide the patient with all accurate information required to make an informed decision. Although each of these principles may support veracity, answers A, B, and E are incorrect because they derive primarily from C. Answer D is wrong because the principle of double effect describes a way to justify a harmful outcome when a beneficial outcome is desired.

17.2 **B.** The justification for invoking the therapeutic privilege is based on avoiding harm to the patient. Answer A may seem correct, but this choice describes more accurately the physician's obligation to promote and act in the patient's best interests, which is a related but ultimately different concept. Answer C is incorrect because therapeutic privilege typically undermines a patient autonomy, although in select cases an argument can be made that nondisclosure may ultimately protect patient autonomy in the long term. Answer E is incorrect because the principle of justice neither strongly supports nor opposes therapeutic privilege.

17.3 **C.** A paternalistic act occurs when a physician, at his or her discretion, withholds information from the patient to avoid harming him or her. Answers A and B are incorrect because withholding information may be either virtuous, compassionate, or neither. Answer D may seem correct because a utilitarian analysis of the potential harms and benefits of disclosure versus nondisclosure must be undertaken, but this is only one part of the analysis. Answer E is incorrect because the principle of respect for autonomy refers to patient autonomy, not the physician autonomy.

17.4 **E.** The physician should perform a thorough analysis before invoking therapeutic privilege. This includes but is not limited to the patient's desire for the information, the emotional/psychological state of the patient, the likely consequence of disclosure and nondisclosure, and his or her own motivations for withholding information.

KEY POINTS

▶ The principle of respect for autonomy creates a strong obligation on the part of the physician to fully disclose information relevant to the patient's decision-making and health.

▶ Nondisclosure jeopardizes the patient's ability to give his or her consent to treatment and may result in assault on the part of the physician.

▶ Empiric data strongly suggest that patients typically want more information that physicians think they want and patients may consider information to be relevant that physicians consider irrelevant.

▶ Therapeutic privilege is the concept where the physician withholds information from the patient in the belief that disclosure would ultimately harm the patient.

▶ In most cases, the patient must be experiencing a psychiatric disturbance to successfully invoke therapeutic privilege.

▶ Successfully invocation of therapeutic privilege requires that the physician pursue a rigorous ethical analysis of the decision.

REFERENCES

Beauchamp TL, Childress JF. *Principles of Biomedical Ethics*. 4th ed. New York, NY: Oxford University Press; 1994:78,126-127,189, 274.

Bostick NA, Sade R, McMahon JW, Benjamin R. Report of the American Medical Association Council on Ethical and Judicial Affairs: withholding information from patients: rethinking the propriety of "therapeutic privilege". *J Clin Ethics*. 2006;17:302-306.

Cannold L. "There is No Evidence to Suggest...": changing the way we judge information for disclosure in the informed consent process. *Hypatia*. 1997;12:165-184.

Faden RR, Becker C, Lewis C, Freeman J, Faden AI. Disclosure of information to patients in medical care. *Medical Care*. 1981;19:718-733.

Hodkinson K. The need to know – therapeutic privilege: a way forward. *Health Care Anal*. 2013;21:105-129.

Mahon JE. The definition of lying and deception. In: Zalta EN, ed. *The Stanford Encyclopedia of Philosophy*. Fall ed. Stanford University Press. Stanford, CA. 2008. http://plato.stanford.edu/archives/fall2008/entries/lying-definition/. Accessed November 28, 2014.

Redline RW, Boyd T, Campbell V, et al. Maternal vascular underperfusion: nosology and reproducibility of placental reaction patterns. *Pediatr Dev Pathol*. 2004;7:237-249.

Richard C, Lajeuness Y, Lussier M. Therapeutic privilege: between the ethics of lying and the practice of truth. *J Med Ethics*. 2010;36:353-357.

Sugarman J, Sulmasy DP. *Methods in Medical Ethics*. 2nd ed. Washington, DC: Georgetown University Press; 2010:13.

Wilson SE, Baker ER, Leonard AC, et al. Understanding preferences for disclosure of individual biomarker results among participants in a longitudinal birth cohort. *J Med Ethics*. 2010;36:736-740.

van den Heever P. Pleading the defence of therapeutic privilege. *S Afr Med J*. 2005;95:420-421.

van Vliet EO, de Kievet JF, van der Voorn JP, et al. Placental pathology and long-term neurodevelopment of very preterm infants. *Am J Obstet Gynecol*. 2012;6:489.e1-e7.

A 45-year-old woman is scheduled to see you in your office for her yearly routine visit. You have been her primary care physician for several years. When reviewing her chart, you notice a radiology report from her visit to the emergency department (ED) where she had presented 10 months ago with fever and cough. Chest radiography was performed at that time to rule out pneumonia. The study was read as showing no parenchymal abnormalities, but there was a suggestion of a retrosternal mass. A follow-up examination was suggested. You do not remember ever having seen this report.

▶ How much detail should be disclosed to the patient when the full extent of the clinical diagnosis is not yet known?
▶ Should you postpone having this conversation until you have spoken to the ED physician? Do you need to first speak with an oncologist so that you can answer the question as to what this mass might be and whether the delay in diagnosis will affect the patient's prognosis?
▶ Is an apology appropriate at this time? If so, for what specifically?

ANSWERS TO CASE 18:

Disclosure and Apology

Summary: A 45-year-old woman is scheduled to see you for an annual routine visit. You noted a radiology report from chest radiography performed 10 months ago at the ED. The study suggested a retrosternal mass, and a follow-up examination was recommended. You do not remember ever having seen this report.

- **Amount of detail to disclose to the patient:** Disclose only what is known to you; do not speculate.

- **Should you postpone having this conversation until you have spoken to the ED physician?** Do not delay speaking with the patient, despite the fact that you do not have all of the answers. Disclose the information that you have and reassure the patient that you will keep her informed as you gather more information.

- **Do you need to first speak with an oncologist?** No, not if there is not time to do so prior to seeing the patient. Provide the patient with the information that you do know. You can speak with the patient again after speaking with the oncologist or after referring the patient for follow-up with an oncologist.

- **Is an apology appropriate at this time? If so, for what specifically?** An expression of empathy is always appropriate and this often uses the language of apology (eg, "I am so sorry that you have to go through this"). In this case, you do know there was a delay in seeing the report, so there should be an apology for that, for example, "I am sorry that I did not see this report until now. I will make sure we get you in to see the appropriate specialist right away."

ANALYSIS

Objectives

1. Identify the principles of transparent and compassionate disclosure.

2. Understand that disclosure is a process, not a single conversation.

3. Recognize the emotional challenges faced by clinicians following an adverse event so that these do not prevent transparent and compassionate interactions with the patient and family.

Considerations

In the case described, a woman is noted to have a retrosternal mass on chest radiography and a follow-up visit recommended. The patient is scheduled for a routine physical examination. In general, always share with the patient the known facts as soon as possible and do not speculate. Do not delay the discussion until you have the answers.

The patient will undoubtedly have many important questions that you will be unable to answer at this time. Acknowledge the importance of these questions and reassure her that you will arrange for her to see an oncologist who will guide her through the next steps. You should not speculate as to why this happened, but do make clear that you will look into why the report did not come to your attention. Be sure to express empathy (eg, "I am so sorry you have to go through this uncertainty"). Acknowledge how difficult it must be to hear this and invite her to express concerns and ask questions. Close by reviewing precise next steps (eg, "I am going to set up an appointment for you with one of my colleagues for sometime this week"). Lastly, be sure to remind her that you will be there for her.

APPROACH TO:
Disclosure and Apology

DEFINITIONS

ADVERSE EVENT: An undesired harmful effect that is not due to the patient's underlying disease process; it may or may not be related to an error.

APOLOGY: A specific acknowledgment and expression of regret for having done something wrong or contributed to an error.

DISCLOSURE: A transparent process in which the known facts of a case are discussed with a patient, family members, or both.

CLINICAL APPROACH

We have a professional ethical obligation to inform our patients regarding their care. This is especially important when there has been an error. However, several research studies have shown that clinicians are not skilled in having discussions with patients and families after medical errors. It seems reasonable to assume that some of the barriers to meeting patient needs after errors might include the clinician's sense of vulnerability and emotional distress.

Grappling with a medical error that caused harm to a patient is one of the most challenging moments of any clinician's career. Many studies have documented the negative emotional impact on clinicians who have made errors. In addition to the sadness at seeing a patient experience suffering, there are professional, personal, and societal expectations of perfection that, although we may know intellectually are unrealistic, we feel deeply on an emotional level. Making an error shatters any illusions of perfection and can result in clinicians feeling ashamed, incompetent, guilty, and sad. The feelings of shame may be particularly strong because of a culture that expects perfection. These emotions may be accompanied by fear of loss of the patient's trust, damaged reputation amongst colleagues, and possible litigation.

The event often involves a series of errors or perhaps someone else's error. Clinicians may be in a position, then, of having to disclose and apologize for a colleague's error. In addition, most clinicians do not have a great deal of experience in this arena, because the incidence of an individual clinician making a clinically significant error is not likely to be high, even over many years of practice. Therefore, it is important for all clinicians to understand some basic principles underlying effective disclosure conversations:

- The most important principle is to do what is best for the patient and family. The question is not "What would I want my physician to do or say in this instance?" Rather, it is trying to understand the needs of the patient and family in the moment and as they evolve.

- The attending physician taking care of the patient when the error is discovered should lead the conversation. If another attending made the error, that physician should ideally be the one to apologize and disclose, but this may be impractical in the immediate aftermath. When appropriate, other team members such as a nurse, social worker or trainee, could be present if this would be helpful to the patient and family.

- Always share with the patient the known facts as soon as possible. It is inadvisable to wait until there has been a root cause analysis or any process that will flesh out all the details.

- Do not speculate. If you know what happened but not why, then all you can share is what you do know. Speculation can inadvertently implicate others or mislead the patient. Because disclosure is a process, not an event, you should explain that you will continue to keep the patient informed if and when more information becomes available.

- Express empathy. One of the most direct ways to do so is to say, "I am sorry this happened. It is not what you or we expected."

- If there has clearly been an error, then apologize. For example, you might say, "I am so sorry we gave you the wrong dose of medication."

- Directly outline the next steps regarding the patient's clinical care, and then pause and solicit the patient's questions or concerns.

- If appropriate, explain that you or your institution is looking into why the event occurred and that you will get back to the patient when you have further information. If there has been an error, then it is important to say that you and your institution are committed to learning from this and working to improve processes to prevent a similar event from happening again.

- Be aware of your emotions so that they do not interfere with your ability to be transparent and compassionate.

Because this process can be emotionally challenging for physicians, it is important for health care institutions to provide both disclosure coaching as well as clinician peer support. Disclosure coaching is needed because few clinicians have vast experience in disclosing errors, and sometimes the circumstances of the adverse event are complicated enough that it is difficult to know what to say and how to say it. In addition, because of the emotions noted above, peer support is essential in helping the clinician be fully present for the patient and his or her family as well as to learn and grow from the experience.

ANALYSIS AND DISCUSSION

Applying these principles to the case above, the following would be a reasonable approach to consider. If the patient has a scheduled appointment the same day you first notice the radiology report, then you would need to tell her about this at that appointment. Delaying the discussion until you have the answers to these questions would likely generate a sense of mistrust. The patient is likely to have several important questions that you will not be able to answer, such as:

- What exactly could this mass be?

- What is going to happen to her?

- If this turns out to be cancer, then will the delay in following-up on the radiograph have harmed her?

All you can say is that these questions are important and that you do not have the answers right now. You are going to arrange for her to see a specialist who will guide her through the process, and you will make sure she gets the best advice and treatment.

Because you know there was an error in not having followed up on the abnormal results on the radiographs, you need to apologize for this. You should not speculate as to why this happened. However, you can say that you are going to look into why the report did not come to your attention.

After pausing and waiting for her to absorb the information, acknowledge how difficult it must be to hear this. Ask how she is feeling and invite her to express any concerns and to ask any questions.

Close by discussing the next steps that you will take, for example, "I am going to set up an appointment with one of my colleagues for sometime this week." Express empathy by saying, "I am so sorry you have to go through this uncertainty." Ask whether she or her family has any other questions right now and remind her that you will be there for her.

Every disclosure situation is unique and challenging. There is no perfect way to have these difficult conversations, but an understanding of some basic principles can be helpful. In addition, it is important that clinicians understand their own emotions so they can manage them and focus on the needs of the patient. Institutional programs that provide disclosure coaching and peer support are invaluable in helping physicians be honest and empathic with their patients.

COMPREHENSION QUESTIONS

18.1 Which of the following is the most common emotion expressed by clinicians that may interfere with a transparent, compassionate disclosure and apology?

   A. Anger

   B. Scorn

   C. Shame

   D. Confusion

18.2 Which of the following is the best approach in disclosure conversations with patients and their families?

A. The use of medical terminology is generally more precise than lay language.

B. When asked why a complication occurred, speculation is wise because it indicates transparency.

C. The physician should allow conversational space for the reactions of the patient and the family.

D. It is best not to give specific details about what we know went wrong because this confuses patients and puts the clinician at risk for malpractice.

18.3 In situations involving the disclosure of medical errors, which of the following statements is most accurate?

A. Whoever caused the adverse event should be the one leading the disclosure conversation; this might be the resident or nurse.

B. One can say "I am sorry" as an expression of empathy without accepting blame.

C. As long as clinicians are honest, patients will not have a negative reaction to errors.

D. The initial disclosure conversation should not be held until all of the facts of the event are known.

ANSWERS

18.1 **C.** Because the culture of medical training and practice emphasizes perfection, there is often an intense feeling of shame when a clinician has been involved in an event that caused patient harm. This may be accompanied by fear of loss of the patient's trust, damaged reputation among colleagues, and possible litigation.

18.2 **C.** Because of the complicated emotions affecting the clinician, there is sometimes an unconscious wish to obfuscate the details of what has gone wrong when discussing them with the patient. It is as if clinicians hope the patient will not understand that we have made an error. Sometimes, especially when pressed for answers by the patient or family, we hypothesize about why the error has occurred. It is a completely natural way for us to communicate; it is what we do when making a differential diagnosis. However, in the setting of a disclosure conversation, speculation can be confusing and destructive when the facts do emerge.

18.3 **B.** The conversation should ideally be led by the attending most involved with the patient. "I am sorry" is an expression of empathy. If the intent is to apologize, then a phrase such as "I am sorry we made this mistake" can be used. Patients sometimes forgive, but at other times they might feel angry, confused, or betrayed. One cannot 'control' the emotions of others. It is important to initiate a disclosure conversation as soon as possible after the event. At that point, one needs to disclose what is known thus far and then reassure the patient that clinicians will communicate with them when they have further information.

KEY POINTS

▶ It is important to initiate a disclosure conversation as soon as possible after the event. The disclosure should include all the information known at the time.

▶ The patient should be reassured that communication will be open regarding relaying further information as it becomes available.

▶ If there has clearly been an error, then apologize. Give assurance that efforts will be made to investigate the reasons for the error and how to prevent a similar occurrence.

▶ Do not speculate, but present what is known.

REFERENCES

Bell SK, Moorman DW, Delbanco T. Improving the patient, family, and clinician experience after harmful events: the "when things go wrong" curriculum. *Acad Med.* 2010;85:1010-1017.

Gallagher TH, Mello MM, Levinson W, et al. Talking with patients about other clinicians' errors. *N Engl J Med.* 2013;369:1752-1757.

Gallagher TH, Studdert D, Levinson W. Disclosing harmful medical errors to patients. *N Engl J Med.* 2007;356(26):2713-2719.

Gallagher TH, Waterman AD, Ebers AG, Fraser VJ, Levinson W. Patients' and physicians' attitudes regarding the disclosure of medical errors. *JAMA.* 2003;289:1001-1007.

Harrison R, Lawton R, Perlo J, Gardner P, Armitage G, Shapiro J. Emotion and coping in the aftermath of medical error: a cross country exploration. *J Patient Safety.* http://journals.lww.com/journalpatientsafety/Abstract/publishahead/Emotion_and_Coping_in_the_Aftermath_of_Medical.99824.aspx.

AR is a 4-year-old boy brought by his parents and grandmother to your emergency department (ED). During a routine visit earlier today, AR's pediatrician palpated an abdominal mass. AR's parents had not noted anything unusual recently, except that his stools had been somewhat smaller. The pediatrician told them she thought AR was likely constipated, but she sent them to the ED to "make sure nothing else was going on." On examination, you note that AR's abdomen is distended and you palpate a right abdominal mass. The examination is otherwise normal. You arrange for abdominal radiographs and ultrasonography, which shows a large right-sided abdominal mass that is likely a Wilms tumor. You contact the pediatric oncologists to evaluate AR in the ED. You must now discuss the imaging findings with AR's parents and inform them that the oncologists will be there shortly. The parents are anxious. The radiology technologists who performed radiography and ultrasonography had made small talk with the patients but advised them to talk to their ED doctor about the findings, which the radiologist would report soon.

▶ What are the barriers to effectively communicating bad news?
▶ How does one overcome such barriers and communicate successfully about bad news?

ANSWERS TO CASE 19:

Communicating Bad News

Summary: A 4-year-old child presents to the ED with a palpable abdominal mass. Ultrasonography demonstrates a probable Wilms tumor. Plans are made to have oncologists evaluate the child in the ED. The ED physician must discuss this information with the child's parents.

- **Barriers:** Lack of adequate time, space, established relationships, and/or support systems; physician emotions and biases.

- **Overcoming barriers:** Skills include: understanding core components of effective communication, including a supportive team member, being agile and improvisational use of nonverbal and verbal skills, and providing training and mentorship.

ANALYSIS

Objectives

1. Understand the key objectives when communicating about bad news with patients and families.

2. Recognize the barriers that make the communication process more difficult for patients, families, and caretakers.

3. Understand the dynamics of effective communication about bad news with patients and families.

APPROACH TO:

Communicating Bad News

DEFINITIONS

BAD NEWS: Information that adversely alters one's expectations for the future.

COMMUNICATION: Sharing or conveying information.

EMPATHY: Recognizing, relating, and responding to the intellectual and emotional experiences of others.

CLINICAL APPROACH

Before entering the room, the ED staff caring for the child should review the pertinent history and clinical information, the communication that has occurred thus far, and any management plans that have been made or communicated. During this "huddle," team members should anticipate the parents' questions and reactions and discuss how to respond. In addition to the primary provider, another individual may be identified to join the conversation to provide support for the primary provider and the family. Effort should be made to find a quiet space, if possible. Immediately before entering the room, providers should regroup to gain a composed and calm demeanor.

Once in the room and introductions are made, efforts should be made to arrange the seating for everyone's comfort. The provider should solicit the parents' current understanding of the situation and provide their own understanding. With careful attention to body language and tone of voice, the probable diagnosis should be conveyed. Ample space should be allowed for questions, processing, and emotional reactions. Patiently repeating information, permitting silence, gently soliciting comprehension and questions, and validating reactions provide such space. At the end of the conversation, salient points and management plans should be reviewed. Even if they are emotionally devastated, the parents should be comfortable that they and their child are in the hands of competent, empathetic, and caring individuals.

ANALYSIS AND DISCUSSION

When communicating about bad news with patients and families, one may consider what one would want for oneself in a similar situation. Would one want the information "delivered" like a pizza? Would one want it "broken" like an egg? "Delivering" bad news connotes a 1-way transaction in which a product or service is provided by one party to another. "Breaking" bad news implies that such a transaction is conducted bluntly, even forcibly. Few would want their child's new cancer diagnosis broken on their heads or mechanistically delivered. Most would want the diagnosis gently and empathetically communicated. We would want substantive, truthful content conveyed in a way that permitted 2-way conversation and established connection and trust between us and the frightening new world into which we had been thrust. We would want to feel invited to process the information, emote, ask questions, and react further. We would want to know what steps had been taken, what may be ahead, and who will be responsible. And, in all likelihood, we would want to feel cared for, confident that we have been heard, and comfortable that our values and preferences will be solicited, acknowledged, and incorporated into care management.

Some may want these elements in varying measures. Some may prefer detailed technical content imparted directly and dispassionately. Others may want empathy or support and may lack the emotional or cognitive capacity to process details at the time of acute diagnosis. How is the doctor to know? This is where practice becomes art.

Conveying unexpected or difficult information presents substantial barriers to effective communication. As with 4-year-old AR, the physician may have met a patient or family only briefly before needing to convey weighty information. Pre-existing relationships help establish connection and trust but may not be possible. Bad news conversations would ideally take place in a private, comfortable environment with minimal distractions and plentiful time. In busy EDs, and many other settings, such an environment is often unavailable. Supportive partners, friends, and other family members may not be available in the acute setting. Conversely, sometimes well-meaning family members or friends create dissonance and distraction. It may be hard for physicians to gauge prospectively what reactions will ensue from any given information. Assumptions about what constitutes "bad news" may prove misguided or perhaps biased. Virtually all parents would react strongly and adversely to a new Wilms tumor diagnosis in their child. A new malignancy in an 85-year-old patient with deep dementia, or a miscarriage in an unmarried medical student may bring relief alongside sadness. Even with unambiguously bad news, patients may sometimes feel relief when a diagnosis has finally been established for a chronic ailment that has been previously dismissed or misdiagnosed.

Indeed, physicians who converse with patients about unanticipated, difficult information must prepare for a wide spectrum of emotional reactions from patients and family members that may include intermingled confusion, guilt, grief, anger, shock, and relief. A physician's own emotions may further confound the process. Even veteran physicians may experience considerable stress. Many physicians may be anxious about their own expertise, or self-conscious about their gender, religion, ethnicity, age, experience, their ability to manage emotions, general communication skills, or their facility with the spoken language. Finally, physicians may bring unrecognized values and biases into the conversations, which may confound the communication. Such barriers come with a cost. Poorly communicated bad news may engender enduring tension, resentment, distrust, and depression.

Practical strategies have been offered to help practitioners approach communication about bad news. One well-known 6-step protocol utilizes the mnemonic **SPIKES**:

Setting and listening skills

Patient's perception

Invite patient to share information

Knowledge transmission

Explore emotions and empathize

Summarize and strategize

Another well-known mnemonic is **ABCDE**:

Advance preparation

Build a therapeutic environment/relationship

Communicate well

Deal with patient and family reactions

Encourage and validate emotions

Such mnemonics are only useful if they are organically internalized. One cannot apply them successfully if the actions are recalled sequentially, like the mnemonic used to recall the anatomical course of the seventh cranial nerve. Numerous internalized actions must be fluidly and sometimes simultaneously performed.

Self-consciousness must be relinquished to allow reflexive, real-time actions that stimulate spontaneity and improvisation. Such is human communication.

Nevertheless, understanding the core elements of effective communication around bad news is crucial. The choreography should be deliberate. Starting well requires advance preparation. Before entering the room, one should glean pertinent clinical information and ascertain whether any relevant language or cultural issues exist. Advance preparation may entail gathering a team to discuss the upcoming conversation, anticipate reactions and questions, formulate optimal responses, and confirm management plans. It may also involve finding a colleague—another physician, nurse, chaplain or social worker—who might join the conversation and support both the physician and the patient. It may involve finding space to converse in quiet privacy. Finally, advance preparation means attending to one's own emotional state. An oft-quoted "law" in Samuel Shem's *House of God* is "at a cardiac arrest, the first procedure is to take your own pulse." The same may be said of providers entering into difficult conversations with patients and family members. Taking a moment to recalibrate, reorient, and relax may enhance the entire process once in the room. So, too, will pausing briefly to remember the patient's name.

In the room, communication commences on 2 planes: verbal and nonverbal. Nonverbal elements may include reconfiguring the seating arrangement comfortably, permitting face-to-face conversation, maintaining eye contact, leaning forward attentively and presenting an empathetic yet professional demeanor. These may all strongly influence the outcome. Physical contact may comfort and establish connections with some patients, but may be uncomfortable and awkward for others. Many providers themselves may be uncomfortable with such gestures. For these physicians and patients, physical contact may undermine efforts to create a comfortable space. No mnemonic will help one negotiate this dynamic, which requires vigilance and sensitivity.

Effective verbal communication is a function of tone and content. Speaking softly attenuates the information's blunt impact. Introductions are, of course, mandatory, and particularly important when caretakers do not know the patient or family well before a conversation, which occurs commonly with ED physicians, radiologists, intensivists admitting acutely ill patients, and surgeons who must operate urgently. Proper introductions include presenting oneself and accompanying personnel, explaining everybody's roles, and directly engaging everybody in the room. Acknowledging the accompanying family members and friends validates their importance and establishes useful alliances. However, it remains important to be attentive to the room dynamics and provide the most latitude to the patient, surrogates, or both to assert themselves privately, if necessary.

After introductions, it is often worthwhile to probe the patient and family about their communication and understanding thus far. Gentle interrogation should also include asking how the patient is feeling, both physically and emotionally. The provider leading the conversation may also find it helpful to summarize his or her own understanding of the history and orient everybody in the room to the same approximate plane. However, this preliminary work may be counterproductive with highly anxious patients. If prolonged, patients may sense that something is wrong and construe anything that delays information transmission as dodging the issue.

The diagnosis must be revealed delicately. It is difficult to overestimate the force of the words and the longevity of their impact. Many physicians have experienced meeting patients whom they do not remember and who recount to them the exact words the physician spoke to them years previously about a jarring new diagnosis. Some providers prefer to convey diagnoses in an immediately straightforward way: "I am afraid I have some difficult news to discuss with you. I have looked at the ultrasound images and spoken with the radiologist. We are very concerned that AR may have cancer in his kidney." Others may prefer a more gradual approach, proceeding step-wise toward more blunt language depending on the understanding imparted at each level: "I have reviewed the images and reports with the radiologist, and it looks like what we are feeling may be related to AR's kidney" may then be followed by, "It looks like there may be a mass" followed by, "Well, it looks like a tumor" and then, "I am afraid it might be cancer" and then, "It seems probable that this is cancer...."

Neither approach is necessarily right or wrong. Utilizing the gradual approach may seem gentler, but it may require the patient or family to work harder to understand the information. It may force them to compel the reticent physician to disclose the information: "What are you saying, doctor; what are you telling us?" It may increase their anxieties and generate tension. Conveying the news more immediately may engender stronger immediate reactions or bring the conversation temporarily to an abrupt halt. On the other hand, once the immediate emotional wave passes, communication may proceed more smoothly, with the patient confident that they are being dealt with honestly. Ultimately, success depends as much on empathy and sensitivity as on words.

Once the diagnosis is imparted, many considerations and questions follow. Along the way, stumbling blocks and opportunities exist either to undermine or enhance the communication process. Technical jargon may impede effective information transfer and distance the physician from the patient. Silent periods seem awkward, but they may allow patients and families space to process information and regain composure. Physicians who are comfortable with silence may find it enhances difficult conversations immeasurably. Mistakes, poor word choices, unintentionally insensitive comments, and misstatements of fact sometimes occur, but earnest acknowledgment, apologies, and rephrasing may strengthen rapport. Another stumbling block is when one does not know the answer to a patient's question. For many young and veteran physicians, admitting that they don't know is as uncomfortable as prolonged silence. Honestly admitting the limits of one's expertise is not a failing, particularly if one offers guidance to the patient about how a question will be answered, whether it regards clinical care, financial matters, or psychosocial support. In all of these circumstances, having a clinical team partner in the room to support both the primary provider and the patient and family may prove invaluable.

Ending the conversation well is crucial. It includes reviewing important information and management plans, and reassuring patients about how unanswered concerns will be addressed. Ending well will help solidify the patient's confidence in their providers' competence and concern for their well-being.

Medical students have ample opportunities to observe mentors and other experienced practitioners engage in difficult patient conversations. Good, bad, or ugly, these are powerful learning moments. Numerous institutions offer innovative educational initiatives to enhance physicians' communication skills. Many such programs effectively utilize actors for simulation-based communication skills training. Unfortunately, it remains unclear whether enhanced skills acquired in such educational settings translate to better communication with actual patients.

Perhaps the best training comes from having received bad news oneself. Such experiences are likely as indelible for physician-patients as for others. Those who have not had had such experiences (and even those who have) may gain insight by talking to patients about their experiences and from reading published patient narratives.

Such is the world physicians introduce patients to when discussing bad news with them. We must proceed with care.

COMPREHENSION QUESTIONS

19.1 A 17-year-old with pelvic pain has returned from ultrasonographic imaging to your clinic. She is in the room with her mother. Ultrasonography shows a normal 6.5-week size intrauterine pregnancy. The ultrasound technologist has not said anything to them and the radiologist did not examine her directly. Barriers to effective communication about the pregnancy may include all except which of the following?

A. Physician anxiety

B. Lack of privacy

C. Incorrect assumptions about what news will be considered "bad"

D. Bringing a nurse or social worker into the room

19.2 A 35-year-old man has suddenly collapsed and is brought into the ED unconscious and intubated. Computed tomography shows a brainstem hemorrhage from a probable ateriovenous malformation (AVM). His pregnant wife and her mother are with him as you enter the ED room with the scan results. Stumbling blocks to effective communication about the information include which of the following?

A. Using technical jargon

B. Allowing silence to pass as you discuss the information

C. Expressing sadness over the situation

D. Introducing yourself to both his wife and her mother

19.3 A 67-year-old long-time smoker, a Vietnam war veteran whom you have not previously met, presents to your urgent care clinic with a highly probable lung cancer on chest radiography that the triage nurse ordered because of a chronic cough. Which of the following describes the model of counseling that most patients would prefer in this setting?

A. "Empathic professional" who communicates with sensitive words and tone of voice, keeps eye contact and shows empathy

B. "Distanced expert" who provides accurate and detailed information, has a confident and straightforward demeanor, but avoids showing or discussing emotions

C. "Emotionally burdened expert" who touches the patient and feels very sad

D. "Rough expert" who ignores the patient's reactions

ANSWERS

19.1 **D.** Bringing a nurse or social worker into the room may help you, the patient, and her mother through the communication process, which may include asking the mother to leave the room. The adolescent may or may not want to be alone when she is told. One's own anxiety about the conversation may make the process more awkward. In some instances, the information may be unwanted; however, in others, it may be embraced.

19.2 **A.** The clinical problem may be difficult to summarize in nonmedical language, but medical terminology may preclude the family's understanding. Silence may help the family process the information and their emotions. Authentic expressions of empathy are appropriate under the given circumstances. The way one introduces oneself prior to conveying the information may be remembered indefinitely.

19.3 **A.** Research has shown that most patients prefer providers who convey both empathy and professionalism. Some patients, although fewer in number, prefer those who are more detached, yet who provide the information straightforwardly. Patients are unlikely to prefer physicians who become exceedingly emotional or who are rough in their approach.

KEY POINTS

▶ Communicating with patients about bad news is a 2-way process between the caregiver and the patient and family.

▶ Effective communication about bad news entails several discreet elements that may be memorized but which must be approached fluidly and naturally within the actual conversations.

▶ Numerous verbal and nonverbal communication techniques may enhance the effectiveness of communication about bad news.

▶ Poor communication about bad news can have long-term negative consequences for patients and families.

REFERENCES

Baile WF, Buckman R, Lenzi R, Glober G, Beale EA, Kudelka AP. SPIKES-A six-step protocol for delivering bad news: application to the patient with cancer. *Oncologist.* 2000;5:302-311.

Brown SD, Callahan MJ, Browning DM, et al. Radiology trainees' comfort with difficult conversations and attitudes about error disclosure: effect of a communication skills workshop. *J Am Acad Coll Radiol.* 2014;11(8):781-787.

Curtis JR, Back AL, Ford DW, et al. Effect of communication skills training for residents and nurse practitioners on quality of communication with patients with serious illness: a randomized trial. *JAMA.* 2013;310:2271-2281.

Fallowfield L, Jenkins V. Communicating sad, bad, and difficult news in medicine. *Lancet.* 2004;363:312-319.

Martins RG, Carvalho IP. Breaking bad news: patients' preferences and health locus of control. *Pat Educ Counsel.* 2013;92:67-73.

Shaw J, Brown R, Heinrich P, Dunn S. Doctors' experience of stress during simulated bad news consultations. *Pat Educ Counsel.* 2013;93:203-208.

VandeKieft GK. Breaking bad news. *Am Fam Physician.* 2001;64:1975-1978.

A 25-year-old woman is admitted to the intensive care unit (ICU) with a diagnosis of sepsis due to acute pneumococcal pneumonia that requires intubation for respiratory support and intravenous (IV) norepinephrine infusion for blood pressure support. The ICU is completely full, and due to difficulty with ICU nurse staffing, the nurse assigned to your patient is also taking care of another patient in the ICU who had a stroke and is in a coma. You are very upset with the staffing due to the severity of your patient's illness, and write an order in the chart: "Please 1:1 nursing to this patient while on ventilator and pressure support."

▶ Is the staffing order on the chart appropriate?
▶ How should a physician handle staffing concerns?

A 78-year-old man was admitted for acute delirium thought to be due to hyponatremia. After fluid restriction, the patient's serum sodium level is corrected, and the attending physician discharges the patient home on hospital day 2. The nurse for the patient notes that the patient still has confusion and a new onset right arm weakness and calls the attending physician about her concerns. The physician states, "Listen, I've been doing this a lot longer than you have, and as the captain of the ship, I am in charge. Discharge the patient like I ordered."

▶ How should the nurse handle the discharge order?
▶ How should nurses deal with the "physician as captain of the ship" doctrine?

ANSWERS TO CASE 20:

Interdisciplinary Issues: Team Conflict

Summary: A 25-year-old woman is admitted to the ICU with pneumococcal pneumonia respiratory failure and sepsis requiring mechanical ventilator and norepinephrine pressure support. The nurse assignment is 1:2, so you write an order in the chart for "1:1 nursing staffing."

- **Is the staffing order on the chart appropriate:** No, because it connotes "arguing in the chart."

- **Physician handle staffing concerns:** Staffing concerns should be addressed with the supervisor or director of the area of concern. In this case, the nursing director of the ICU should be contacted and concerns discussed. If there is continued concern, then the physician may appeal to the physician director of the ICU.

Summary: A 78-year-old man is discharged home by the attending physician; however, the nurse caring for the patient is concerned about continued confusion and new onset right arm weakness. When the nurse contacts the physician, he instructs the nurse to discharge the patient as per his order, and states that, "As the captain of the ship, I am in charge."

- **How should the nurse handle the discharge order:** The nurse should go up her chain of command, which most likely will be the floor charge nurse. As an advocate for the patient, the nurse should continue to go up the chain of command to get appropriate care for the patient.

- **Dealing with the "physician as captain of the ship" doctrine:** Nurses and physicians are members of the same team in caring for patients and work collaboratively; however, nurses are not blind "followers" of physicians but have an independent duty to the patient. When a nurse makes the assessment that the patient is in jeopardy, that nurse has a duty to intervene for the patient. This usually means activating the nursing chain of command.

ANALYSIS

Objectives

1. Describe the appropriate method of addressing concerns about hospital or patient care staffing concerns.

2. Describe the principles of team-based health care.

3. Discuss the ways to handle patient management conflicts between members of the health care team.

Considerations

The situation in Scenario 1 is a common source of concern for physicians as well as nurses. In this situation, a 25-year-old woman is admitted to the ICU with acute and complex medical needs, including mechanical ventilation and norepinephrine infusion.

The physician caring for the patient is concerned about the appropriate level of nursing care because of the patient complexity and level of illness. However, because of the number of patients in the ICU, and due to the difficulty with ICU nurse staffing, the nurse assigned to the physician's patient is also taking care of another ICU patient with a stroke and coma. Rather than writing an order on the chart requesting "1:1 nursing to this patient while on ventilator and pressure support," the first avenue of appeal should be to dialogue with the charge nurse of nursing director of the ICU to explain the medical and nursing needs of the patient. The nursing director could very well be working on freeing up a nurse or recruiting a nurse from the back-up pool, and the current 1:2 staffing is only temporary. By contrast, if dialogue with the ICU nursing director is unfruitful, then an appeal to the medical director of the ICU may be a proper next step. Although these situations can be difficult and frustrating, the best approach involves being calm yet firm, factual rather than emotional, including an explanation of the patient's clinical care requirements, the sharing of national guidelines or hospital specific policies, working collaboratively, and avoiding arguing in the chart or in front of patients or their families.

The situation in Scenario 2 is also a common one, in which an assessment by the nurse is in conflict with that of the physician. In this case, an elderly man is discharged home by the attending physician after fluid restriction normalized his serum sodium level; however, the nurse caring for the patient is concerned about continued confusion and new onset right arm weakness. When dealing with these cases, it is helpful to consider the change in the physician–patient relationship over the last 30 years. Previously, under a paternalistic model, the patient sought the advice of the physician, and the physician determined what was best, and all members of the health care team reinforced that plan. In addition, historically, nurses were primarily hired by physicians in the past, reinforcing the nurse as "an agent" of the physician. However, the current physician–patient relationship has shifted to be a patient-centered model, and the health care members use a team-based approach. In this new model, each team model has an independent and primary role of advocating for the patient. Thus, the nurse has a duty to advocate for this patient despite the attending physician's orders. The nurse should do so in a respectful, private, and appropriate manner. The next step for the nurse would be to express the concerns to the charge nurse of the unit.

APPROACH TO:
Interdisciplinary Issues: Team Conflict

DEFINITIONS

PATERNALISM: Model in which the physician believes he or she knows what is best for the patient and steers the patient through medical decisions with little or no patient input.

TEAM-BASED HEALTH CARE: A model in which various members of the health care team, including the patient and family, work together to help the patient achieve his or her goals.

NURSING DUTY: A nurse's primary commitment is to the health, well-being, and safety of the patient.

CLINICAL APPROACH

Physician–nursing conflicts are fairly common due to the stressful high-stakes environment, differences in training and perspective, limitations of resources, and simple human personality issues such as ego, culture, and expectations. However, these conflicts impact the working environment negatively and can also compromise patient care. A national survey on patient safety provided to more than 600 institutions revealed that the biggest contributor to problems with patient safety was disruptive behavior, with 82% of respondents noting that disruptive behavior had been reported. Respondents who noted disruptive behavior replied that 46% of the time patient safety or patient care was affected. These observations have caused The Joint Commission to require a new leadership standard for these accredited institutions:

EP4: The hospital/organization has a code of conduct that defines acceptable and disruptive and inappropriate behaviors.

EP5: Leaders create and implement a process for managing disruptive and inappropriate behaviors.

Conflicts between doctors and nurses happen for a variety of reasons. One of the most significant reasons is different role expectations. The physician–nurse relationship has undergone tremendous changes, especially over the past 30 years. In the 1902 treatise, *The Household Physician*, McGregor-Robertson writes, "A nurse must begin her work with the idea firmly implanted in her mind that she is only the instrument by whom the doctor gets his instructions carried out; she occupies no independent position in the treatment of the sick person." Physicians who trained in "the past" may still have this "doctor is captain of the ship" philosophy. In the past, there was limited recognition of the nurse's ability to independently assess and advocate for the patient; today, however, the nurse is recognized as having the education, training, and status to be able to make independent assessments, and with advanced training, to be able to make management decisions (Table 20–1).

Nursing Duty

The nurse's primary duty is to the patient. There may be other allegiances, such as loyalty in the role of employee, whether those be to a hospital, a clinic, or other health care facility. Friendships or allegiances inevitably also exist with other health care professionals. Nevertheless, the nurse's first and foremost obligation is to advocate for the patient's health, well-being, and safety.

Table 20–1 • FACTORS OF CHANGE IN THE PHYSICIAN–NURSE RELATIONSHIP
Workplace context
Multidisciplinary relationships
Status and experience of the doctor and nurse
Patient and family expectations
Nursing training and education
Institutional norms and expectations
Professional norms and expectations

When the nurse is aware of questionable or unsafe practice, he or she should first discuss the issue with the person initiating the questionable practice. For instance, if a physician puts an order on the chart that may be detrimental (ie, ordering an antibiotic when the patient is allergic to that medication), then the first avenue should be to communicate with the physician. When such communication does not lead to resolution of the concern, then the nurse is obligated to report to the appropriate supervisor or administrator. This is sometimes called the nursing chain of command.

Physicians may have conflicts with nursing when there is lack of understanding about the nurse's independent ability to make assessments and independent duty to the patient. Instead of welcoming a "second pair of eyes," the physician may have the expectation that all orders will be carried out without question. The patient-centered, team-based health care model instead values every team member's perspectives and input. The physician is well equipped to be the team leader by virtue of the education and trainings he has received. The effective team leader would look for input from different viewpoints, keeping the best interest of the patient as the primary goal. In this team model, the physician leader values dissenting voices. In fact, each team member is held to the duty to raising the concern with firmness until there is a satisfactory resolution, not simply speaking the concern only once.

Staffing Issues

With the financial pressures on every health care institution, there is continued scrutiny of staffing ratios, necessitating practices to optimize staffing for both cost-containment and patient safety. Perhaps nowhere is this issue as acute as in nursing care in the hospital setting. However, hospitals that are overly frugal on staffing can promote nursing dissatisfaction and burn-out. A cross-sectional study in Pennsylvania showed that there was an increased risk of 30-day mortality with higher patient:nurse ratios and higher risk of nurse burn-out. This is a universal, worldwide issue that is not limited to the United States alone. In a study conducted in the United Kingdom and Canada in 2000 involving 303 hospitals, a total of 10,319 nurses were surveyed. There was a three-fold increased rate of perceived low quality of patient care and a five-fold increased job dissatisfaction and burn-out in hospitals of low staffing and support as compared with those with high staffing.

Clearly, there is validity to the position that some health care facilities are purposely understaffing their facilities for cost-containment. Adequate staffing levels have been shown to reduce medication errors, improve patient satisfaction, decrease mortality, and decrease patient complications. Nevertheless, sometimes the staffing issue is a dynamic one that cannot be predicted or scheduled. An ideal staffing model allocates to the acuity and number of patients, as well as those ancillary personnel, such as licensed or unlicensed assistive personnel, and the skills and training of nurses. This is a collaborative model that simultaneously reviews the needs of the entire unit or hospital, as well as the individual patient, and the resources available.

When the physician is unhappy with the staffing ratio, the appropriate next step to take is to discuss the issue with the nurse manager of the unit. This should be in private, nonemotional, and should deal with the factual issues of the case. Having information such as recommendations from national nursing associations on the recommended staffing for various acuity levels can be helpful. Behaviors that are counterproductive include public rants of frustration, threats, blaming or inflammatory comments on the chart, or unwarranted discussions with the patient or family about these concerns.

At times, the staffing issue may be temporary. For instance, if a large number of patients suddenly are admitted, no amount of scheduling or planning can anticipate and provide "perfect staffing." In these cases, the nursing director and nursing team should be working on a solution, reviewing personnel resources and individual patient needs. For instance, in the first scenario involving the patient with sepsis and respiratory failure, the nursing director may be working on calling in a nurse from home to help to relieve the shortage issue. In that case, the physician's order on the chart specifying "1:1 nursing" is unnecessary and inflammatory. When the immediate nursing director is unable to resolve the issue, then the physician may need to appeal to the physician director or chief nursing officer.

Communication Issues

Clinical communication that is effective should be direct, clear, and respectful. Furthermore, effective communication encourages input from all team members, and there is an openness to new information or new ideas. One of the key areas for physicians to focus on is listening skills. The physician should not view inquiry as challenges to his or her expertise or proficiency, but instead view them as protective. In fact, the leader who is willing to admit that the initial course of action may not have been best, or who is willing to consider new information, is typically highly admired and esteemed. When both parties appreciate a different point of view, patient care becomes more fluid and well-rounded, and just like in any working relationship, a foundation of mutual respect between physician and nurse goes a long way.

Sometimes prior experiences, training, or cultural exposure may impact the expectations of the health care member or their communication approach. For instance, physicians or nurses who may be foreign-educated may have biases or unspoken preconceptions that interfere with bidirectional communication. Multidisciplinary weekly conferences allowing each member of the team to receive the input and contribution from others may lead to positive changes.

On some occasions, communication is rocky because staff are unsure how to address or resolve an issue. In these cases, it is helpful to consider the key aspects of timing, setting, people involved, and wording. Timing of a discussion may be variable depending on the urgency of the issue. For example, a questioned medication order may require immediate attention, while other issues may be minor and can wait until both parties are free from pressing tasks. However, conflict resolution should not be delayed for days/weeks, especially if it pertains to direct patient care. Next, it is important to decide what the proper setting is, such as whether a discussion should take place at the nurses' station or in private, etc. Third, involving the appropriate people can help avoid confusion and frustration. As in the case of the staffing issue, knowing the right person to talk to (nursing director) contributed to quicker, more direct problem solving. Lastly, being aware of word choices, tone of voice, and one's own emotions and biases before attempting to resolve an issue helps ensure the conveyed message is the same as the intended message. Taking a moment to ask, "Is this the right time, the right place, and the right person, and the right wording to address this issue?" can go a long way to lead to more effective communication and conflict resolution.

Barriers to good communication often occur because the parties are unwilling to admit that there is an issue. It is easier to ignore problems than confront them, a fact that discourages nurses from asking physicians for the rationale for questionable orders or try to understand possible discrepancies in management. It also discourages physicians from raising concerns about staffing issues even when patient care may be jeopardized, because it is "easier to go with the flow" rather than "fight the tide." In summary, the institution must put into place strategies that enhance and reward physician–nurse communication, using measurable outcomes such as communication competency, surveys on satisfaction on communication among the health care team, and team-based communication.

COMPREHENSION QUESTIONS

20.1 A 22-year-old woman at term gestation is admitted to the hospital in labor. The nurse assesses the fetal heart rate pattern as normal and reassuring. The obstetrician comes in to evaluate the patient and notes that the fetal heart rate pattern to his evaluation shows repetitive late decelerations and is alarming. He bellows to the nurse in front of the patient, "How can you be so incompetent so as not to see these late decelerations? Get this patient ready for a cesarean delivery immediately. And if there is any oxygen compromise to the baby or brain damage, I will hold you personally responsible!"
How should the labor and delivery nurse handle the situation?

A. Do not say anything and get the patient ready for cesarean delivery because the physician would likely not be receptive anyway.

B. Challenge the physician regarding the fetal heart rate tracing and ask that another physician review the tracing.

C. Apologize to the patient and family for the outburst and ask to speak to the physician in private.

D. Report the incident immediately to the charge nurse and request to never be assigned to this physician's patient.

20.2 Your community hospital is examining nursing staffing ratios in the general medical and surgical ward. In-patient hospital payments have been decreasing and expenses have been increasing, putting tremendous pressure on hospital staffing. Which of the following is the most accurate statement that you can give for higher nurse:patient staffing?

A. Higher nurse:patient staffing has been shown to improve medication errors but has not impacted 30-day mortality rates.

B. Higher nurse:patient staffing leads to higher nursing satisfaction but does not impact patient satisfaction.

C. Higher nurse:patient staffing leads to less medical errors and decreased patient length of stay but increases cost.

D. Higher nurse:patient staffing leads to less decubitus ulcers, less medication errors, but increases in 30-day mortality risk.

ANSWERS

20.1 **C.** During times of disruptive outbursts, the nurse's first priority should be to the patient and her family. Understandably, this nurse will feel personally attacked and possibly humiliated. The natural reaction will be to either strike back in retaliation or have an emotional reaction, whether that be in the form of anger, fear, or inadequacy. However, rather than reacting, the nurse must consider the devastating effect the physician's behavior is having on the patient, and the nurse must get the doctor to a private location away from the patient immediately. The incident does need to be reported to the charge nurse, but doing so is a secondary priority.

20.2 **C.** Higher nurse:patient staffing has been shown to improve medication errors, lower 30-day mortality rates, achieve higher nursing satisfaction, increase patient satisfaction, and decrease patient length of stay; however, it does increase cost. There also have been fewer decubitus ulcers associated with higher nursing ratios.

KEY POINTS

► The appropriate method of addressing concerns about hospital or patient care staffing is initially with the nursing director of the unit, in private, and in an objective manner.

► Team-based health care means putting the patient takes priority and all the input from all members of the team must be valued.

► Nurses have the duty to make independent assessments of the patient and act as advocates of the patient. They are also obligated to question treatment that may be detrimental to the patient.

► Patient management conflicts between members of the health care team are best handled in private rather than in front of patients, with openness and respect, and with the understanding that differences of opinion are encouraged.

REFERENCES

Aiken LH, Clarke SP, Sloane DM, Sochalski J, Silber JH. Hospital nurse staffing and patient mortality, nurse burnout and job dissatisfaction. *JAMA*. 2002;288:1987-1993.

Kaba R, Sooriakumaran P. The evolution of the doctor-patient relationship. *Int J Surg*. 2007;5:57-65.

Fagin L, Garelick A. The doctor-nurse relationship. *Adv Psych Treat*. 2004;10:227-286.

Johnson C. Bad blood: doctor-nurse behavior problems impact patient care. *Physican Exec*. 2009;35:6-11.

Rosenstein Ah, O'Daniel M. Disruptive behavior and clinical outcomes: perceptions of nurses and physicians. *Am J Nurs*. 2005;105:54-64.

Stecker M, Epstein N, Stecker MM. Analysis of inter-provider conflicts among healthcare providers. *Surg Neurol Int Spine*. 2013;4:375-380.

The Joint Commission. Behaviors that undermine a culture of safety. *The Joint Commission*. 2008;40-43.

A 74-year-old man presents to the emergency department (ED) complaining of weakness and dizziness. He is having trouble maintaining consciousness. The patient's electrocardiogram (ECG) reveals third-degree heart block with a heart rate of 34 beats/minute and a blood pressure reading of 90/55 mm Hg. The patient's cardiac instability calls for immediate intervention. As the attending physician and senior resident are attempting to place a transvenous pacemaker, the attending physician orders the medical student on the team to consult the critical care unit (CCU) service. The medical student proceeds to the nearest telephone. CCU fellow: "CCU." Student: "Uh, hi, I'm a student in the ED. We have a patient down here with third-degree heart block. They're placing a transvenous pacemaker right now." CCU fellow: "I'm extremely busy right now. What do you need?" Student: "Well, I'm supposed to call you, right?" The CCU fellow sighs and hangs up the phone and arrives in the ED 45 minutes after hanging up. He approaches the team workstation and yells angrily, "You had a student consult me again!"

▶ How would you characterize the consultation?
▶ How does the consultant's behavior affect the patient?

ANSWERS TO CASE 21:
Difficult Consultation

Summary: An elderly patient in the ED is unstable with third-degree heart block. The attending physician requests that the medical student on the team places a CCU consultation. The student did not use the proper consultation technique while on the phone with the CCU fellow. The CCU fellow inappropriately hung up on the student. He arrives in the ED 45 minutes later and yells at the health care team.

- **How would you characterize the consultation?** This was a difficult consultation that was disruptive.

- **How does the consultant's behavior affect the patient?** The consultant's behavior puts the patient's health and well-being at risk and could have lead to the patient losing trust in the health care professionals.

ANALYSIS

Objectives

1. Understand what needs to be taken into consideration when requesting physician consultation.

2. Describe the 5 Cs model for a proper physician consultation.

3. Identify ways in which to deal with a difficult or disruptive physician.

Considerations

Unfortunately, the consultation interaction between the medical student and the CCU fellow did not go well and can best be characterized as difficult. As a result of this interaction, the patient is not receiving appropriate care, the medical student is left demoralized, and the fellow is angry. Interpersonal skills and effective communication between providers are often overlooked in the stressful environment of the medical setting. Providers may have different cultural backgrounds, training experience, and personality differences, which only add to the chaos in communicating patient information. The Accreditation Council for Graduate Medical Education formally recognizes interpersonal skills as a required core competency for residents in all fields. Proper communication of medical information requires effective interpersonal skills. Suboptimal communication of patient information threatens both patient and medical staff safety. The Joint Commission on Accreditation of Healthcare Organizations has shown that communication failure was the major cause of studied preventable sentinel events that led to patient harm between 2004 and 2012. Patients view physicians as calm, collected, confident, compassionate, respectful, mature, and strong individuals. It is expected that medical providers overcome personal distractions and stress when caring for others. Failure to maintain these standards threatens patient care and safety. When a provider exhibits disruptive emotion in the health care setting, he or she also places stress on the entire team. Moreover, one provider's emotional instability can affect more than just a single patient.

APPROACH TO:
The Medical Consultation

Medical resource and specialty expansion makes physician consultation a daily activity for most providers. It has been shown that consultations are performed on up to 40% of patients presenting to the ED. The modernization of medicine itself further complicates the effective communication of medical information. When does one acquire the skills to effectively consult another provider? For the most part, these critical skills are developed through observation during one's undergraduate medical education and further honed during residency training.

The consultation process requires attention to skill, attitude, and behavior. The approach begins with a proper introduction and identification of all involved parties. This is not only essential for documentation, but it exemplifies respect and cooperation. The reason for consultation should not be excluded under the assumption that the consultant's experience eliminates the need for step-by-step case description; this information can always be communicated in a manner that is not condescending when the objective to attain a consultation, not a service, is kept in mind. The urgency of the consultation must be made clear early in the process, allowing the consultant to better organize their approach to the case. The case should be formally presented and include all pertinent information, as if the consultant knows nothing about the patient. An organized consultation report should follow the conversation, as anyone can always refer back to documentation. Lastly, preparation is the key. Be prepared to provide any of the patient's information and answer questions prior to calling in the consultation. All learners should be prepared to ask questions of their team prior to engaging in the consultative process if any uncertainty as to the purpose of the consult is present.

Multiple communication models have been developed and adapted to the medical profession to bridge gaps in communication during hand-offs and consultation requests. Two of the most commonly used techniques are the 5Cs and the situation, background, assessment, and recommendation (SBAR) technique, which was originally developed by the US military (Table 21–1). Its use became widespread in the health care industry in the 1990s. Similarly, the 5Cs model has been shown to significantly improve the quality of communication during consultation (Table 21–2). Both are appropriate approaches to physician consultation.

Application of the 5Cs Model
CCU fellow: "CCU."

5Cs Student (**Contact**): "Hello, my name is John Doe. I am a third-year medical student on service in the ED. My supervising attending is Dr Jane Smith. With whom am I speaking?"

CCU fellow: "This is Dr Davis; I'm the CCU fellow on service. I'm extremely busy right now. What do you need?"

5Cs Student (**Communicate**): "We have a 74-year-old man with symptomatic bradycardia who was brought to the ED complaining of weakness and dizziness.

Table 21–1 • SBAR MODEL FOR PHYSICIAN CONSULTATION

Situation	Requires all parties identify themselves, establish the relationship, and provide a brief summary of the issue to be addressed	• Identification of the speaker and his or her role on the team • Identification of supervising attending • Identification of consulting physician • Identification of the patient, including name, location, and medical record number • Recitation or brief description of the patient's medical issue necessitating consultation
Background	Provides context for the consultation	• Identification of any relevant patient history including past medical/surgical history
Assessment	Provides further details and reveals the speaker's understanding of the patient's status	• Identification of pertinent physical examination findings, including any abnormalities in vital signs • Identification of the provider's clinical impression (eg, that the patient is in heart failure) and severity of that condition (eg, decompensating, placed on Biphasic positive airway pressure [BiPAP]) • Identification of relevant laboratory and radiographic findings supporting the clinical impression • Explanation of actions being taken to stabilize or treat the patient
Recommendation	Provides the listener with a summary of the goals of consultation	• Identification of specific suggestions or questions regarding the further evaluation and treatment (eg, additional laboratory tests, medications to be started) • Explanation of what action is required from the consulting physician (eg, to come and evaluate patient, provide telephone recommendations or clinic follow-up)

Table 21–2 • THE 5Cs MODEL FOR PHYSICIAN CONSULTATION

Contact	Requires introduction of all parties and establishes the relationship	• Identification of the speaker • Identification of supervising attending • Identification of consulting physician
Communicate	Present the patient's case and all relevant information including location within the hospital, patient history, physical examination findings, as well as any relevant laboratory and radiographic information	• The story should be accurate and concise • Speak clearly
Core Question	Prepare a question for the consultant	• This specifies the need for consultation • Should include a consultation timeframe
Collaboration	The discussion should lead to a planned course of action	• This incorporates the consultant's recommendations • Discuss any alteration in patient management and testing
Closing the Loop	Both parties should agree with the management plan	• Repeat the patient management plan • Agree to communicate changes in the patient's status • Thank the consultant

He is located in Shock room 3. He is unstable as he is having difficulty maintaining consciousness. Telemetry and ECG demonstrates third-degree heart block. He was given atropine and transcutaneous pacing was attempted by emergency medical services prior to arrival without electrical or mechanical capture. His heart rate is currently 34 beats/minute and his blood pressure is 90/55 mm Hg. Dr Smith and her resident, Dr Mark, are currently intubating the patient and setting up to place a transvenous pacemaker."

CCU fellow: "Well, what exactly do you need from me?"

5Cs Student (**Core question**): "Based on the information I provided over the phone, do you have any recommendations or instructions such as additional laboratory or radiographic testing or medication or equipment orders that I may pass on to the team to facilitate your consultation? Also, if you could please let me know when the team should expect you to arrive, we can make sure to have everything you need either already completed or at the patient's bedside."

CCU fellow: "Thank you. I'll be available to evaluate the patient within 20 minutes. In the meantime, please proceed with transvenous pacemaker placement. I'd like cardiac enzymes, a BMP (basic metabolic panel) and BNP (brain natriuretic peptide) and a chest radiograph ready for me when I arrive if they have not already been ordered."

5Cs Student (**Collaboration and Closing the loop**): "Okay, we will see you here in the ED in 20 minutes. I will check to see if cardiac enzymes, a BMP, a BNP, and a chest radiograph have been ordered. If not, I will notify Dr Smith of your request for laboratory studies and imaging. I will also notify Dr Smith of your recommendation to continue with the transvenous pacemaker placement. We will alert you immediately with any change in patient status. Thank you, Dr Davis."

APPROACH TO:
The Disruptive Physician

What is a disruptive physician? The American Medical Association's *Code of Medical Ethics* defines disruptive physician behavior as "personal conduct, whether verbal or physical, that negatively affects or that potentially may negatively affect patient care." Verbal behaviors include, but are not limited to, yelling and profanity.

Medical students are commonly abused by disruptive physicians. Many students are unwilling to report such behavior due to their fear of retaliation. Student abuse has consequences extending beyond the student's embarrassment, depression, and guilt. Physicians serve as role models for students and provide examples of appropriate or inappropriate behavior as learners advance through their career.

Disruptive physicians breach their duties and violate codes of medical ethics and professionalism. Medicine is a team effort, and medical students are members of the team. As stated in the ethics manual of the American College of Physicians, "Physicians share their commitment to care for ill persons with a broad team of health professionals. The team's ability to care effectively for the patient depends on the ability of individual persons to treat each other with integrity, honesty, and respect." They go on to say that particular attention should be paid to relationships with inherent power imbalances due to the potential for abuse. Most institutions have developed protocols aimed to manage disruptive physician behavior. Reporters should be reassured not to fear retaliation, because these protocols are instrumental in protecting patient and staff safety and staff wellness.

The CCU fellow is an example of a disruptive physician. Even with the medical student's poor initial consultation technique, it was unethical and abusive to hang up on the student. If the fellow was actively engaged in caring for another patient at the time of the consultation call, then it would have been acceptable for him to be brief and direct with the student in providing his recommendations. However, there is often a fine line between being direct and to the point when communicating with medical personnel, patients, or family members and being perceived as short or rude. Such perceptions can be colored based on cultural backgrounds and training norms but a wise practitioner will always air on the side of being polite and professional. In addition, by hanging up on the student, the fellow failed to gather the details of the patient's case in order to prepare for the encounter and determine patient priority. Personal frustrations, even when justified, cannot be permitted to interfere with the quality of patient care. Furthermore, yelling is disruptive and inappropriate in any medical setting. The fellow's overall demeanor was not conducive to a multidisciplinary collaboration in medicine.

Disruptive behavior results in a breakdown of effective communication and may stem from a physician's significant emotional or physical stress, including exhaustion or illness. Repeat episodes of disruptive behavior are often a hallmark of drug or alcohol abuse and represent opportunities to intervene and assist the impaired provider and protect the public.

In the case above, the fellow's actions should be reported to the attending ED physician. The attending physician can then address the fellow's behavior at such a time as not to compromise patient care. Patient care must take priority to addressing lapses in medical ethics and professionalism. In other words, it would be inappropriate for the attending physician to chastise the fellow for his treatment of the medical student immediately upon arriving at the patient's bedside. However, once the patient is stabilized, the attending physician should privately speak to the fellow to address the lapse, with one goal being an apology to the student. A private conversation will also allow the fellow an opportunity to express his frustration at the poor quality of the initial consultation by the student and give the fellow and the attending physician an opportunity to teach the student more effective consultation techniques.

If the matter is not satisfactorily resolved or represents a pattern of behavior by the consultant, the attending ED physician should report the fellow's behavior to the cardiology department because remediation may be necessary. If the fellow's supervisors fail to curb his disruptive behavior, then the fellow's actions should be brought to the attention of hospital administrators.

COMPREHENSION QUESTIONS

21.1 Which of the 5Cs is missing out of the following telephone consultation?

CCU fellow: "CCU."

Student: "Hello, my name is John Doe. I am a third-year medical student on service in the ED. My supervising attending is Dr Jane Smith. May I ask whom I have reached?"

CCU fellow: "This is Dr Davis; I'm the CCU fellow on service. I'm extremely busy right now. What do you need?"

Student: "We have a 74-year-old man with symptomatic bradycardia who was brought to the ED complaining of weakness and dizziness. He is located in CCU room 3. He is unstable as he is having difficulty maintaining consciousness. Telemetry and the ECG demonstrate third-degree heart block. He was given atropine and transcutaneous pacing was attempted by emergency medical services prior to arrival without electrical or mechanical capture. His heart rate is currently 34 beats/minute and his blood pressure is 90/55 mm Hg. Dr Smith and her resident, Dr Mark, are currently intubating the patient and setting up to place a transvenous pacemaker."

CCU fellow: "Well, what exactly do you need from me?"

Student: "I was told to contact you for consultation for this patient. When will you be available for consultation?"

CCU fellow: "I'll be available to evaluate the patient within 20 minutes. Please proceed with transvenous pacemaker placement. I'd like cardiac enzymes, a BMP and BNP, and a chest radiograph ready for me when I arrive."

5 C's Student "Okay, we will see you here in the ED in 20 minutes. We will alert you immediately with any change in patient status. Thank you, Dr Davis."

A. Communicate

B. Closing the loop

C. Contact

D. Core question

E. Collaboration

21.2 When might it be appropriate to report a disruptive physician's behavior to his or her superior or supervisor rather than addressed directly with the physician?

A. When the medical students are present and the disruptive physician is providing a poor role model for the students

B. When there is a suspicion of drug or alcohol abuse on the part of the disruptive physician

C. When the patient's health or well-being is at risk

D. When the morale of the team is negatively impacted

ANSWERS

21.1 **B.** The student should have included all components, including repeating the patient's management plan, agreeing to communicate changes in the patient's status, and thanking the consultant. The portion the student omitted was repeating the management plan: "I will check to see if cardiac enzymes, a BMP, a BNP, and chest radiograph have been ordered. If not, I will notify Dr Smith of your request for laboratory studies and imaging. I will also notify Dr Smith of your recommendation to continue with the transvenous pacemaker placement."

21.2 **B.** If the patient's well-being is not jeopardized and there is time to safely obtain a consultation, it may be appropriate to address concerns about the physician's disruptive behavior with the physician's supervisor or superior where there is concern for drug or alcohol abuse. When the medical students are witnessing unprofessional behavior, the patient's health is at risk, or the morale of the team is negatively impacted, the disruptive physician's behavior should be immediately addressed with the physician. If no satisfactory response is obtained, then the physician's supervisor should be notified.

KEY POINTS

▶ Physicians who display disruptive behaviors (eg, verbal or physical abuse) not only violate the codes of medical ethics but erode team morale, undermine the delivery of quality medical care, and threaten both patient and staff safety.

▶ Strong interpersonal communication skills are essential to the practice of medicine.

▶ Interpersonal communication skills are influenced by a physician's personality and culture as well as their training environment and past experiences. Medical providers display a wide range of communication styles, some of which may conflict, particularly in the context of busy environments or otherwise stressful situations.

▶ 5Cs and SBAR are two models designed to ensure consistent, efficient, and professional communication while minimizing conflicts or misunderstandings between medical providers.

REFERENCES

American Medical Association (AMA). *E.9.045 Code of Medical Ethics: Current Opinions with Annotations: 2006-2007.* Chicago, IL: AMA; 2006.

Council on Ethical and Judicial Affairs (CEJA) American Medical Association. "Physicians with disruptive behavior." Report 106. June 2000. https://com-psychiatry-pep.sites.medinfo.ufl.edu/files/2014/06/AMA-Physicians-and-Disruptive-Behavior-Policy.pdf. Accessed September 22, 2014.

Kessler C, Chan T, Loeb JM, Malka ST. I'm clear, you're clear, we're all clear: improving consultation communication skills in undergraduate medical education. *Acad Med.* 2013;88:753-758.

Kessler C, Kalapurayil, P, Yudkowsky R, Schwartz A. Validity evidence for a new checklist evaluating consultations, the 5Cs model. *Acad Med.* 2012;87:1408-1412.

Mueller P, Snyder L. Dealing with the "disruptive" physician colleague. Medscape Multispecialy Education Online. Published 2009. http://www.acponline.org/running_practice/ethics/case_studies/disruptive.pdf. Accessed February, 2014.

Sibert L, Lachkar A, Grise P, et al. Communication between consultants and referring physicians: a qualitative study to define learning and assessment objectives in a specialty residency program. *Teach Learn Med.* 2002;14:15-19.34.

The Joint Commission. Sentinel event data: root causes by event type, 2004-2012. http://www.jointcommission.org/assets/1/18/Root_Causes_Event_Type_04_4Q2012.pdf. Accessed February 22, 2014.

A 34-year-old woman on the inpatient floor is admitted for an infected wound on her right foot. The patient has a past medical history of type 2 diabetes mellitus. She has had overnight temperature spikes to 101°F, but she has otherwise been asymptomatic with stable vital signs. Her blood cultures and wound culture are still pending. Late last night she was placed on empiric intravenous (IV) antibiotics for her wound. At admission, the medical student, the surgery intern, and the attending physician examined her. Aside from her infected wound, her entire physical examination was unremarkable. Today, the medical student's examination reveals a harsh 3/6 holosystolic murmur at the cardiac apex, along with expansion of the wound's surrounding erythema. On rounds, the surgery intern presented the patient's case, accurately describing the wound changes, but described the cardiac examination as "regular rate and rhythm, with no murmurs." The medical student knows that the intern arrived late this morning and rushed through his examination without a stethoscope.

▶ What has the surgical intern done wrong?
▶ What is the next step for the surgical intern?
▶ What is the next step for the medical student?

ANSWERS TO CASE 22:

Clinical Dishonesty

Summary: A 34-year-old woman presents to inpatient service with a lower extremity wound infection. The following morning, the medical student notes a new cardiac murmur and increased erythema surrounding the wound. During rounds, the surgical intern falsifies his physical examination by reporting a normal cardiac examination. The medical student knows that the surgery intern did not fully examine the patient as he arrived late and was without a stethoscope.

- **What has the surgical intern done wrong?** He has shown clinical dishonesty.

- **What is the next step for the surgical intern?** The trainee should assume responsibility for the clinical dishonesty and inform the team of the error in the physical examination.

- **What is the next step for the medical student?** The student has a responsibility to address the issue by performing an accurate cardiac examination.

ANALYSIS

Objectives

1. Understand what defines dishonesty and how it may affect patients in a clinical setting.

2. Understand the appropriate response when encountering a dishonest team member.

Considerations

The surgical intern came unprepared to their clinical duties, which resulted in the inadequate examination of a patient. Compounding matters, the intern falsified his cardiac examination findings during rounds, which painted an incorrect picture of the patient's clinical status and risked the team missing the diagnosis of bacterial endocarditis. As uncomfortable as it may be to confront a superior, the medical student must advocate for the patient. As a patient advocate and team member, the student must reveal the true physical examination findings and, if the intern is not forthcoming in admitting that he did not listen to the patient's chest, the student should report the intern for a breach in medical ethics and clinical dishonesty.

APPROACH TO:

Clinical Dishonesty

The road to medical school is long and arduous, and, to stay competitive for a coveted spot, students may feel compelled to cheat, lie, or both to improve their chances at admission. Cheating and acts of personal and professional dishonesty often continue throughout undergraduate medical education as the curriculum intensifies and competition for the residency selection process ensues. Residency, fellowship, and daily medical practice can also be tainted by ethical lapses and clinical dishonesty. Indeed, this behavior notoriously resurfaces when medical awards and positions or promotions are at stake.

Studies have shown that anywhere between 27% and 58% of medical students have cheated during medical school. It is not a surprise that students who cheat on examinations more often exhibit clinical dishonesty while completing their clinical clerkships when it is more difficult to prove lying or cheating than on a multiple-choice/computer-based test. The fact that there are more seniors than freshman who cheat in medical school contributes to the prevalence of dishonesty in a clinical setting, because students are exposed to this throughout the latter half of medical school.

Unsurprisingly, students who engage in clinical dishonesty to "survive" the rigors of medical school are more likely to face disciplinary action by state medical boards throughout their careers as their clinical dishonesty and unprofessional behavior is uncovered by coworkers and peers. In this regard, unprofessional behavior was defined as poor reliability and responsibility (clinical dishonesty), lack of self-improvement and adaptability, and poor initiative and motivation.

Testimony has shown that the false reporting of physical findings on an examination is commonplace for many students and practicing physicians. The pressure to see and juggle more patients within strict time limits, the increasing administrative burdens and documentation requirements, the odd work hours, and infrequent encounters with abnormal physical findings make it easy to find blank or copied and pasted reports within the physical examination portion of the medical record. These pressures also enable the practitioner to justify cutting corners. In essence, the busy physician abdicates his or her responsibility and convinces himself or herself that he or she is merely doing the "best I can in an otherwise dysfunctional system."

Hospital-based practitioners who see the same patients on a daily basis for many days in a row also do not expect or anticipate abrupt changes in the patient's physical examination and, as a result, may be particularly vulnerable. This mental anchoring often makes it easy for a practitioner to miss a critical finding by forgoing the necessary daily physical examination.

It has been suggested that the "herd mentality" in the medical environment enables students and practitioners to follow this trend as we learn from one another through observation. Copying progress notes and history and physical examination findings between students and residents without an independent examination and verification exemplifies the same dishonest principles as falsifying physical examination findings. Busy practitioners may find these practices convenient and even attempt to justify their use, but they are never in the patient's best interests and may be detrimental to a patient's well-being.

One may ask: Where does the lying stop? In the context of professional or academic misconduct, dishonesty takes many forms, including, but not limited to, fraud or deceit, cheating, plagiarism, false representation, and alteration of medical records. In fact, becoming complicit in someone else's deceit, even if it is only remaining silent, is also a form of dishonesty. The intern's false report of the patient's cardiac examination is an example of clinical dishonesty. Incomplete examination of the patient puts the patient at risk, especially if the patient has underlying medical problems. It is the medical student's responsibility to ensure the well-being of the patient by disclosing the patient's new examination finding. If the attending is not already aware, then the student should privately notify the attending physician of the resident's dishonesty.

It is both unethical and unprofessional for a health care professional to hide the dishonesty of another health care professional, especially if it endangers patient's well-being. The student could be held liable to the same degree as the intern if he chooses to say or do nothing. As stated in the American Medical Association's *Principles of Medical Ethics*, "A physician shall deal honestly with patients and colleagues, and strive to expose those physicians deficient in character or competence, or who engage in fraud or deception."

Failure to report ethical breaches by superiors is often predicated on fear of retaliation. For medical students, this fear typically manifests as fear of poor clinical evaluations or recommendations that adversely impact the grade that they will receive for their clerkship, which potentially impacts their class ranking and overall competitiveness for the residency selection process. For resident physicians (when the lapse is on the attending physician's part), this fear manifests itself as concern for poor evaluations, failure to secure a fellowship recommendation, or future employment. Most medical schools and health care agencies have specific policies in place designed to protect the so-called whistle-blower from retaliatory practices and to uphold the public's faith in the medical profession.

Failure to properly police and punish those in our ranks who do not safeguard the public's health, safety, and trust is one of the factors that resulted in the marked increase in medical malpractice law suits and governmental regulation of the health care industry. The right to practice medicine and the right to learn medicine is a privilege. There is no room for malpractice in the form of clinical dishonesty, gross negligence, or malfeasance. Practitioners should not stand idly by and say nothing when others engage in such behavior. It is our duty to investigate and, whenever possible, correct all unprofessional behaviors that we encounter during our medical practice. Repeat offenders should face disciplinary action, which may include expulsion from school or residency, or license revocation or suspension.

COMPREHENSION QUESTIONS

22.1 What is the next best step for the surgical intern after presenting the falsified cardiac examination findings to the team on rounds?

A. Examine the patient after rounds.

B. Tell the medical student to examine the patient after rounds.

C. Ask the medical student if the patient had a normal cardiac examination.

D. Admit to the team that he has made a mistake because he forgot his stethoscope.

E. Ask to borrow the medical student's stethoscope and examine the patient in front of the team.

22.2 What is the medical student's best next step after hearing the surgical intern's cardiac examination report during rounds?

A. Confront the surgical intern to say that he noticed that he did not bring his stethoscope.

B. Report the intern's clinical dishonesty to his program director and hospital administration.

C. Speak out to the team explaining that you heard a murmur on cardiac examination and point out that the intern does not even have a stethoscope.

D. Ignore the situation because it is none of the medical student's business.

E. Speak out and present the abnormal cardiac examination findings.

22.3 What is the next best step for the attending physician as he notices a cardiac murmur upon his own examination of the patient?

A. Immediately contact the state medical board to report the intern's clinical dishonesty.

B. Immediately contact the intern's residency program director without discussing the matter with the intern.

C. Ask the intern where their stethoscope is and if he completed a cardiac examination.

D. Continue with rounds and give the intern a failing grade on his evaluation.

ANSWERS

22.1 **D.** To document or recite a physical examination finding inaccurately is considered clinical dishonesty. All of the other choices support the falsified physical examination report. If any member of the team were to ask the surgery intern about his physical examination findings before or while proceeding with any of the other answer choices, the intern would be forced to resort to admit to the team that he has made a mistake because he forgot his stethoscope. Not doing so is a breach of the Hippocratic oath and the code of medical ethics and is subject to disciplinary action.

22.2 **E.** The team must be aware of the new murmur present on cardiac examination. Any abnormal finding must be incorporated into the patient's history and patient plan, if necessary. In this case, additional empiric antibiotics to cover for infective endocarditis may be required. Echocardiography may also need to be obtained to assess for cardiac vegetations and valvular dysfunction. A detailed neurologic examination may also help rule out septic emboli. In addition, intensive monitoring of vital signs may be considered. All of these steps require prompt action, which is why answers B and D are inappropriate. Answers A and C are confrontational and may further interfere with the team's dynamic and could possibly further compromise patient care.

22.3　**C.** The attending physician should make no assumption as to whether the intern's cardiac examination was actually performed. Medical students and resident physicians may miss subtle or even critical history and physical examination findings as they have limited experience with complex examinations. Indeed, it is the duty of the attending physician to meticulously examine the patient himself to ensure appropriate treatment and care and to ensure that his team members are developing the requisite clinical skills as they progress with their clinical training. All other choices do not follow this guideline. After being questioned by the attending physician, if the surgical intern were to lie and again falsify the cardiac examination results, the incident should be reported to the intern's residency program director. The attending physician should have proof, such as the intern's lack of a stethoscope, direct observation by the medical student during pre-rounds, or both.

KEY POINTS

▶ Up to 58% of medical students report having cheated at some point during medical school.

▶ Cheating in medical school is a predictor of clinical dishonesty.

▶ Those who engage in clinical dishonesty in medical school are more likely to face disciplinary action by state medical boards throughout their careers.

▶ It is unethical and unprofessional for a health care professional to hide the dishonesty of another health care professional, especially if it endangers patient's well-being.

▶ Those who cover up clinical dishonesty on the part of a colleague may be held liable to the same degree as the dishonest clinician, should the patient be harmed.

REFERENCES

American Medical Association (AMA). *Principles of Medical Ethics.* http://www.ama-assn.org/ama /pub/physician-resources/medical-ethics/code-medical-ethics/principles-medical-ethics.page. Accessed September 22, 2014.

Fred HL. Dishonesty in medicine revisited. *Texas Heart Inst J.* 2008;35:6-15.

Teherani A, Hodgson C, Banach M, Papadakis M. Domains of unprofessional behavior during medical school associated with future disciplinary action by a state medical board. *Acad Med.* 2005;80(suppl):s17-s20.

Young T. Teaching medical students to lie. *Can Med Assoc J.* 1997;156:219-222.

CASE 23

You are a senior medical student on the emergency department (ED) medicine rotation. A 50-year-old homeless man is brought in by ambulance to the ED having been found unresponsive on the street. His medical history is unknown. The paramedics diagnosed him as being in cardiac arrest without any shockable rhythm. He is unresponsive on arrival, with no spontaneous heartbeat or breathing. Resuscitation is attempted with cardiopulmonary resuscitation (CPR), intubation, and vasopressor administration. A central line kit is opened; however, before the line is placed, the team recognized that further attempts at resuscitation would be futile. The patient is declared dead after 25 minutes in the ED and the endotracheal tube is removed. A senior resident with whom you are working would like to ask permission from the attending so that the two of you can practice intubation and central line insertion on the fresh cadaver. There is no medical simulation center available at your institution, and any chance to practice these procedures is highly prized. The patient has no known friends or family from whom to obtain consent. The resident assures you that practicing on the newly deceased is common practice in your medical institution and suggests that you take advantage of this opportunity.

▶ What are some ethical arguments for and against practicing procedures on the recently deceased?
▶ Under what conditions, if any, should consent regarding the procedure be obtained?
▶ What are strengths and weaknesses of educational alternatives to practicing procedures on the newly deceased or unconscious patients?

ANSWERS TO CASE 23:

Student Issues: Procedures on Patients

Summary: A 50-year-old homeless man is brought into the ED, and, after attempts are made at resuscitation, he is declared dead. He has no family or friends available. The senior resident is asking whether you as a fourth-year medical student would like to participate in practicing intubation and central line placement on this recently deceased person.

- **Ethical arguments for and against practicing procedures on the recently deceased:** Practicing procedures on recently deceased patients, as well as on those who are unconscious, has been common practice in several medical centers, but the practice raises important issues of autonomy and consent. Medical trainees are often hesitant to practice procedures on patients who might experience discomfort or be harmed due to the trainee's relative inexperience. Practicing on recently deceased patients or unconscious patients with exceedingly low chances of recovery circumvent these concerns and have been seen as invaluable opportunities to learn skills that can be used to help others. However, consent should be obtained from family members or friends.

- **Conditions for obtaining consent:** Consent should be obtained from friends and family members whenever possible prior to practicing procedures on someone who cannot consent for themselves, even when there is no risk of harm, as in the case of a deceased patient.

- **Strengths and weaknesses of educational alternatives:** Although there are several educational alternatives to practicing procedures on the newly deceased, none of them are perfect. Working with living patients exposes them to an increased risk of discomfort and possible harm due to trainee inexperience. The preservation process alters the tissue of volunteered cadavers. Simulation technology continues to improve, but it cannot precisely replicate both the exact pliancy and variety of human tissue.

ANALYSIS

Objectives

1. List the ethical arguments for and against practicing procedures on the recently deceased.

2. Describe how and when to approach friends and family about performing procedures on patients who cannot consent for themselves.

3. Explain the strengths and weaknesses of alternatives to practicing procedures on the recently deceased or unconscious patients with low chances of recovery.

Considerations

Consent should be obtained prior to any procedure, whether on the living, nearly dead, or newly deceased. Despite the unique benefits of practicing procedures under these conditions, procedures should not be performed if such consent cannot be obtained. It is important to approach this issue with appropriate delicacy, as friends and family members are likely to be grieving. If possible, such discussions are best managed by an attending with training and experience in discussing issues surrounding end-of-life care. To not approach the issue at all, however, not only deprives the trainee of an experience that could help other patients in the future, but may also deprive friends and family of the knowledge that their personal tragedy may have some benefit to the good of society.

APPROACH TO:
Student Performing Procedures

DEFINITIONS

MEDICAL PROCEDURE: A course of action intended to somehow benefit a patient, often by means of invasive techniques requiring specialized training to perform.

SIMULATION TRAINING: The use of artificial scenarios to replicate a medical experience, such as the use of a specially designed mannequin, to practice procedures.

CLINICAL APPROACH

It is essential that physicians be skilled in several procedures, which, when quickly and capably performed, can save patient lives. However, the acquisition of these unquestionably important abilities can be challenging. Opportunities to practice can be scarce, and students may be insecure about approaching a patient to request a chance to perform a procedure that might be painful or even harmful if improperly performed.

There are several ways for medical trainees to learn about procedures. Lectures and videotapes can provide instructions and visual guidance, and students may have the opportunity to watch procedures being performed by others as they rotate in the hospital; however, it is widely recognized that learning how to actually perform any procedure requires actual hands-on practice. Having a procedure performed by a novice, however well supervised, likely increases the risks of harm to the individual patient. Therefore, there is an inherent ethical dilemma in medical training in which the societal need for well-trained physicians is juxtaposed with the desire to provide optimal medical care to each patient as an individual.

Medical simulation technology offers one way for trainees to practice important procedures without increasing risks to patients in their care. Simulation technology has been shown to be effective in teaching several important procedural skills, including advanced cardiac life support, central venous catheterization, lumbar puncture, and thoracentesis. Although simulation technology is becoming increasingly lifelike, it cannot be expected to perfectly duplicate the experience of working with actual human anatomy. Working with cadavers is a time-honored and highly valued practice in medical education and is irreplaceable in gaining experience with detailed human anatomy and variability. However, cadavers become less lifelike with the passage of time, as human tissue loses pliancy and other expected post-mortem changes occur. Alternatively performing procedures on the newly deceased permits trainees to practice in the most lifelike of settings without fear of harming a living patient.

Due to this unique opportunity to practice on human tissue without the risk of causing undue pain or other damage, it has been argued that performing medical procedures on the newly dead is an ethical imperative. However, unlike situations in which people have volunteered their bodies to medical education after their death, practicing on the newly dead often raises ethical questions regarding consent. The dead, being unable to exercise choice, do not have the same kind of autonomy as the living. This has led some to justify practicing on fresh cadavers by claiming that any possible costs to the deceased are outweighed by the benefits of well-trained physicians for the living. That being said, efforts are generally made in medicine to respect the wishes of what a person would have wanted were he or she able to choose. Such is the rationale behind legal wills, for example, and the reason we demand consent for organ donation despite the clear benefits to the living of that procedure.

However, the same kind of consent obtained for organ donation has been less frequently obtained for practicing on the recently deceased. According to surveys, between 39% and 47% of hospitals and up to 63% of ED medicine programs stated that procedures had been performed on the recently deceased. The range of procedures practiced ran the gamut, including intubation, cut downs, central line insertions, and many more. Nevertheless, 76% of program directors in one study stated they almost never obtained consent before practicing procedures on fresh cadavers. The frequency of requesting consent has been described as being as low as 10%.

Some practitioners have argued that the patient essentially consented to this practice by coming to a teaching hospital in the first place. Such an argument may overstate the general public's knowledge of the workings of an academic medical center. One survey revealed that almost 48% of people with medical problems who enter a training hospital are not aware that a student or trainee may be involved with their care.

Others have argued that, while obtaining consent from family members would be preferable, this is often impractical due to the frequency that friends or family were not present at the time of death. However, such an argument is seldom used to justify organ donation. If family members are present, then providers may neglect to gain their consent due to the seeming impropriety of asking grieving loved ones whether the body could be used immediately for educational gain. Studies that have examined whether people would consent to educational practice on a recently deceased loved one have shown that, while responses vary by culture, the majority of people do consent. This is akin to the majority of people who consent to being the first to receive a minor medical procedure performed by a trainee, despite the fears of many trainees about revealing their relative inexperience. Alternatively, angry responses to being asked about procedural practice on the newly dead were also not uncommon in the United States. As with other discussions surrounding death, the dialog is best directed by someone, preferably an attending physician, with dedicated training in holding such conversations.

Some medical educators have attempted to circumvent the societal or legal constraints regarding practicing on the newly deceased by running "slow codes" in which enough time is spent with an unconscious patient in whom death is certain to permit residents to practice techniques that while medically futile are educationally valuable. However, without consent, this practice is also morally questionable. It also potentially represents fraud if clinicians subsequently bill for such procedures.

Like performing procedures on a cadaver, procedural practice without consent on those in whom death is certain could erode future patient confidence and risks violating cultural values. Truth telling is an important component of the physician–patient relationship, which, if eroded, degrades society's trust in the medical community as a whole. Moreover, survivors are not allowed a sense of altruism by consenting, which might help them cope with their loved one's passing.

In addition to purely ethical considerations, there are practical concerns when performing procedures on a cadaver without adequate precautions and consent. For example, if a postmortem examination is to be performed, then this could be complicated by small injuries that occurred after death. Furthermore, legal action for postmortem manipulation has been successfully pursued in some states.

The code of medical ethics of the American Medical Association (AMA) specifically states that doctors "should inquire whether the deceased individual had expressed preferences regarding handling of the body or procedures performed after death." If attempts to find someone with authority to gain permission fail, "physicians must not perform procedures for training purposes on the newly deceased patient." Two other medical organizations, including the Society for Academic Emergency medicine (SAEM) and the American Heart Association's Emergency Cardiac Care (ECC) committee, recommend informed consent to use the newly dead for training.

Although it is not common practice, it may be worthwhile to explore the inclusion of procedural practice after death within other discussions commonly held regarding someone's death. Some have even suggested that a symbol could be included on a driver's license in a similar manner to organ donation. However, as with many aspects of end-of-life care, ensuring that a clear understanding exists between the patient and family will be of utmost importance.

COMPREHENSION QUESTIONS

23.1 Which of the following most closely represents the AMA's position on practicing procedures on the newly deceased?

    A. Procedures should never be performed on the newly deceased.

    B. Procedures may only be performed on the deceased if consent was obtained from the individual beforehand.

    C. Procedures may only be performed on the deceased if consent was obtained either by the individual or someone else with authority to grant permission for the procedure.

    D. Procedures may be performed without consent of the deceased or his or her family.

23.2 Which of the following statements justifying the practice of procedures on the deceased has most factual merit?

A. The right of autonomy cannot legally be applied to the dead as it is to the living.

B. Asking for consent unfairly traumatizes the family.

C. It is not necessary to ask consent because most patients have consented by virtue of consenting to be cared for in an educational hospital.

D. Asking for consent is impractical due to the high chance of refusal.

23.3 Which of the following statements about educational opportunities to learn procedures is most accurate?

A. Simulator technology is an ideal replication of performing procedures on actual patients.

B. Practice on something other than a conscious person is critical, as most patients would refuse to consent to someone performing even a minor medical procedure on them for the first time.

C. "Slow codes" are a clear ethical alternative to practicing on the newly deceased.

D. Practicing on the newly deceased provides a valuable opportunity to learn procedural skills.

ANSWERS

23.1 **C.** The AMA has stated that attempts should be made to determine whether the deceased patient had "expressed preferences regarding handling of the body or procedures performed after death," or attempt to obtain consent from someone else with authority to grant permission for the procedure. Without such consent, the procedure should not be performed.

23.2 **A.** Although it is true that notions of autonomy cannot be applied to the dead in the exact way as they are to the living, trust between patients and physicians demands that respect be paid to the wishes of patients and their families regarding the remains of the deceased. While asking for consent from family members during a moment of grief may feel like a traumatic intrusion, such paternalistic protection may actually prevent some families from sublimating their grief through altruism. The idea that people consent to having procedures performed on them after death simply by being in an educational hospital is undermined by the high percentage of people who do not even realize that being cared for in an academic medical center may mean that trainees are involved with their care. A high predicted likelihood of refusal is not only an unethical reason to avoid asking for consent, but it may not even be accurate regarding discussions of procedural practice on the newly deceased. The majority of families consented when asked. However, many did respond emotionally, highlighting the need for a skillful approach to the conversation.

23.3 **D.** Although simulator technology has demonstrated impressive results in teaching many procedural skills, it cannot perfectly replicate human anatomy and tissue characteristics and will therefore be always somewhat less than ideal. While practicing procedures on something other than a conscious person is ideal to minimize patient discomfort and risk, most patients actually consent to being the first person on whom a trainee has performed at least a minor medical procedure, although this does decline with perceived procedural invasiveness. While some practitioners have practiced slow codes in which a code situation is prolonged in a patient who is certain to die so that procedures can be practiced, such blurring of educational and therapeutic motives leads to ethical quandaries and may occasionally even meet criteria for fraud unless consent is obtained from family to practice procedural skills. Despite the ethical nuances involved, however, practicing on the newly deceased does provide a precious opportunity to practice procedures, whereby the dead can assist young doctors in being better able to serve the living.

KEY POINTS

▶ Practicing procedures on newly deceased patients or unconscious patients in whom death may be inevitable can be a valuable way for medical trainees to learn without fear of causing patient discomfort or cause.

▶ This practice has often been performed without gaining consent either of patient or family, although this behavior raises strong ethical concerns.

▶ Concerns about increasing family distress by asking for consent or a high likelihood of refusal may not be well founded.

▶ Conversations regarding consent for procedural practice in the newly deceased are delicate and best managed by an attending with training and experience in discussing issues surrounding end-of-life care.

▶ The AMA, SAEM, and the American Heart Association's ECC committee recommend that physicians ascertain the deceased patient's preferences, if possible, and otherwise obtain permission from the family or others with the authority to grant permission, prior to practicing procedures on the newly dead.

REFERENCES

Council on Ethical and Judicial Affairs. *Code of Medical Ethics of the American Medical Association: Current Opinions with Annotations.* http://www.ama-assn.org/resources/doc/ethics/ethics-in-hand-student-version.pdf. Accessed January 25, 2014.

Iserson KV. Law versus life: the ethical imperative to practice and teach using the newly dead emergency department patient. *Ann Emerg Med.* 1995;25:91-94.

Jones JW, McCullough LB. Ethics of rehearsing procedures on a corpse. *J Vasc Surg.* 2011;54:879-880.

Karczewska M. Ethical issues in the emergency department: consent for procedure training on newly deceased patients. *McGill J Med*. 2009;12:116-119.

Morag RM, DeSouza S, Steen PA, et al. Performing procedures on the newly deceased for teaching purposes: what if we were to ask? *Arch Intern Med*. 2005;165:92-96.

Santen SA, Hemphill RR, Spanier CM, Fletcher ND. 'Sorry, it's my first time!' Will patients consent to medical students learning procedures? *Med Educ*. 2005;39:365-369.

During the microbiology laboratory of the second year of medical school, you note that your laboratory partner has been exhibiting some unusual behavior over the last 2 months. He has been missing quite a few classes and labs, even the ones that are mandatory; previously, he had attended all lectures and labs, even the ones that were optional. You note that he is irritable, appears tired, and that the quality of his work has dramatically deteriorated. You have asked him twice if there was a problem and whether there is a reason for his absences. Upon questioning, he became even more irritable and defensive. Today, your laboratory partner arrives late again to microbiology. His hair is uncombed, and his shirt is wrinkled and stained.

▶ What is the most likely explanation for the laboratory partner's behavior?
▶ What is the best next step in this situation?

ANSWERS TO CASE 24:

Fellow Addicted Student

Summary: A second-year medical student colleague begins to exhibit unusual erratic behavior such as tardiness, decline in academic performance, and decreased attention to personal hygiene.

- **Likely explanation:** Substance abuse.

- **Next step:** Compassionate and ethical intervention to protect the safety of patients as well as the physical, psychological, and professional well-being of your colleague.

ANALYSIS

Objectives

1. List the characteristics of an individual who exhibits substance abuse.

2. Describe the risk factors for substance abuse.

3. Describe the best course and duty of the student who suspects that a fellow student has a problem with substance abuse.

Considerations

A second-year medical student colleague begins to exhibit erratic behavior inconsistent with his previously high level of functioning. He arrives late to required activities at the microbiology laboratory without regard to the consequences for himself and others, his academic performance and personal hygiene suffer, and he becomes defensive and evasive when questioned about his behavior. He is exhibiting classic signs and symptoms of substance abuse. Substance abuse is a common problem among health care professionals. The best approach to this situation is to ensure early detection and reporting, formal treatment, professional support, and ongoing monitoring to protect patient safety as well as the physical, psychological, and professional well-being of your colleague.

APPROACH TO:

The Addicted Colleague

DEFINITIONS

BENEFICENCE: The ethical principle in which physicians have a fiduciary duty to act in the best interest of the patient, regardless of the physician's personal interests or the interests of third parties (eg, hospital systems, insurers).

NONMALEFICENCE: The ethical principle in which physicians have a fiduciary duty to refrain from providing services or treatments that are ineffective or situations in which the risks outweigh the benefits.

SUBSTANCE ABUSE: A maladaptive pattern of substance use manifested by recurrent and significant adverse consequences related to the repeated use of such substances.

SUBSTANCE DEPENDENCE: A cluster of cognitive behaviors and physiologic symptoms indicating that the individual continues use of the substance despite significant substance-related problems.

CLINICAL APPROACH

Contrary to popular opinion, substance abuse is equally common among health care professionals as it is in the general population; in fact, it estimated that between 10% and 12% of physicians experience some kind of substance use disorder. Although physicians are less likely than the general population to abuse cigarettes and street drugs such as heroin, cocaine, and methamphetamine, they are more likely to abuse alcohol and prescription drugs, especially stimulants such as dextroamphetamine and methylphenidate, benzodiazepines, and opioid analgesics. Although physicians of all specialties are at risk for the development of substance use disorders, one study found that 5 particular specialties account for more than 50% of addicted physicians: family medicine (20.0%), internal medicine (13.1%), anesthesiology (10.9%), emergency medicine (7.1%), and psychiatry (6.9%).

There are a variety of commonly abused substances among health care professionals, and it is important to be able to identify the psychiatric and physiologic signs and symptoms of intoxication and withdrawal from these substances. These signs and symptoms are summarized in Table 24–1.

In addition to recognizing acute intoxication and withdrawal, it is important to pick up on the signs and symptoms of substance use disorders in general. **Any deterioration from a student or physician's baseline level of functioning could be an indication of a developing substance use disorder; however, it is important to differentiate between this and other causes due to the extremely sensitive nature of the issue and the potential for harm to the person in question's relationships, livelihood, and professional reputation.** In the above case, the student exhibits warning signs, such as deterioration in academic performance, loss of conscientiousness toward scholastic obligations, and decline in personal hygiene. In addition, he demonstrates defensiveness, evasiveness, and irritability when his behavior is brought into question. All of these behaviors serve as red flags for the presence of substance use in this individual.

When substance abuse is suspected in a student or physician, it is a concerned colleague's ethical responsibility to further explore the situation. The diagnosis of a substance use disorder is a historical one; a thorough history comprising reliable reports of substance use correlated with behavioral change from a number of sources (eg, family members, colleagues, friends) is the most useful diagnostic tool. Results from urinalyses can be helpful, but they are not adequate on their own; for example, highly potent substances (eg, fentanyl, opioid analgesics) have a short half-life and their use may not be detected. Moreover, samples for urinalyses are easily tampered with and results are commonly altered.

Table 24–1 • INTOXICATION AND WITHDRAWAL SYNDROMES OF COMMONLY ABUSED SUBSTANCES		
Substance	**Intoxication**	**Withdrawal**
Alcohol	**Early:** Apparent central nervous system S stimulation (via depression of inhibitory control in the RAS* and cerebral cortex) Euphoria Increased verbal communication, aggression **Intermediate:** Loss of motor coordination Sedation Impaired judgment and memory Decreased psychomotor activity **Late:** Stupor Coma Death	**Mild:** Anxiety Restlessness Irritability Insomnia Tremor Increased reflexes **Moderate:** Tachycardia Hypertension Diaphoresis Hyperthermia Fasciculations Anorexia Nausea Vomiting **Severe:** Seizures Delirium Hallucinations Death
Benzodiazepines	Similar to alcohol Death extremely unlikely except when combined with alcohol/other central nervous system depressants	Similar to alcohol, however severe withdrawal symptoms are uncommon
Cannabinoids	Initial euphoria followed by drowsiness and sedation Altered perceptions of time Sensory distortion Dissociative experiences Impaired cognition Decreased coordination Impaired reaction time and motor coordination Conjunctival injection Tachycardia Paranoia Hallucinations Agitation	**Difficult to characterize, but may include:** Insomnia Irritability Depression Anxiety Anorexia Nausea Tremor

(Continued)

Table 24–1 • INTOXICATION AND WITHDRAWAL SYNDROMES OF COMMONLY ABUSED SUBSTANCES (*CONTINUED*)		
Substance	Intoxication	Withdrawal
Opioids	Euphoria Warmth Facial flushing Pruritus Dry mouth Pupillary constriction Sedation Respiratory suppression Hyporeflexia Hypotension Tachycardia Apnea Cyanosis Death	Hyperalgesia Photophobia Piloerection Abdominal cramping and diarrhea Tachycardia Hypertension Myalgias Arthralgias Anxiety Depression
Stimulants	Tachycardia Hypertension Vasoconstriction Pupillary dilation Diaphoresis Tremor Anorexia Hyperactivity	Depression Dysphoria

*RAS: Reticular Activating System

Once a colleague is reasonably suspected of substance abuse, it is important to confront that person in a firm yet compassionate way. The ultimate goal for this meeting should be for the physician in question to accept that he or she has a problem and to agree to a treatment protocol with the goal of returning to safe practice. This is a difficult conversation to have because people with substance abuse (especially people with previously high levels of functioning) can have enormous burdens of guilt, fear, and denial with respect to their problem. It is important to emphasize the gravity of the situation, while offering support and hope for future success in the medical field.

In most states, physicians suspected of substance abuse are required to undergo formal evaluation as specified by a physician health program (PHP) that has been sanctioned by a state medical board. It is the job of these PHPs to manage the treatment of medical and psychiatric conditions that may threaten the livelihood of a physician in that state. Physicians that voluntarily enter these substance abuse programs may remain anonymous from their state medical board; physicians who are mandated to complete such a program risk the revelation of their identities. This functions as an incentive for impaired physicians to complete treatment. Once a treatment program has been successfully completed, the physician is allowed to return to practice without further disciplinary action on the part of the hospital or the state. A probationary period follows that involves counseling, drug testing, and close follow-up.

Although there are many mechanisms in place that provide compassionate, career- and perhaps life-saving care for impaired physicians, there are still many barriers to the reporting and treatment of those affected. Dealing with an addicted colleague is an extremely delicate and emotionally charged situation; many professionals find it easier to remain in denial about the situation, or feel the need to invoke a kind of professional solidarity in order to protect their colleague. If the physician in questions occupies a position of power within the workplace hierarchy, then colleagues may fear for their jobs or professional reputations when weighing a decision about reporting. This is especially true of students who may fear their grades or clinical evaluations will be altered when they are suspicious of a supervising physician.

Lack of education about the nature of substance abuse and its diagnosis and treatment also poses a large barrier to reporting, even in the medical world. Students and doctors can experience substance addiction for long periods of time before their colleagues suspect them, and misconceptions about the nature of the disease can lead to unwarranted destruction of reputations and fears of legal sanctioning. Improvement in education about substance abuse and available resources starting early in medical school and continuing into postgraduate training could help to alleviate these problems and to improve early detection rates.

In conclusion, substance abuse is a common problem among physicians and medical students that often escapes notice until it is too late. It is the ethical obligation of a suspicious colleague to make his or her concerns known; patient safety is at risk, as well as the safety of the physician or student in question. Most hospitals and medical schools, in conjunction with state medical boards and PHPs, have protocols in place to compassionately address and effectively treat physicians and students who experience substance abuse. Increased education about these disorders and the available resources for those who experience them could significantly improve early detection and successful treatment of medical professionals with a substance abuse disorder.

COMPREHENSION QUESTIONS

24.1 You are taking overnight call on your general surgery rotation during your third year of medical school. At 3:00 am, you are called by your resident to scrub in on an emergent appendectomy. Before scrubbing in, you notice that the on-call anesthesiologist, who has just arrived at the hospital, appears disheveled and bleary-eyed. When you approach him to introduce yourself, he grumpily waves you off, and you are sure you smell alcohol on his breath. What is the next best course of action?

A. Do not say anything, since he is probably just tired.

B. Wait until tomorrow to say something to a superior in private.

C. Pull a trusted upper-level resident aside immediately and voice your concern in a tactful way.

D. Confront the anesthesiologist directly about his alcohol abuse.

E. Try to find out from nursing and surgical staff whether or not this has ever happened before with this particular doctor.

24.2 You are a chief resident enjoying your new favorite privilege of at-home call. A nonmedical friend whom you have not seen in a while because of your busy schedule invites you out to dinner and you accept. Midway through the meal, you stand up to use the restroom and realize that you have had 1 or 2 more glasses of wine than you had planned. Inevitably, your pager goes off and you are needed at the hospital to manage an emergency with one of your sicker patients. What is the next best course of action?

   A. Ignore the page and pretend that you did not notice it because your battery on the pager is running out.

   B. Call another one of the chief residents to cover for you.

   C. Do a quick check of your memory and mental capability, and then go in to the hospital to take care of your patient.

   D. Call the resident back and explain the situation.

   E. Call the attending on call and explain the situation.

24.3 One of your classmates during her second year of medical school begins to exhibit bizarre behavior in the library while studying for a pharmacology examination. She appears anxious and hyperactive; her pupils are dilated and she is diaphoretic. You notice that her clothes seem to fit much more loosely than they did at the beginning of class 2 weeks ago. Which of the following substances is she likely to be abusing?

   A. Dextroamphetamine

   B. Fentanyl

   C. Marijuana

   D. Lorazepam

   E. Cocaine

ANSWERS

24.1 **C.** If you have concerns about this physician's ability to do his job, you should let a superior know immediately. Waiting until the next day is inappropriate because it does not take into account patient safety. Confronting the physician directly is unlikely to be helpful because it will lead to unnecessary and unproductive conflict in an already stressful situation. Asking incriminating questions of multiple staff members is also inappropriate because the action could lead to unfounded rumors and damage the physician's professional reputation without helping to resolve the situation at hand.

24.2 **E.** If there is a problem with impaired house-staff, that physician's supervisor should be notified immediately. Ignoring the page would be unprofessional and would leave the service without medically and legally integral personnel. Calling in a favor to another chief resident puts that physician in an awkward position; he or she might be torn between loyalty to their colleague and ensuring patient safety and house staff responsibility. Although the lower-level resident would have an ethical responsibility to report the chief for alcohol abuse while on the job, it is not that person's job to handle this situation. The supervising physician on-call should be notified of the problem immediately to ensure patient safety and adequate hospital coverage.

24.3 **A.** This student is most likely abusing prescription stimulants (eg, dextroamphetamine) as a study aid during a stressful examination week. She is exhibiting classic signs of stimulant intoxication, which can include hyperactivity, anxiety, sweating, pupillary dilation, and weight loss. Cocaine use might present similarly, but the highly functioning medical student during examination week is more likely to abuse prescription stimulants than recreational cocaine. Opioid, benzodiazepine, and marijuana intoxications do not present like this.

KEY POINTS

▶ The prevalence of substance abuse is equal in physician and nonphysician populations.

▶ Substance use disorder is a clinical diagnosis that requires reliable reports of substance use correlated with behavior change from multiple trustworthy sources.

▶ It is a colleague's ethical obligation to report suspected substance abuse in a fellow student or physician.

▶ The vast majority of hospital systems and medical schools have career-saving protocols in place that treat addicted physicians and medical students.

▶ Barriers to reporting include fear of legal action, fear of retaliation (eg, bad grades, evaluations, employment termination), instinct to protect a colleague, and lack of education about substance use and available resources.

REFERENCES

Federation of State Medical Boards. *Federation of State Medical Boards' Policy on Physician Impairment*, Washington, DC, 2011. http://www.fsmb.org/pdf/grpol_policy-on-physician-impairment.pdf. Accessed April 1, 2014.

Hughes PH, Brandenburg N, DeWitt BC, Storr CL, Williams KM, Anthony JC, et al. Prevalence of substance use among US physicians. *JAMA*. 1992;267:2333-2339.

Lo B. Ethical issues in clinical medicine. In: Longo DL, Fauci AS, Kasper DL, Hauser SL, Jameson J, Loscalzo J, eds. *Harrison's Principles of Internal Medicine*. 18th ed. New York, NY: McGraw-Hill; 2012.

Martin PR. Substance-related disorders. In: Ebert MH, Loosen PT, Nurcombe B, Leckman JF, eds. *Current Diagnosis & Treatment: Psychiatry*. 2nd ed. New York, NY: McGraw-Hill; 2008.

McClellan TA, Skipper GS, Campbell M, DuPont RLl. Five year outcomes in a cohort study of physicians treated for substance use disorders in the United States. *BMJ*. 2008;337:a2038.

Seppala MD, Berge KH. The addicted physician: a rational approach to an irrational disease. *Minn Med*. 2010;93:46-49.

A third-year medical student is assigned by the chief resident of the internal medi-cine service to give a short presentation on ulcerative colitis versus Crohn disease for the next day. In the course of putting together the presentation, the student copies various sections of a website on inflammatory bowel disease, putting whole paragraphs from the webpages into his report. After the presentation is over, the chief resident asks whether the presentation was copied from a website, because the sentence structure seemed different from what the medical student would use. The student states that he researched the material from websites, but the words he used were his own.

► Has this student committed an act of plagiarism or is this action acceptable?
► If you were a fellow student on the service and aware of this student's research methods, how should you respond?

ANSWERS TO CASE 25:

Student Cheating and Plagiarism

Summary: A third-year medical student gives a short presentation on ulcerative colitis versus Crohn disease. The student lifts entire paragraphs from a website. When confronted about the unusual structure and syntax, the student states that he researched his presentation using the Internet, but the words he used were entirely his own.

- **Plagiarism or not:** This is a case of plagiarism.

- **How should a fellow student respond:** One has an ethical duty to confront this lapse in professionalism of a fellow student.

ANALYSIS

Objectives

1. Define plagiarism and cheating.

2. Describe the duty of each student and fellow students in upholding the highest ethical and professional standards.

3. Describe the reasons that cheating and plagiarism are harmful.

Considerations

A third-year medical student passes off the work of another as his own by copying and pasting entire paragraphs from a website on inflammatory bowel disease. Definitions of plagiarism differ from academic institution to institution. Although students may be aware of the ethical duty not to plagiarize, many students may not understand exactly what constitutes plagiarism or how to define the offense. Cheating and plagiarism in academia is often hard to identify or define. Knowledge of an institution's standards of plagiarism and the consequences of committing plagiarism is vital to the assessment of the cheating student and a fellow student aware of the academic infraction. Although committing plagiarism is inexcusable, the learning outcomes or perceived learning outcomes must be considered.

APPROACH TO:

Student Cheating And Plagiarism

DEFINITIONS

CHEATING: Violating ethical and professional codes by acting unfairly or dishonestly.

PLAGIARISM: A form of cheating; claiming the work of another as one's own; copying work (including one's own work) without proper acknowledgment or citation.

PROFESSIONALISM: This is the commitment to carrying out one's professional responsibilities, and adhering to ethical principles, while being sensitive to a diverse patient population.

CLINICAL APPROACH

Cheating is a widespread phenomenon within academia, and the problem has worsened with technological development and the increase in available information to students. One study found that 43% of undergraduate and graduate students surveyed admitted to some kind of cheating. Another survey found that more than one-half of surveyed medical students reported cheating during medical school. The phenomenon of academic dishonesty is not a recent phenomenon but continues to spread and affect a large population of students at all levels of education.

There are many reasons for cheating, but the principal reasons for academic dishonesty are fear of failing and of falling behind fellow students. Definitions of cheating include any form of academic dishonesty. Copying off another student in a test and bringing notes into closed-book tests are forms of cheating, but plagiarism is the most common type of cheating among today's students. Plagiarism is claiming the work of another as one's own. Technological ease, discomfort with writing ability, and a generational gap in perceptions of plagiarism all come into play when students consider plagiarism. The ease of cheating does not excuse the behavior. Medical students are expected to be professional, which includes being honest and ethical in their academic work. Although it may be a failure of the academic institution to have clearly defined the expectations and regulations of academic integrity, a student should know and understand the professional expectations of his or her institution by the third year of medical school. At this stage in his or her career, a third-year medical student should be serving as an exemplary academic model for other students.

Plagiarism is especially easy with the abundance of information online. Plagiarism occurs any time a student claims the work of another. In addition, a student can self-plagiarize, turning in previously completed course work, or autoplagiarize, which is failing to cite oneself. The ease of the copy/paste function in word processors of sentences and even paragraphs from online sources tempts students to claim this work as their own, whether explicitly or implicitly, by not providing a citation or reference. Research has demonstrated that acts of plagiarism have significantly increased with the ease of copying and pasting from online sources.

Reasons for Cheating

When confronted, students give several reasons for cheating. The first reason is fear of falling behind their peers or failing. Especially in competitive academic environments, students worry about failing out of school or about losing academic standing. A second reason is that some non-native English-speaking students are not confident in their ability to write in English. Not wanting to appear incompetent or uncomfortable with communicating in English, some students feel a temptation to copy material directly from a native English speaker. A third reason that students plagiarize is they may be unclear on what exactly constitutes plagiarism. Although most students know that plagiarism is wrong in theory, when it comes to the actual practices and concrete examples, students are less certain of what constitutes dishonest academic practices. For example, a student may be able to articulate that cheating and plagiarism are wrong, but he or she may not be able to describe what practices are considered academically dishonest. Students may also not see the harm in cheating, viewing the act as a victimless offense.

Harm of Cheating

Students are often confused about the harm of cheating because, on the surface, cheating does not seem to bring harm to anyone. Despite this feeling, cheating is not a victimless offense. There are at least 3 parties offended in any case of cheating. The first is the instructor. When a student who turns in work completed in a dishonest manner, he or she is intentionally deceiving the instructor regarding the assignment. The second offended party is made up of the cheating student's peers. Academic dishonesty creates an imbalance in equality: It is not fair to the students who put in the energy and time to complete assignments or tests in an honest manner. The third party harmed by cheating is the offending student. By cutting corners through cheating, a student ends up harming himself or herself because he or she is not learning the material or he or she is not putting the work into assignments or studying the material. Students who cut corners by cheating or plagiarizing do themselves an academic disservice. Instructors design assignments and tests with specific goals in mind. Learning goals often include the demonstration that a student can re-present material covered in a course and be actively engaged with the material. When bypassing this step, the student disservices himself or herself by not accomplishing the desired learning goals. These are the three parties harmed in every case of cheating, and in the case of plagiarism there is a fourth party harmed, and that is the uncited source. By plagiarizing another source, a student does not give proper credit or acknowledgment to the owner of the content who did put in the time and effort to publish his or her own work. The medical profession has a possible fifth party harmed, and that is the future patient. If a student fails to learn the material necessary to his or her medical education, then this action has a possibility of affecting that student's ability to care for his or her patients.

Duty to Report

Students are often hesitant to report fellow students of cheating for a variety of reasons. Students do not want to be perceived as a "tattletale" or a "snitch." Students are especially hesitant to turn in other students in academic environments where expulsion is the consequence for cheating. Despite the hesitance, if a student knows that another student is cheating, then he or she has a duty to report the infraction. The reason a student must report academic dishonesty of another student, even if it seems harmless, is that the offending student is performing an ethical infraction. When one observes an ethical infraction by a peer, one has a duty to take action. By reporting a cheating student, one protects the equality of the academic system and upholds the values of honesty and integrity. Furthermore, if a student fails to learn material necessary in the medical education, then those who suffer from this action are future patients.

Summary

Cheating is any form of academic dishonesty. A common form of cheating is plagiarism, which is the act of failing to acknowledge the source of ideas or words by claiming them as one's own. Students have a variety of reasons they give for cheating; however, no matter the pressures of academia, cheating is never an acceptable solution. Though on the surface it may seem like a victimless offense, cheating is a serious ethical violation that does harm others and often oneself. If a student observes a fellow student cheating, then he or she has an ethical duty to report that student.

COMPREHENSION QUESTIONS

25.1   As a second-year medical student, you have been given an orientation on academic honesty and cheating. Which of the following constitutes the best example of plagiarism in its strict definition?

A.   Turning in the same document for multiple courses.

B.   Copying from an online document but citing the website.

C.   Copying a few sentences from a document one has turned in to another course.

D.   Copying a paragraph that is "common knowledge" in the field.

25.2   You are a first-year medical student. During an anatomy examination, you see that the student sitting next to you is using a cheat sheet on the test. You are good friends with the student and believe that she has the intellect and diligence to succeed, but you know she is anxious about the workload. If you have an opportunity to speak to her after the examination, then you believe you will be able to reassure her of her ability. However, you have signed an honor code requiring that you report any suspected cheating. What is your next step?

A.   Warn the student not to cheat again, or you will report her.

B.   Go directly to the instructor.

C.   Confront the student, telling her that if she does not turn herself in, you will.

D.   Do nothing, because cheating is its own punishment.

25.3   It is acceptable to copy information from the Internet into one's own coursework as long as which of the following?

A.   You include the website name in the reference list.

B.   It is never acceptable.

C.   You include the website name in a footnote or in-text citation as well as in the reference list.

D.   You clearly indicate where your own words end and the words of another begin with proper citation and the use of quotes around the other person's work.

ANSWERS

25.1 **B.** In its strict definition, plagiarism is claiming work from another as one's own. The answers in the question may indicate "self plagiarism", the strict definition is using another's work and representing it as one's own.

25.2 **B.** Although this is a difficult situation, and one can have personal alliances, it is important to adhere to a "no tolerance" policy regarding cheating. Reporting on cheating may have negative implications for personal relationships such as friendships, and doing so may be emotionally troubling. It is not an easy decision. Nevertheless, it has been shown repeatedly that cheating early in one's career can lead to more severe lapses in behavior and judgment, which can affect patient care. Thus, it is more than one "simple test."

25.3 **D.** Citation involves indicating what work is original and what work is another's by listing the author of that work.

KEY POINTS

▶ Clarity is necessary in defining expectations and standards in academic institutions.

▶ Cheating and plagiarism, although widespread, are not acceptable.

▶ Students have a duty to report ethical infractions of fellow students.

REFERENCES

Accreditation Council of Graduate Medical Education (ACGME). *Core Competencies Definitions*. Chicago, IL. www.acgme.org. Accessed May 1, 2014. http://www.gahec.org/cme/Liasions/0)ACGME%20Core%20Competencies%20Definitions.htm. Accessed December 23, 2014.

Carroll J, Appleton J. Plagiarism: a good practice guide. *Joint Inform Syst Comm*. 2001.

Cole AF. Plagiarism in graduate medical education. *Fam Med*. 2007;39:436-438.

Coverdale J, Henning M. An analysis of cheating behaviour during training by medical students. *Med Teacher*, 2000;22:582-584.

McCabe D. Cheating among college and university students: a North American perspective. *Int J Educ Integrit*. 2005;1:1.

Sierles F, Hendrickx I, Circle S. Cheating in medical school. *J Med Educ*. 1980;55:124.

A 25-year-old man who is an organ donor has been assigned to the intensive care unit (ICU). He was pronounced brain dead after undergoing closed head trauma following a motorcycle collision. He was intubated on assist-control mode with a rate of 16/minute, tidal volume of 450 mL, and a fractional inspired oxygen concentration (FIO_2) of 35%. Arterial blood gas data were as follows: pH of 7.36, $PaCO_2$ 36 mm Hg, and PaO_2 150 mm Hg. The transplantation and operating room teams were alerted. The blood pressure reading was 110 mm Hg systolic and 60 mm Hg diastolic, heart rate was regular at 110 beats/minute, and his temperature was 96°F. The man weighed 70 kg, and his height was 157 cm (62 in). Electrolyte values were sodium 155 mEq/L, potassium 4 mEq/L, chloride 105 mEq/L, and bicarbonate 20 mEq/L. His urine output is 150 mL/hour.

▶ How is a pronouncement of brain death performed?
▶ If his family members insist that cardiopulmonary resuscitation (CPR) be performed in the event of cardiac arrest, what should be your response?
▶ How should the issue of organ donation be introduced to the family?

ANSWERS TO CASE 26:

Organ Transplantation and Do Not Resuscitate Orders

Summary: A 25-year-old patient is pronounced brain dead following a motor vehicle collision and massive closed head trauma. He is physiologically stable.

- **Diagnosis of brain death:** Clinical ascertainment of irreversible absence of brain function, including brain stem function.

- **Response if the family members insist that CPR be performed in the event of cardiac arrest:** In general, a family's wishes should be honored unless an advanced directive exists in the absence of irreversible signs of death (rigor mortis, decapitation, dependent lividity).

- **How the issue of organ donation should be introduced to the family:** The issue should be brought up after the questions about the patient's status and prognosis are discussed, and optimally together with someone well versed in organ donation.

ANALYSIS

Objectives

1. Describe how to diagnose brain death.
2. Describe possible dilemmas with do not resuscitate (DNR) orders.
3. List the ethical issues surrounding organ donors.

Considerations

This case describes a young man who was involved in a motorcycle collision and was declared brain dead. The diagnosis of brain death is dependent on the diagnosis of irreversible loss of all brain function, including brain stem function. **Brain death** must be distinguished from **brain damage.** Possible confounding variables such as medications or drugs may interfere with brainstem function and must therefore be identified. The diagnosis of brain death is a clinical one and depends on the presence of coma, absence of brainstem function, and absence of apnea. In this case, a massive closed head injury was noted. The patient was likely observed for level of consciousness and then for brainstem function, such as pupillary reflex, corneal reflex, gag reflex, spontaneous movement, movement, or response to voice or painful stimuli, and tested for spontaneous respirations when taken off the ventilator. After the initial evaluation, a secondary evaluation is often needed to allow for brain injury to subside; typically, a 6- to 8-hour period of observation is needed. Head imaging procedures can also be useful. After declaring the patient brain dead, the patient's next of kin should be notified. The discussion must be careful, compassionate, and with thoughtfulness. The topic of organ transplantation may occur at this time. Depending on state regulations, a second physician may need to certify brain death before the transplantation process is initiated.

> ## APPROACH TO:
> ## Organ Transplantation and Do Not Resuscitate Orders

DEFINITIONS

ADVANCE DIRECTIVE: The advance directive is a document that details the kinds of decisions the patient would like be made if he or she was unable to participate at the time when a critical medical decision must be made. This document may list or indicate specific decisions (eg, living will); otherwise, it may designate a specific person to make health care decisions for him or her (eg, durable power of attorney, health care proxy). There is some controversy of how literal living wills should be interpreted. Preferences expressed in a living will are the most compelling when they reflect long held, consistently stable views of the patient. These preferences can often be determined by conversations with family members, close friends, or health care professionals who have had a long-term relationship with the patient.

SURROGATE DECISION MAKER: In the absence of a written document, the law recognizes a hierarchy of family relationships in determining which family member should be the official "spokesperson" or health care proxy.

BRAIN DEATH: Breath death refers to the irreversible loss of all brain functions, including brainstem function.

CLINICAL APPROACH

Brain Death

Brain death and organ donation are difficult topics for the caregiver and family. In this situation, common sense judgments of critical care must be applied. Guidelines generally include optimizing cardiovascular and pulmonary functions, fluid and electrolyte balance, treatment of infection, and the administration of hormones.

Donor organs are influenced by the prevailing systemic physiology (eg, oxygen delivery, blood electrolyte composition, regional and systemic cytokines). General parameters of optimal care are addressed in Table 26–1 as well as individual factors that may affect a transplantable organ.

Donor care is often a complex undertaking. Providing the best possible organs to awaiting recipients demands careful attention to multiple variables. The paucity of evidence-based data that could be helpful in providing clinical guidance is a challenge to the critical care, organ procurement, and transplantation teams. In the ICU, DNR orders are common and should be clearly displayed on the patient's chart or in the electronic health record. If such orders are not present, then the patient can be preemptively asked if he or she wants resuscitation following cardiac arrest or life-threatening arrhythmia. Like many other medical decisions, deciding whether or not to resuscitate a patient experiencing cardiopulmonary arrest involves careful consideration of the potential likelihood for clinical benefit balanced with the patient's preferences for the intervention and its likely outcome. Decisions to forego cardiac resuscitation are often difficult because of real or perceived differences in these considerations.

Table 26–1 • RECOMMENDATIONS FOR DONOR CARE GUIDELINE PARAMETERS	
Central venous pressure, 4–12 mm Hg	Glucose, 70–150 mg/dL
Pulmonary artery occluded pressure, 8–12 mm Hg	pH, 7.40–7.45
Cardiac index, > 2.4 L/min	PaCO2, 30–35 mm Hg
Cardiac output, > 3.8 L/min Urine output, 1–3 mL/kg/hr	PaO2, > 80–90 mm Hg
Mean arterial pressure, 60 mm Hg	Hemoglobin, > 10 g/dL
Systolic blood pressure, > 90 and < 120 mm Hg	Hematocrit, > 30%

When Should CPR Be Administered?

CPR is a set of specific medical procedures designed to establish circulation and breathing in a patient. CPR is designed to maintain perfusion to vital organs while attempts are made to restore spontaneous breathing and cardiac rhythm by implantable cardioverter defibrillation. If the patient stops breathing or cardiac arrest occurs in the hospital, then standard care involves CPR in the absence of a valid physician's order to withhold it. Paramedics responding to an arrest in the field are required to administer CPR.

Hospitals have policies that describe circumstances under which CPR can be withheld. Some general situations arise that justify withholding CPR:

- When CPR is judged to be of no medical benefit

- When the patient has the capacity to make serious decisions and clearly indicates that he or she does not want CPR, with signed documents confirming these wishes written in medical—rather than legal—language

- When the patient displays an impaired decision making capacity, a health care proxy can make the decisions for the patient. The proxy can indicate that the patient does not wish to receive CPR

CPR is futile when it offers the patient no clinical benefit. In these situations, physicians are ethically justified in withholding resuscitation. It is important to define what it means to "be of benefit." The distinction between providing measurable effects (eg, normalizing the serum potassium) and providing significant health benefits is helpful in this deliberation. One approach to defining benefit examines the probability of an intervention that leads to a desirable outcome. CPR has been prospectively evaluated in a wide variety of clinical situations. Knowledge of the probability of success with CPR could be used to determine its futility.

CPR might also seem to lack benefit when the patient's quality of life is so demonstrably poor that no meaningful improvement is expected with resuscitation. Judging "quality of life" tempts prejudicial statements about patients with a chronic illness or disability. There is substantial evidence that patients with such chronic conditions may rate their quality of life much higher than would healthy people.

Patients in a permanent unconscious state possess a quality of life that few people would accept; therefore, CPR is typically considered "futile" for such patients.

If CPR is judged to be medically futile, then the health care professional has no obligation to provide it. Nevertheless, the patient, his or her family members, or all parties should still have a role in the decision about a DNR order to preserve the principle of autonomy. In many cases, the patient and his or her family, upon being given a caring but frank understanding of the clinical situation, will agree with the DNR order. In such cases, a DNR order can be written at that time. Each hospital should have specific procedures for writing a valid DNR order. In all cases, the order must be written or cosigned by the attending physician. A decision to withhold CPR may also arise from a patient's expressed wish that CPR not be performed. If the patient understands the existing medical condition and possesses an intact decision-making capacity, then the DNR request should be honored.

Ethicists and physicians are divided about how to proceed if family members disagree. A DNR order can only be written with full agreement by the patient or family member. Every reasonable effort should be made to explain all details of the medical situation with involved parties, which usually will lead to a resolution of the conflict. In difficult cases, an ethics consultation can prove helpful. Nevertheless, CPR should generally be provided to patients, even if the procedure is judged to be futile.

So-called "slow-codes," where half-hearted efforts at resuscitation are made, are not ethically justified. Such actions undermine a patient's rights and violate the code of physician–patient trust. In most instances, the decision to initiate or deny CPR occurs at a time when the patient is unable to participate in the decision-making and his or her preference may be unknown. There are 2 general approaches to this dilemma, advanced directives and surrogate decision-makers, which are discussed in more detail below.

Advance Directive

The advance directive is a document that details the kinds of decisions a patient would like to have made if he or she is unable to participate in a particular decision at a critical time. This document can specify or indicate specific decisions (eg, living will), or it may designate a person to make health care choices for the patient (eg, durable power of attorney for health care, surrogate). In the absence of a written document, the law generally recognizes a hierarchy of family relationships in determining which family member should be the "official spokesperson" for the patient, although court battles have be waged to determine who truly has the best interest of the patient and knows what the patient would have wanted. These include the following individuals:

- Legal guardian with health care decision-making authority, also called the health care proxy

- Spouse

- Parents of patient

- Individual given durable power of attorney for health care decisions

- Adult children of patient (all in agreement)

- Adult siblings of patient (all in agreement)

Organ Donation

During the time of a tragic and unexpected death, the family members are often emotionally and psychologically devastated. Thus, a sensitive, culturally aware, and supportive approach is best in broaching the topic of organ donation. **Studies have shown that health care professionals with special training on the issue are more likely to be successful in obtaining familial permission; the optimal approach is for organ procurement personnel to talk to the family together with the patient's health care team.** Although the timing of organ donation discussion is not well studied, experts recommend "decoupling" the discussion about brain death and talking about the possibility of organ donation (unless the family brings it up spontaneously).

Whether the counseling occurs at separate times, the initial discussion must be focused on the patient's condition, reasons why the patient has been assessed as brain dead, the reasons that the physicians believe this with certainty, and the allowance of time to absorb and process this information. Although time is of the essence in organ procurement and survival, the family's emotional health and understanding is a higher priority. Many times it is best to ask if someone from the organ procurement team can give them some information to allow the family to spend time asking questions, clarifying misconceptions about issues such as funeral costs after procurement, or physical appearance for a funeral or viewing. Above all, psychosocial support for the family must be the priority.

Conclusions

Basic medical treatment should not be withheld, but established medical and ethical practices should be performed. Respect for personal autonomy and informed consent are important when confronted with decisions regarding interventions with CPR. Issues such as whether to perform CPR or "do not resuscitate" are best resolved with prior discussion and documentation such as advance directives.

COMPREHENSION QUESTIONS

26.1 You are on duty at the emergency department. A patient is brought in by ambulance and the paramedics state: "Got no pulse." In which of the following clinical scenarios would it be appropriate to withhold CPR?

A.   A 28-year-old drowning victim with apnea and no spontaneous movement.

B.   A 32-year-old man with pinpoint pupils and tract marks on arm.

C.   A 46-year-old woman with breast cancer whose advance directive states no CPR desired, but her daughter tells you to do "everything possible."

D.   A 19-year-old man brought out of a burning building with no movement and no spontaneous respirations.

26.2 An 82-year-old woman with colon cancer and liver metastases was admitted for chemotherapy. Because of her poor prognosis, she is asked about a DNR order, but she requests to be a "full code." Which is the most appropriate management of this patient's condition?

A. Explain to the patient that signing a DNR order means she will need to be placed in hospice care.

B. Emphasize to her with compassion that a decision should be made in the next several hours in the event that cardiac arrest occurs.

C. Sharing this decision with family members is rarely helpful because guilt is often a complicating factor.

D. Discuss with the patient that a DNR order will not mean she will receive less care.

ANSWERS

26.1 **C.** Withholding CPR is generally performed in compliance with an advance directive, obvious signs of irreversible death, and with clear physiologic futility (which often takes time to evaluate completely). The 46-year-old woman with breast cancer and an advance directive is the most appropriate patient to withhold CPR, even though the daughter is insisting that everything be done. The patient's wishes generally take priority over family members' instructions. The other scenarios describe situations of potentially reversible brain dysfunction. Drowning victims may be successfully resuscitated even after being submerged for 30 minutes and sometimes even longer. A patient with possible heroin overdose may outwardly show absence of brain function, but may gain function with resuscitation and opiate reversal. A patient who has been in a burning building can experience smoke inhalation or carbon monoxide poisoning, but he or she should be resuscitated before a conclusion is drawn about possible brain death or physiologic futility.

26.2 **D.** This patient is elderly and has metastatic cancer. Out-of-hospital survival would not be expected should this patient require CPR. Thus, CPR for MW could be described as being a futile effort. The patient does not meet other criteria for futility. It is important that she is of sound mind. A DNR order should not be written even if CPR would be judged to be futile unless the patient or family members concur. Patients must be given time to understand the seriousness of their diagnosis. Periodically readdressing the question of CPR with patients and their family should be done on a continual basis. This is best performed in the context of other medical decisions that occur during patient care. The health care professional should emphasize that a DNR order does not mean that the patient will be abandoned or receive a lower standard of care.

> ## KEY POINTS

> ▶ Brain death is defined as the irreversible loss of brain function, including brain stem function, and is different from brain injury.

> ▶ Brain death is a clinical diagnosis and depends on the absence of spontaneous movement, brain stem function, and apnea.

> ▶ CPR can be withheld due to a valid advanced directive or when there is clear evidence of irreversible death (rigor mortis).

> ▶ Discussions about organ donation should be approached with sensitivity and only after dealing with the questions about brain death.

REFERENCES

Annas GJ. Standard of care — in sickness and in health and in emergencies. *N Engl J Med*. 2010;362: 2126-2131.

Cherniack EP. Increasing use of DNR orders in the elderly worldwide: whose choice is it? *J Med Ethics*. 2002;28:303-307.

Deutschman C, Neligan P. *Evidence-Based Practice of Critical Care*. Philadelphia, PA: Saunders Elsevier; 2010.

Holmquist M, Chabalewski F, Blount T, et al. A critical pathway: guiding care for organ donors. *Crit Care Nurse*. 1999;19:84-98.

Loscalzo J. *Harrison's Pulmonary and Critical Care Medicine*. New York, NY: McGrawHill; 2010.

Wood KE, Becker BN, McCartney JG, et al. Care of the potential organ donor. *N Engl J Med*. 2004;351:2730-2739.

A 63-year-old woman is afflicted with widespread metastatic ovarian cancer that has recurred despite surgery, radiation therapy, and chemotherapy. She has extensive pelvic and peritoneal tumor burden. The tumors are affecting her stomach and small bowel and encase her sigmoid colon. As a result, she has frequent bouts of small- and large-bowel obstruction and near-obstruction. These episodes are painful and cause severe nausea and vomiting. Her condition thus far has been managed by decompressing the upper gastrointestinal (GI) tract using a nasogastric tube, but the bouts are becoming more frequent, more painful, and more distressing to the patient. Furthermore, hepatic metastases are causing early liver failure. There are no surgical solutions for her obstructions, because her upper and lower GI tracts are severely affected. It is predicted that within 3 to 6 months, but most likely within 3 to 6 weeks, she will die of complications related to her tumor no matter what interventions are attempted. At this time, the patient is recovering from the latest and most severe episode of obstruction. She is just starting to take liquids by mouth, and she may be able to remove the nasogastric tube in the next few days. Everyone involved agrees that the patient seems mentally sharp, and no one questions whether she has the capacity to make medical decisions for herself. In discussions with her oncologist, the patient points out that the end of her life is almost certain to be characterized by severe pain and suffering, and, in her view, a lack of dignity. She asks the physician to prescribe a medication such as a barbiturate that will end her life painlessly at a time of her choosing.

- ▶ If the physician were to prescribe a medication for the patient to administer herself, the intent of which is to end her life, what should the act of prescribing most properly be called?
- ▶ Would such an act be ethical?
- ▶ Would it be legal?
- ▶ What are the alternatives in this situation?

ANSWERS TO CASE 27:
Physician-Assisted Suicide

Summary: A woman is facing the prospect of a death preceded by pain and indignity. She has requested a lethal prescription that she plans to administer to herself at a time of her choosing. The physician must evaluate the ethics and the legality of providing her with a lethal prescription.

- **The act of prescribing a lethal medication for the patient to administer herself with intent of death:** This is called physician-assisted suicide (PAS) or physician aid in dying (PAD).

- **Would such an act be ethical?** The ethics of PAS are controversial and unsettled. However, public and professional attitudes toward PAS appear to be shifting in favor of its permissibility as experience grows in the states that have legalized the action.

- **Would it be legal?** As of publication, legislatures have passed laws in 3 states that authorize PAS and describe preconditions and procedures for its implementation. These are Oregon, Washington, and Vermont. In Montana and New Mexico, courts have ruled in particular cases that state laws do not prohibit PAS.

- **Alternatives in this situation:** Alternatives to PAS include continued psychological support and adequate palliation of physical and emotional suffering, voluntary stopping eating and drinking (VSED), and palliative sedation.

ANALYSIS

Objectives

1. Define PAS.

2. Distinguish PAS from palliation of suffering at the end of life and from euthanasia.

3. Understand the ethical arguments for and against the permissibility of PAS.

4. Understand the legal status of PAS in the United States.

Considerations

When a dying patient requests a lethal prescription that he or she plans to administer to himself or herself, physicians must recognize this as an example of a request for PAS. Physicians must evaluate the competence of the patient and explore the reasons for the request. Whether PAS is legal or illegal in the physician's state, physicians should carefully investigate alternatives to PAS. Physicians must be able to distinguish PAS, which is legal only in some jurisdictions, from the palliation of symptoms, which is legal, and in fact required, in all jurisdictions, and from euthanasia, which is illegal in all US jurisdictions.

> # APPROACH TO:
> ## Physician-Assisted Suicide

DEFINITIONS

EUTHANASIA: When a physician administers a fatal medication or performs a fatal procedure for the purpose of causing a patient's death earlier than the death would have otherwise occurred.

PALLIATIVE SEDATION: Formerly called "terminal sedation," it occurs when physicians sedate a patient into unconsciousness for the purpose of alleviating suffering (whether physical or emotional) at the end of life. While this can result in death occurring sooner than it would otherwise have happened, the earlier death is not intended, nor is it required to achieve the palliative effect. Thus, palliative sedation is not the equivalent to euthanasia.

PHYSICIAN AID IN DYING OR PHYSICIAN-ASSISTED SUICIDE: These interchangeable terms refer to physicians who provide the medical means for a patient to cause his or her own death earlier than the death would otherwise have occurred.

VOLUNTARY STOPPING OF EATING AND DRINKING: Occurs when a competent patient voluntarily chooses to stop taking in enough hydration and nutrition to sustain life.

CLINICAL APPROACH

When clinicians receive a request for aid in dying, they must evaluate the request to fully understand what is being requested. Is the patient asking for PAS, euthanasia, or something else? The clinician must also be aware of the legally permissible options where he or she practices. With these facts in mind, one can evaluate whether the request can be honored both ethically and legally. Whatever the result of these deliberations, physicians must always attempt to understand the reasons for a request for aid in dying, and they must try to identify alternative strategies for addressing the patient's concerns without hastening death. In jurisdictions in which PAS is legal, there are some important procedural safeguards that must be observed, which are described further in the discussion below. Clinicians contemplating PAS should consult other colleagues as a way to ensure clarity of thinking and justifiability of their actions. In the section that follows, these issues are considered in more detail.

ANALYSIS AND DISCUSSION:

If the physician were to prescribe a medication for the patient to administer himself or herself, the intent of which is to end life, what should the act of prescribing most properly be called?

This would usually be described as PAS. This is sometimes called PAD to avoid any unwarranted connotations of the word "suicide."

When a physician provides access to a medical technique or medication that the patient will administer to himself or herself, the physician is not directly (or most proximately) causing the death; thus, this would not be considered an act of killing. One might describe such a prescription as "allowing to die," but this description is usually used when withdrawing or withholding a life-sustaining measure such as mechanical ventilation or tube feedings. Some would not consider "allowing to die" a plausible use of the phrase when physicians aid patients in causing their own death. Euthanasia occurs when a physician acts as the proximate cause of death, for example, by injecting a lethal medication intravenously or into a feeding tube.

Would such an act be ethical?

The ethics of PAS are controversial and unsettled. Much has been written on both sides of the issue. Arguments defending the permissibility of PAS rely on widely accepted principles in biomedical ethics. The following types of argument can be made:

1. **Respect for autonomy:** Since we all must die, we should allow each other some control over the timing and manner of death.

2. **Beneficence or compassion**: Suffering comes in many forms, both physical and emotional or psychological. Pain can often, but not always, be treated without intentionally causing death earlier than it would otherwise occur. The existential pain some experience with the loss of independence, loss of sense of self, and loss of function, can be as intense as physical pain. These types of suffering might not always be "treatable" without hastening death; thus, PAS may be viewed by some as a compassionate response to suffering.

3. **The diminishing duty to prolong life:** For a terminally ill patient, who, by definition, will die soon in any case, the duty to prolong life diminishes as death approaches. For some, the duty to alleviate suffering and respect autonomy will outweigh the duty to prolong life at a point before death would occur in the absence of PAS.

4. **Honesty and professional integrity:** There is evidence that PAS already occurs, even in jurisdictions where it is illegal. Physicians who violate the law by participating in PAS have an incentive to do so in secret and cannot discuss their activities without fear of legal repercussions. Legally permitting PAS would allow the practice to be done openly, with scrutiny by the public and by legal and professional bodies, so that it can be regulated properly to minimize mistakes or abuses.

5. The mere availability of PAS might help patients even if they do not go on to take the lethal medication. Patients who fear loss of control or unbearable suffering at the end of their lives are often comforted by the knowledge that PAS is available. Many who receive lethal prescriptions continue to live as long as possible, dying without ever using the lethal prescription.

The following types of arguments are often made that PAS is morally impermissible:

1. **Professional integrity:** Some believe that because historical ethical traditions in medicine, such as the Hippocratic oath, have forbidden the intentional administration of fatal medications, it should not be permitted. Some major professional bodies, including the American Medical Association, oppose PAS, due to the public perception of an erosion of the professional integrity of physicians.

2. **Potential for abuse:** Some worry that vulnerable individuals, including the elderly or those who lack access to ordinary care, will be pressured into pursuing assisted death.

3. **Sanctity of life:** This type of argument is usually rooted in religious traditions that claim that intentionally causing death is a violation of the "sanctity" of life.

4. **Fallibility of medical professionals:** Some are concerned with the possibility of error, because it is well known that both diagnoses and prognoses are sometimes given in error. Furthermore, physicians cannot always detect the factors that should indicate that a patient is not able to provide voluntary competent informed consent to PAS. For example, coercion by family members or severe depression might not always be easy to detect.

There is a deep literature on the defensibility of PAS and the issue is far from settled. However, PAS is increasingly perceived as permissible by both the public and by medical professionals. This is reflected in the gradual adoption of laws permitting PAS in various states.

Would it be legal?

In the United States, PAS has been legal in Oregon since 1997, in Washington since 2009, and in Vermont since 2013. The laws in these states are similar, and they have a number of preconditions and procedural requirements meant to ensure that PAS is performed properly, and only in appropriate patients. In Montana, a 2009 court ruling found that there is no public policy or law that would prohibit PAS, so PAS is considered legal but there is no statute describing the proper procedure. In New Mexico in January 2014, a state trial court ruled that PAS was permissible; however, at the time of this writing, the ruling was subject to reversal on appeal.

In the three states that have passed laws explicitly permitting PAS, the following conditions are set. Patients must be state residents older than 18 years of age and must be competent to make medical decisions. They must have a terminal illness (an incurable condition expected to be fatal within 6 months as determined by two physicians). They must be able to voluntarily express a wish to die. The decision must be informed—that is, the patient must be fully informed about the medical diagnosis, the prognosis, the potential risks of the prescription for PAS (usually a barbiturate), the probable result of taking the medication (death), and alternatives including palliative care, hospice care, and counseling. The patient's reasons for the request must be evaluated carefully, and alternatives to PAS that might help the patient achieve their goals must be discussed. A consulting physician must review the medical facts, confirm the diagnosis, and confirm that the patient is competent and is voluntarily requesting a lethal prescription. If either the original or the consulting physician has concerns about psychiatric factors that might impair the patient's judgment, then the physicians must refer to a counselor.

What are the alternatives in this situation?

Even in states in which PAS is legal, physicians must be familiar with the alternatives to a lethal prescription. It is likely that many patients contemplating PAS do so because they are afraid of conditions that have not yet materialized, but can be predicted to do so. If those conditions can be ameliorated without a lethal prescription, then, generally speaking, it is preferable to do so. Examples include treating pain or physical suffering with appropriate medications and palliative techniques; treating fear of abandonment with more engagement and perhaps counseling or support groups; treating the fear of loss of control with engagement or perhaps with hospice care; and reassuring the patient that he or she will not be alone at the end.

Many patients can hasten their own death without taking a medication to do so and instead act by VSED. By most accounts, this is a painless method that gradually results in unconsciousness and death over a period of days or up to a couple of weeks. Because this does not require a physician's direct aid, physicians cannot be accused of participating in PAS even if they remain engaged in the care of a patient dying after VSED. Indeed, physicians have an obligation to remain engaged to palliate any symptoms that occur.

Another option is palliative sedation. This is a procedure whereby suffering patients are sedated into unconsciousness to palliate their suffering. Because they are unconscious, they are not eating or drinking, and will necessarily die sooner than they otherwise would have. Palliative sedation is a preferred term for this practice, which is sometimes called terminal sedation. However, the word *terminal* implies that the purpose of the sedation is to cause death, whereas the procedure should only be performed as a way to palliate suffering that cannot be alleviated any other way. The fact that death will occur sooner as a result of the sedation is an unintended (though foreseeable) consequence. In other words, if the procedure did not hasten death, it would still be performed because it would still have the primary benefit of alleviating suffering.

COMPREHENSION QUESTIONS

27.1 JW is a 65-year-old man dying of advanced esophageal cancer. He is fed via gastrostomy because of his esophageal disease. His cervical spinal cord was injured after an epidural abscess formed in the context of his illness, and he is quadriparetic, having only minimal use of his limbs. He lives in Oregon, meets all the requirements for access to PAS, and requests a lethal prescription from his physician Dr Hansen. Dr Hansen, after JW pursued consultation with another physician, writes the prescription for a lethal dose of barbiturates. Because James cannot swallow and cannot effectively use his arms, Dr Hansen administers the prescription to JW via his gastrostomy tube. Which of the following is the best way to describe Dr Hansen's actions?

A. Dr Hansen merely allowed JW to die of his esophageal cancer.

B. Dr Hansen participated in PAS, also known as PAD.

C. Dr Hansen participated in the euthanasia of JW.

D. Dr Hansen provided palliative care to JW.

27.2 In states in which PAS is not yet legal, which of the following is not an obligation that a physician has toward a dying patient?

A. The provision of medication intended to alleviate physical suffering such as nausea, constipation, dyspnea, or pain.

B. Continued access to the physician's expertise and counseling.

C. Referral to appropriate providers who have the expertise to manage suffering at the end of life, such as psychologists/psychiatrists, palliative care specialists, and hospice programs, among others.

D. Provision of medication intended to cause a painless death.

27.3 A 9-year-old boy underwent surgery for mandibular hypoplasia. The anesthesiologist could not ventilate after induction of anesthesia and the boy experienced cardiac arrest. After 2 weeks in the intensive care unit, he remained comatose and ventilator dependent. Magnetic resonance imaging showed laminar necrosis, suggesting widespread death of cortical neurons. After long conversations with his parents, the decision to withdraw the ventilator and allow him to die is made. Which of the following represents good end-of-life care? (This case is adapted with permission from unpublished work of Robert D. Truog.)

A. The endotracheal tube is removed. The patient develops gasping respirations (8 breaths/minute). The mother asks the physician to do something, but the physician says he cannot do anything to hasten death. After 45 minutes of gasping respiration, the patient dies.

B. The physician administers 0.1 mg/kg of morphine sulfate and then removes the endotracheal tube. Every 5 to 30 minutes, he administers another 0.1 mg/kg of morphine, titrated to patient comfort. The patient appears comfortable. After about 2 hours, the patient develops bradycardia and then circulatory arrest.

C. The endotracheal tube is removed. The patient develops gasping respirations (8 breaths/minute). The mother asks the physician to do something. The physician administers 50 mEq of KCl by rapid intravenous push, resulting in immediate cardiac arrest.

D. The physician administers 2 g of morphine sulfate intravenously, which is a large dose that would cause an otherwise healthy child to die of respiratory depression. The endotracheal tube is withdrawn. The patient appears peaceful, makes no respiratory effort, and is pronounced dead 5 minutes later.

ANSWERS

27.1 **C.** When Dr Hansen administered the lethal prescription directly, he intentionally served as the proximate cause of JW's death. Because Dr Hansen administered the drug himself, his action is described as euthanasia. He cannot describe this as physician aid in dying because PAS requires that the patient himself or herself administer the medication. Answers A and D are not plausible descriptions of Dr Hansen's actions. Although it may be true in a sense that Dr Hansen was providing palliative care to JW, he was not just providing palliative care. Likewise, although esophageal cancer was the underlying, or ultimate, cause of JW's death, Dr Hansen did more than allow JW to die. In theory, Dr Hansen might have been able to arrange things so that JW could administer the drug himself (eg, using an electronic device that JW could activate to administer the medication via the gastrostomy tube), but this would be logistically challenging and might still put Dr Hansen in danger of being accused of too-direct involvement under Oregon state law. Physicians in Dr Hansen's position would be well advised to consult with legal and ethical experts before attempting to provide a lethal prescription.

27.2 **D.** Providing a medication for the purpose of causing death is considered PAS, and, at the time of this writing, cannot be performed legally in the United States except in Washington, Oregon, Montana, and Vermont. All of the other answers are obligations physicians have to their dying patients, regardless of jurisdiction.

27.3 **B.** The physician anticipates the possibility of air hunger or suffering after removing the endotracheal tube, providing a dose of morphine designed to eliminate the symptoms. Subsequent morphine doses are given for the purpose of alleviating any suffering. If the morphine doses in answer B hasten death at all, then this action is an unintended but foreseeable consequence, and, thus, is ethically permissible. In answer A, the physician fails to fulfill his duty to alleviate suffering, incorrectly believing that physicians can never hasten death. As the explanation above shows, as long as an earlier death is an unintended consequence of alleviating the suffering, it is not necessarily ethically prohibited. In answer C, the physician initially fails to alleviate suffering. He then does so, but only by acting in a way that can only be described as administering a lethal medication because KCl at these doses could have no other purpose than to hasten death. In answer D, the physician administers morphine, which definitely alleviates and prevents any suffering. However, the dose is so large that the physician cannot plausibly claim that her main or only purpose in choosing that dose was to alleviate suffering.

KEY POINTS

▶ PAS, also called PAD, is performed when a physician provides a lethal prescription to a patient who then administers the medication to himself or herself.

▶ PAS is legal in Oregon, Washington, and Vermont where legislatures have passed laws that permit PAS and specify preconditions and procedures for it. In Montana, courts have ruled that PAS is legally permissible but statutes that specify procedures for PAS have not been passed.

▶ Euthanasia is performed when a physician administers a lethal medication or performs a lethal procedure.

▶ VSED is an option for patients with a terminal condition who wish to hasten death without resorting to PAS or euthanasia (or when PAS or euthanasia are unavailable).

▶ Palliative sedation is a procedure whereby a patient is sedated into unconsciousness for the purpose of relieving otherwise untreatable symptoms. When this prevents patients from accessing hydration and nutrition, it will hasten their death; however, when PAS is performed for the purpose of alleviating otherwise untreatable suffering, it is permissible and is not considered euthanasia or PAS/PAD.

REFERENCES

Eddy D. A conversation with my mother. JAMA. 1994;272:179-181.

Nicolaidis C. My mother's choice. JAMA. 2006;296:907-908.

Orentlicher D, Pope TM, Rich BA. The changing legal climate for physician aid in dying. JAMA. 2014. 2014;311(19):1961-1962.

Quill TE, Lo B, Brock DW. Palliative options of last resort - a comparison of voluntarily stopping eating and drinking, terminal sedation, physician-assisted suicide, and voluntary active euthanasia. JAMA. 1997;278:2099-2104.

A 55-year-old lawyer collapsed and is unconscious in the courtroom, and he was rushed to the emergency department. There, computed tomography (CT) of his head revealed a large (> 100 cm³) intracerebral hemorrhage, extending into the lateral ventricles and associated with hydrocephalus. An external ventricular drain (EVD) was placed, and he was found to have elevated intracerebral pressure (ICP). Over the first 48 hours, the patient's ICP was difficult to control. After 6 days the patient remained in a coma and dependent on a ventilator, but with some brainstem reflexes (eg, gag reflex, blink reflex) intact. All of the caregivers involved, including the patient's wife, who is his legally designated health care proxy, recognized that there was no meaningful chance for a good neurologic outcome. A decision is made by all involved to stop the patient's ventilator, intravenous fluids, and medications, understanding that he would die shortly thereafter. The patient's wife then asks about organ donation, observing that the patient had long expressed an interest in organ donation and was registered with the Department of Motor Vehicles as an organ donor.

▶ Is it ethically and morally permissible to discontinue this patient's life support, knowing that he will die as a result? If so, how should such a decision be made?
▶ Would the analysis be different if the patient did not need a ventilator but only was receiving tube feedings?
▶ Would the analysis be different if the patient was in a coma and lacked all brainstem reflexes, including the drive to breathe?
▶ Can this patient be an organ donor?

ANSWERS TO CASE 28:

End-of-Life Ethics

Summary: A previously healthy man has experienced a devastating brain injury as a result of an intracerebral hemorrhage. Medical providers and surrogates must make a decision about life-sustaining therapy (LST)—in this case, mechanical ventilation. After a decision is made to withdraw LST, the question of organ donation arises: Can this patient be an organ donor?

- **Is it ethically and morally permissible to discontinue life support?** It is ethically and morally permissible to withdraw LST from a patient who has lost decisional capacity (or competence) when it is judged that the patient would prefer to forego LST.

- **If so, how should such a decision be made?** When a previously competent person becomes decisionally incapacitated, clinicians first consult any specific advance directives the patient made, and then ask a designated health care proxy to exercise substituted judgment on the patient's behalf. When no clear answer can be arrived at with these standards, the best interests standard is used.

- **Analysis if the patient did not need a ventilator but only tube feedings:** Tube feedings, whether administered through a nasogastric tube or a gastric tube, are considered medical therapies. As such, patients have a right to refuse them, and incapacitated patients can refuse tube feeding by way of advance directives, substituted judgment, or a best-interests analysis.

- **Would the analysis be different if the patient was in a coma and lacked all brainstem reflexes, including the drive to breathe?** In this case, the patient would be considered dead as measured by brain death criteria. In this case, physicians would not be obliged to continue LST, and the patient would be legally declared dead.

- **Can this patient be an organ donor?** If the patient were brain dead, then he might be a so-called heart-beating donor. If not brain dead, then he might be able to donate using donation after cardiac death (DCD) protocols, whereby his ventilator support is withdrawn, physicians wait for his heart to stop, and then organs are procured for transplantation. Eligibility to donate also depends on consent, either from the patient or a surrogate, and also requires that there not be any contraindications (eg, some infections, some types of cancer).

ANALYSIS

Objectives

1. Understand that competent patients have the right to refuse LST.

2. Understand that incapacitated patients also have the right to forego LST, although others must make that decision.

3. Become familiar with decision-making standards for the incapacitated patient.

4. Understand the different types of vital organ donation (beating heart donation using a brain dead donor, or DCD by a patient forgoing ventilator support but who is not brain dead).

Considerations

The patient in this scenario has lost decision-making capacity and has suffered a severe brain injury from which he is not likely to recover. Many would consider life in such a cognitively devastated state not worth living, and so a decision must be made about whether to continue LST. Because he cannot make decisions for himself, a process of decision-making must be followed. If he had any advance directives that specifically addressed his situation, then these would take highest priority in estimating what should be done. If there are no advance directives that help with the decision, then health care proxies must be asked to exercise substituted judgment on his behalf in an effort to make the decision he would have made. If neither advance directives nor someone who could exercise substituted judgment was available, then a decision must be made about what is in the patient's best interests, all things considered. In all such cases, it can be very helpful to enlist the aid of ethics consultants and others who can help direct the decision-making process in a fair and unbiased manner.

APPROACH TO:

Discontinuing Life Support

DEFINITIONS

ADVANCE DIRECTIVES: Instructions that a formerly competent patient left regarding his or her medical care in the event he or she was to become incompetent. Examples include living wills, designating a health care proxy, or even conversations with family, friends, or health care professionals.

BEST INTEREST STANDARD: This is used to supplement advance directives or substituted judgment in decision-making for an incompetent patient. Under this standard, decision-makers try to estimate what is in the patient's best interests, all things considered.

SUBSTITUTED JUDGMENT: This is when a health care proxy attempts to make the decision that the patient would have made, based on knowledge of his or her values, preferences, and approach to decision-making. Only surrogates who knew the patient prior to losing his or her capacity can exercise substituted judgment.

CLINICAL APPROACH

When making important decisions for an incompetent patient, clinicians must understand the various standards for making decisions and their ethical priority. When decisions are difficult or contentious, clinicians should consult widely, most importantly with ethics consultants, to help with decisions and to provide an independent check of their thinking. When a decision to withhold or withdraw LST is being considered, then clinicians must also understand ethical and moral norms regarding LST. In the discussion below, standards for decision-making and moral norms about LST are discussed in detail.

DISCUSSION

Is it ethically and morally permissible to discontinue this patient's life support knowing that he will die as a result?

Yes. Properly selected or designated health care proxies can withhold or withdraw LSTs on behalf of an incapacitated patient. This conclusion is widely accepted in the practice of medicine, biomedical ethics, and in the law, and can be defended fairly straightforwardly by recognizing following two principles:

1. Competent informed patients have the right to refuse any medical interventions, life-sustaining or not, even if it would result in their death coming sooner than it otherwise would.

2. Incompetent patients do not lose this right (but it must be exercised by others on their behalf).

These two principles are generally quite uncontroversial. The first is recognition of the competent patient's right to self-determination (also expressed as respect for the patient's autonomy). The second reflects recognition that patients without decision-making capacity should have access to all the options that competent patients would have, including the right to refuse LST. This reflects a deep respect for the rights of disabled or incompetent patients.

The tricky part is exercising the right to refuse LST on behalf of an incapacitated patient. There are some decision-making standards that should be applied in such situations. The following standards are arranged in a rough order of priority, from highest to lowest. When a higher-priority standard is unavailable, decision-makers must rely on a lower-priority standard.

1. **The patient's previously expressed wishes (advance directives):** This could be in the form of a specific document that details what should be done in certain medical situations (eg, a living will), or it could simply be knowledge of pertinent prior conversations with physicians, family, or friends.

2. **The substituted judgment standard:** Substituted judgment occurs when family or friends who knew the patient attempt to make the decision that the patient would have made, based on their knowledge of his or her values, preferences, and approach to decision-making. Only persons who knew the patient before he or she lost decision-making capacity are in a position to

exercise substituted judgment. Physicians cannot exercise substituted judgment on behalf of a patient they did not know previously. There is a rough order of priority when it comes to deciding who is in the best position to exercise substituted judgment. The order can vary somewhat from state to state, and not every state specifies an order in statutes. But in case law or in statutes, most states respect something like the following priorities, listed from highest to lowest:

a. Anyone that the patient previously designated as a decision-maker. This is usually done officially by way of assigning someone durable power of attorney for health care, or in some states executing a health care proxy that assigns a decision-making agent. When the patient did not previously designate someone, the remaining persons in this list are generally involved.

b. Spouse

c. Adult children

d. Parents

e. Siblings

f. Extended family members

g. Acquaintances

3. **Best interests standard:** Under this standard, decision-makers who do not know the patient's prior values or priorities try to make a decision about what would be best for this patient, all things considered. This standard is applied for patients who have never had capacity (children or the cognitively disabled), or when no one is available who knows the patient well enough to exercise substituted judgement on his or her behalf.

In the case described above, we are unaware of any advance directives that apply to this situation. The patient did designate his wife as his health care proxy, which reassures us that he made the conscious decision that his wife would be the best individual to exercise substituted judgment on his behalf. This patient's wife has to exercise substituted judgment on her husband's behalf.

Physicians and other medical professionals can help her by describing her role (eg, "Your job is to help us make the decision that your husband would have made") and by helping her to explore her husband's preferences and values through discussion and questioning. For example, clinicians might say things like, "Help us understand your husband as a person. What did he value most in life? How did he feel about medical care? About disability? About being dependent on others?" Such a conversation achieves several important goals. First, it helps clinicians better understand their patient as an individual. It also signals to family and friends that clinicians care about the patient as an individual, which can be very helpful in establishing trust that clinicians have the patient's interests firmly in mind. It helps focus the surrogate on the right questions—for example, "Would my husband want to be kept alive with LST, given the prognosis?"—rather than focusing on minutiae—for example, "How difficult or painful is the procedure for placing a gastrostomy tube?"—that only distract from the important questions.

After such a conversation, it is perfectly permissible for clinicians to make a specific recommendation if it seems clear what the patient would have wanted.

For example, if the conversation revealed that the patient was someone who highly valued his personal bodily integrity, his independence, and intellectual and interpersonal pursuits, it might be clear that he would not want to continue LST. If so, it would be reasonable for a clinician to say something like, "Based on our discussions, it sounds to me like your husband would not want to continue LST. I think what we should do is change the focus of our care to simply make him comfortable, and we should stop the things we're doing that are only prolonging his life, like the ventilator. Does this sound to you like a decision he would have made?"

Contrast this with an impersonal approach, employed all too commonly, in which clinicians simply describe the medical situation and the prognosis, and then ask the surrogate, "What do you want us to do?" This approach has one (somewhat dubious) advantage, which is that it allows clinicians to feel like they are "off the hook" in terms of moral responsibility for withdrawing or withholding LST, and it doesn't require a sometimes emotionally challenging conversation about the patient as an individual. It has major disadvantages, however. It can signal to surrogates that the clinician is indifferent to the outcome ("We'll do whatever you tell us to do"). It fails to remind the surrogate that her job is to make the decision that the patient would have made, rather than the decision that she prefers. Perhaps most importantly, it places all of the decision-making burden on surrogates, which can make it psychologically impossible for some to authorize the withdrawal of LST, even when it may be clear to all that the patient would have wanted it.

Would the analysis be different if the patient did not need a ventilator but only tube feedings?

Imagine that the patient was breathing adequately on his own but remained unconscious or minimally conscious, such that he could not be fed safely and adequately by mouth. In this situation, the only LST required by the patient is tube feedings (initially through a nasogastric tube, or later through a gastrostomy). Are surrogates permitted to withhold tube feedings on behalf of an incapacitated patient? Tube feedings (including water for hydration) are sometimes called artificial hydration and nutrition (AHN), or medically administered hydration and nutrition (MHN).

Again, the answer is yes. It is now well established in Western law, ethics, and the medical profession that AHN is no different than any other life-prolonging medical therapy. Competent patients have the right to refuse AHN even if would mean that they will die, just as they have a right to refuse ventilator support or any other medical intervention. Because respect for the incompetent patient requires that he or she has the same right, exercised through a surrogate, the wife in this case has the right to refuse AHN on her husband's behalf.

Would the analysis be different if the patient was in a coma and lacked all brainstem reflexes, including the drive to breathe?

Patients who have experienced an irreversible whole-brain injury that eliminates consciousness and all the brainstem reflexes, including the drive to breathe, can and should be pronounced dead on the basis of brain death criteria. In all the states of the United States and in most developed Western nations, death can be diagnosed in two ways. The first is using cardiorespiratory criteria. Perhaps obviously, a patient who has irreversibly lost the ability to circulate blood and/or exchange gases through respiration is dead. The second is by way of brain death criteria. There are formal procedures for pronouncing death by brain criteria. The brain injury must be irreversible. There must be no reversible conditions that could mimic brain death (eg, drugs, hypothermia, neuromuscular conditions producing paralysis). The patient must be comatose—having no signs of interaction with the external or internal environment. All brainstem reflexes must be absent. Finally, the drive to breathe, mediated by the lower brainstem, must be absent, as determined through an apnea test. Once these criteria are satisfied, then the patient is pronounced brain dead.

If the patient in this case were brain dead, then this would no longer be a case involving end-of-life decision-making, because no decisions remain, apart from the timing of discontinuing the ventilator and other medical interventions. Physicians are under no legal or moral obligation to continue LST for patients pronounced dead, because no therapy can sustain life in these circumstances. It should be noted that in two US states (New Jersey and New York), limited exceptions exist for families who do not accept the concept of brain death on religious grounds.

Naturally, after pronouncing death by brain death criteria, obligations to the family do not cease. Physicians are obliged to explain brain death carefully and sensitively. It is permissible to continue LST for a brief period even after brain death has been declared to allow families to understand the situation and say their last goodbyes. Pronouncing death by brain death criteria has implications for organ donation as well. This is discussed further in the following section.

Can this patient be an organ donor?

If the patient in the case were brain dead, then he could potentially donate all of his vital organs, including his heart and lungs. This is possible because brain-dead donors can serve as so-called beating heart donors. They may have their vital organs (eg, whole liver, pancreas, both kidneys, and portions of the gastrointestinal tract) removed even while circulation and respiration continue. This does not violate the dead donor rule (DDR), which states that patients must not be killed by the process of organ donation, because persons pronounced brain dead are already dead before the process of organ retrieval begins.

The patient in the original case is not brain dead. Although he is comatose, he still has some brainstem reflexes. Therefore, it would violate the DDR to retrieve his vital organs while his heart is still beating. However, he might be a candidate for DCD. In other words, after his LST has been discontinued, and after he is pronounced dead on the basis of cardiorespiratory criteria, it might be possible to procure some of his vital organs. In our case, DCD would play out roughly as follows:

1. The patient's wife and clinicians agree that the patient would want to withdraw LST.

2. Representatives of the organ donation system (not the clinical team) would discuss the possibility of DCD.

3. If a decision is made to pursue DCD, then the ventilator is discontinued while the patient is monitored for evidence of death by cardiorespiratory criteria.

4. If death (absence of circulation and respiration) occurs within approximately 60 minutes, organ procurement can begin.

DCD necessarily involves a period of hypoperfusion of the organs, which has two important consequences. First, DCD can only be performed for donors who are on ventilator support, because death by cardiorespiratory criteria must happen within 60 minutes (some institutions have a slightly longer limit, up to 90 minutes). Patients on tube feedings alone cannot donate using DCD protocols, because they will usually take days to die after tube feedings are discontinued, which would render their organs unsuitable for donation. The second consequence of the period of hypoperfusion is that the heart and lungs cannot generally be donated, and the organs that are donated have a slightly lower chance of graft survival in the recipient.

For some patients who die too slowly for DCD, tissue donation may still be possible. Tissues that can be donated may include bone, heart valves, veins, skin, ligaments, and tendons.

COMPREHENSION QUESTIONS

28.1 John, aged 49 years, had a stroke that rendered him incapable of making decisions for himself. Of the following, who is in the best position to exercise substituted judgment on his behalf?

A. His wife.

B. His parents.

C. His friend Steven, to whom John assigned durable power of attorney for health care.

D. His 22-year-old son.

28.2 Which of the following interventions cannot be refused by a surrogate on behalf of a patient?

A. Mechanical ventilation

B. Food and water administered through a gastrostomy tube

C. Antibiotics

D. None of the above (they can all be refused)

28.3 A 23-year-old woman has experienced a traumatic brain injury, and her family has decided to withdraw artificial hydration and nutrition, her only LST. Assuming she is a viable organ donor and made it known in the past that she wished to donate her organs, which of the following organ donation options may be possible for her?

A. All vital organs can be donated.

B. Most vital organs can be donated (eg, liver, kidneys, pancreas), but heart and lungs will not be possible.

C. No donation is possible.

D. Some durable tissues (tendons, heart valves, bones) could be donated.

ANSWERS

28.1 **C.** When a patient has not appointed a health care proxy, his or her spouse usually receives the highest priority. However, when a patient has specifically designated another person as his or her health care proxy, this suggests he or she had a reason to believe that that person would best represent his or her interests. After spouses, adult children usually receive priority, followed by parents.

28.2 **D.** Any and all medical interventions can be refused by a surrogate acting on behalf of an incapacitated patient. This includes artificial hydration and nutrition administered through a feeding tube.

28.3 **D.** The patient described is not brain dead; thus, she cannot be a beating-heart donor, which would allow for the potential to donate her heart and lungs. She is not on ventilator support, and so would not die quickly enough after withdrawal of LST to qualify for DCD. Once her tube feedings are withdrawn, she will most likely take days, sometimes up to two weeks, to die, which means her organs would not be suitable for donation. However, she could possibly donate some durable tissues that can remain useful even after a fairly prolonged period of hypoperfusion.

KEY POINTS

▶ Surrogates are permitted to withhold or withdraw LSTs on behalf of incapacitated patients (or patients who have never had decision-making capacity).

▶ The major decision-making standards for incapacitated patients are (in order of priority): (1) advance directives such as living wills, (2) substituted judgement, whereby people who knew the patient try to make the decision that the patient would have made, and (3) best interests, whereby people who didn't know the patient try to make the decision that best serves the patient's interests, all things considered.

▶ Hydration and nutrition administered through a feeding tube is considered a medical intervention and can be refused by a surrogate acting on behalf of a patient.

▶ Vital organs may be donated in 1 of 2 ways: (1) the beating-heart donor is a patient who has died, as determined by brain death criteria, and (2) patients withdrawing from ventilator support may donate some of their vital organs, but only after their heart has stopped in a process known DCD.

REFERENCES

Beauchamp TL, Childress JF. *Principles of Biomedical Ethics*. 5th ed. Oxford: Oxford University Press; 2001.

Bernat JL. *Ethical Issues in Neurology*. 2nd ed. Boston: Butterworth-Heinemann; 2002.

Meisel A, Cerminara KL. *The Right to Die: The Law of End-of-Life Decision-making*. 3rd ed. New York, NY: Aspen Publishers; 2005.

A 32-year-old woman slips and falls from a 10-foot ladder at work. Her coworkers find her awake and attempting to mouth words, but she is not capable of moving her limbs, and she is barely breathing. When paramedics arrive, she is unconscious and still barely breathing, so they intubate her. At the hospital, she opens her eyes spontaneously and appears to attend when spoken to. She can blink when asked but she cannot move her limbs. She appears to have no sensation below the neck. She is on ventilator support but is generating no spontaneous respiratory movements. When asked about pain, she indicates using blinks and facial gestures that her neck is very painful.

She is then medically sedated in order to obtain imaging studies. Computed tomography (CT) of the cervical spine reveals a burst fracture of the atlas, with bony fragments and soft tissue within the spinal canal. Magnetic resonance imaging (MRI) reveals severe edema of the upper cord from the level of the first cervical vertebra to the third. She is admitted to the surgical intensive care unit (ICU). Because she is sedated, the ICU attending and neurosurgeon approach the patient's husband and parents. The neurosurgeon indicates that the patient is very likely to be permanently quadriplegic and dependent on ventilator support. She recommends surgery as soon as possible to stabilize the upper spine to minimize pain and maximize the likelihood of some neurologic recovery.

To the physicians' surprise, the patient's husband and her parents unanimously refuse surgery. Moreover, they explain that they are certain that the patient would refuse all life-sustaining therapy (LST). The patient's husband has durable power of attorney for health care, also sometimes called a health care proxy, for his wife, and specifically requests that ventilator support be stopped and that she be allowed to die. The husband and parents all indicate that they have had prior discussions about spinal cord injury and disability with the patient, and that she has specifically stated that she "would rather be dead than [quadriplegic]." When the surgeon suggests waking the patient and discussing the matter with her, the family refuse, claiming that, "We know what she would want, and we're not going to put her through that. She would definitely not want to go through the trauma of finding out about her condition."

- ▶ Can the patient's family, acting as the patient's surrogates, refuse LST on her behalf, knowing that she will die as a result?
- ▶ If the patient were awake and refusing LST for herself, should her clinicians stop it, knowing that she will die as a result?

ANSWERS TO CASE 29:
Withholding Life Support

Summary: A young woman experiences a high cervical spinal cord injury and is quadriplegic and ventilator-dependent. She is extremely unlikely to ever regain motor independence or breathe without the ventilator. At the moment she is sedated for acute evaluation of her injuries, but we know of no reason she would lack decision-making capacity if she were awoken. Her husband and her parents state that she (1) would not want to be kept alive in such a state, and (2) would not want to be woken up to be informed of her situation or make decisions for herself.

- **Can the patient's family refuse LST?** Although it is usually the case that surrogates can refuse LST on behalf of an incapacitated patient, there are 2 strong arguments against honoring their request to stop her ventilator. The first is that this patient only lacks decision-making capacity because she is being medically sedated. Because she is able to make decisions for herself (at least as far as the clinicians and family know), then generally speaking, she should be consulted about decisions that will have major and irreversible impact on her life. The second is an argument that decisions to withdraw LST in the first hours, days, or weeks after a high cervical cord injury should be postponed.

- **If the patient were awake and refusing LST for herself, should her clinicians withhold LST?** Many experts in neurology and rehabilitation medicine argue that decisions to forego LST after a high cervical cord injury resulting in quadriplegia should be postponed until (1) some time has passed to allow the acute emotional and psychological trauma of the event to subside somewhat, and (2) the patient has had a chance to learn more about what their quality of life will be like in his or her new debilitated state. This amounts to denying the request of a patient who meets our usual standards for competence, which cannot be done indefinitely without unacceptably infringing her right to self-determination. Most commentators on this issue recommend a period of 6 months or more in a rehabilitation program before clinicians honor a request to stop LST.

ANALYSIS

Objectives

1. Recognize the settings in which decisions should be made by patients and distinguish from settings in which surrogate decision-making is appropriate.

2. Understand the arguments for and against honoring a request to forego LST in the acute time period after a high cervical cord injury.

Considerations

When approaching a difficult case one should try to identify the decision-making standards that should be used. Is this a case of a competent patient who should decide for herself? It would seem so in this case, but this requires recognizing that the sedated patient is *capable* of decision-making. If the patient has lost decision-making capacity, has she made any advance directives that apply to the situation? Has she designated someone as the best surrogate?

One must also identify the *range* of ethically permissible courses that could be pursued. If it would not be ethically permissible to withdraw LST, then this should not be an option offered to the patient or her surrogates. If the patient or her surrogates ask to pursue an ethically impermissible course, then clinicians can and should resist the temptation to simply acquiesce. Clinicians should ask for help in the form of ethics and, in some cases, legal consultations.

APPROACH TO:
Withholding Life Support

DEFINITIONS

COMPETENCE: This is used interchangeably with decision-making capacity to refer to a patient's ability to make medical decisions for himself or herself.

LIFE-SUSTAINING THERAPY: This phrase is typically used to refer to mechanical ventilation and artificial hydration and nutrition. However, it can also be used to refer to any therapy that is currently needed to keep the patient alive (eg, pressors, antibiotics, dialysis).

SUBSTITUTED JUDGMENT: The standard of decision-making wherein surrogates attempt to make the decision that the patient would have made, based on the surrogate's knowledge of the patient's values, preferences, and decision-making style.

CLINICAL APPROACH

In a difficult case in which patients or surrogates are requesting to pursue a course of treatment that the clinicians think is ethically impermissible, it is usually best to continue talking rather than take an action that cannot be easily reversed. Obviously, in this case, removing the ventilator would very rapidly become irreversible. Alternatively, if the clinicians insist on continuing LST, and even on pursuing surgery for the spinal fracture, the patient will still have the option later to discontinue LST. Continuing LST and performing surgery over the objections of the patient or her surrogates could obviously be contentious and lead to conflict between the parties. Clinicians should anticipate this, by being prepared to patiently explain their actions, and by consulting with others who can help the patient and family understand why the usual practice of honoring the request of patients, surrogates, or both to forego LST is not being pursued. This might include social workers, patient–family relationship professionals, ethics consultants, and, if necessary, legal counsel.

DISCUSSION

To decide on the most ethically defensible course of action in a difficult case, it is best to start by trying to identify the ethical principles at stake. By identifying the type of question we are facing, we make it much easier to identify the principles we should rely on when choosing a course of action. This also allows us to draw on experience from other cases sharing similar ethical features, and helps ensure that we reason consistently from case to case.

At first glance, this case appears to be a case of deciding for others, in which family members or surrogates who know the patient have to make medical decisions on the patient's behalf. If it is a case of deciding for others, then perhaps all we have to do is to ensure that the surrogates are well informed and are exercising substituted judgment (trying to make the decision they think the patient would have made, based on knowledge of the patient's premorbid values and preferences). If those conditions are met, and the family agrees that the patient would not want LST, perhaps the most appropriate course is to cease ventilator support and allow the patient to die, while also ensuring to palliate any pain or suffering that might occur as a result.

However, there are a number of problems with this approach. One very important problem is that the patient described here potentially has the cognitive capacity to make decisions for herself. As far as we can tell, the only reason she is unconscious right now is because she is being medically sedated. If she is only temporarily incapacitated, especially if we the clinicians are the ones incapacitating her, then we should not think of her as lacking decision-making capacity. If she *can* participate in important medical decisions, then generally speaking she *ought* participate in those discussions. This is all the more important when the decisions come with such stark and irreversible consequences.

Perhaps, then, the clinicians should wake up the patient and discuss LST with her? If she wanted to continue LST, then she would need the cervical fusion, but the main topic of discussion would be about whether she wants to continue living, knowing that she is very likely (though it's not absolutely certain) to remain a ventilator-dependent quadriplegic. Assuming she has capacity, discussing LST with her certainly seems like an important way to respect her autonomy as an individual. But, first we need to consider some important arguments against waking her up and letting her decide. One is the family's argument that waking her up and discussing the situation with her would be horribly traumatic to the patient, and could only result in the same decision. Another is a more general point about when medical providers should allow patients, or surrogates on their behalf, to refuse LST after a sudden traumatic and life-altering event such as traumatic high cervical quadriplegia.

In this case, the parents argue quite plausibly that, if the patient were to be awakened and learn of her situation, then she would be emotionally devastated. Furthermore, they say that they are absolutely certain that they know what her decision will be in the end. Regarding the decision to wake her up, they also claim that they know she would not want to be woken up to learn of her situation. So what purpose would be served by discussing it with her?

In a sense, they are arguing that *the decision to wake her up* is a decision that can only be made by her surrogates. And, because they know the patient best, they should be allowed to exercise substituted judgment on her behalf regarding the question of whether to wake her up. This may well strike some readers as a plausible and perhaps even a persuasive argument. Other readers will probably disagree, believing that surrogates should only be permitted to make decisions for patients when they are incapacitated by their injury or their disease. (Though perhaps such a reader would allow an exception when surrogates make decisions that can later be reversed. For example, one might say that it is permissible for the surrogates to consent to the fusion surgery on behalf of the patient rather than wake her up, because the surgery does not commit her to indefinite LST, but it would not be permissible for the surrogates to refuse LST, because this is obviously an irreversible decision.)

There are reasonable arguments on either side about what role the surrogates should play in making decisions for a patient like this one. So let us set this problem aside for a moment and consider the second problem: when, if ever, should we allow "competent" patients to refuse LST after a sudden and severely debilitating injury like traumatic high cervical quadriplegia? Imagine that the family consented to the cervical fusion. The surgery is performed without complication, and it is now 4 days after her fall. We wake her up. We manage (with some difficulty, of course) to establish reliable communication with her using communication boards with eye movements and lip-reading, and all are in agreement that she is fully awake and able to understand what is being said to her. Imagine that she is appropriately emotionally distraught, but able to pass any cognitive tests that anyone proposes, and she is able to understand her medical situation and prognosis, at least as it is conveyed to her by her care providers. Finally, imagine that she indicates that she wants the ventilator turned off. Should the attending physician immediately honor this patient's competent refusal of LST?

Generally speaking, physicians ought to honor competent patients' informed voluntary refusal of any therapies, even life-sustaining therapies. For many, however, this type of case is the exception that proves the rule. Many but not all clinicians and ethicists argue that patients who suddenly lose their physical capabilities should not be permitted to refuse LST until (1) a period of time has passed to allow the acute emotional upset to subside, and (2) the patient has enough experience with her new disability to consider her perspective to be informed.

This argument, it should be noted, is not an all-or-none argument. No mainstream ethicist would argue that competent and informed vent-dependent quadriplegics must be forced to continue living on a ventilator *indefinitely*. Rather, the argument is that some amount of time should pass, and some amount of information-exchange and learning should occur before a decision to discontinue LST. Most who take this position will recommend at least a few months before such a decision, and some argue that as long as 2 years are required before patients have sufficient emotional capacity and relevant information about life with their disability. It is well known that patients' perception of quality of life gradually changes after a sudden disability, and it is also true that nondisabled persons systematically underestimate quality of life with disability when compared with disabled persons' perceptions of their own quality of life.

There appears to be a tension between the principle of beneficence on one hand and the principle of respect for autonomy on the other. Beneficence suggests that patients should be kept alive for a time because at least some of them will come to view life as a quadriplegic as acceptable and worth living. Respect for autonomy suggests that competent informed patients should not be subjected to medical interventions that they refuse. Early on in such a case, the principle of beneficence has strong persuasive power—should we at least give her a *little* time to think about her situation before withdrawing support? Later on, the principle of respect for autonomy gains more and more force: "You can't keep me on LST against my wishes forever."

Whenever we draw a line (a few days, a few weeks, a few months, a few years), it will be arbitrary and will not fully resolve the tension between the principles. So now we see that there aren't any clear lines we can draw that will 'solve' the case, but we can identify some guiding principles:

1. Potentially competent patients should be permitted to participate in important medical decisions for themselves, particularly when the decision being contemplated is irreversible and consequential.

2. Whenever possible in the immediate aftermath of a devastating injury, decisions to discontinue LST should only be made in a deliberate fashion, after the relevant parties have had time to adjust emotionally and learn more directly about what life will be like after the injury. Most ethicists and clinicians recommend a waiting period from a few months to a few years after a high cervical cord injury before discontinuing LST. Ideally, patients in this situation should be allowed to learn about rehabilitation, and should meet other survivors of high cervical quadriplegia.

Both principles strongly suggest that the clinicians in this case should not simply honor the request of the family to turn off the ventilator within the first few days of the injury. Withdrawal of LST should only be seriously contemplated after the patient can be consulted, and only after an adjustment and information-exchange period has passed.

These conclusions are not uncontroversial. Some readers may even disagree strongly. This is a perfect opportunity to point out the importance and utility of consultation with parties who might have differing perspectives on such a case. Ethics consultation services are particularly helpful. Legal counsel might reasonably be sought. Experts in rehabilitation can be very useful, as can psychiatrists and neurologists, social workers, therapists, and others. No matter what decision is reached, when the stakes are high and there are widely divergent opinions among the stakeholders, it is wise to be slow and deliberate, making use of wide consultation.

COMPREHENSION QUESTIONS

29.1 A patient experienced a traumatic high cervical cord injury 1 week ago and is quadriplegic and ventilator-dependent. He is requesting that the ventilator be stopped and that he be allowed to die. The attending physician refuses to withdraw the ventilator until the patient is in rehabilitation and at least 6 months have passed. Which pair of ethical principles is most directly in conflict?

A. Justice and nonmaleficence

B. Respect for autonomy and beneficence

C. Nonmaleficence and beneficence

D. Beneficence and justice

29.2 Which of the following decisions should surrogates *not* be permitted to make on behalf of a patient?

    A. An elderly woman experienced a large stroke that renders her unable to speak or move the right side of her body. She cannot swallow without aspirating food or liquids. Surrogates believe she would not want a feeding tube placed and request that she be made comfort-measures only.

    B. A 6-year-old boy was hit by a car and experienced a devastating traumatic brain injury, with no reasonable hope of a good cognitive recovery. His parents decide to withdraw LST and allow him to die.

    C. A 37-year-old mother of 2 young children suffered a brainstem hemorrhage 2 weeks ago and she is almost completely "locked in" (awake and aware, but unable to move her limbs or her face, apart from small movements of her eyes and eyelids). She currently is on a ventilator using an endotracheal tube. Communication with her is extremely difficult, although she appears to understand what is said to her fairly well. If she is to survive and go to a rehabilitation hospital, she will need tracheostomy and gastrostomy. Once in a rehabilitation setting, it might be possible to improve communication with her dramatically, although probably only after weeks of effort and training. Her family wants to forego the tracheostomy and gastrostomy and allow her to die.

    D. An elderly man has advanced and untreatable cancer, and has now developed pneumonia. He needs to be intubated if he is to survive the acute illness; however, even if he survives and the pneumonia is successfully treated, he will probably only live a handful of weeks or maybe a few months more. His adult daughter has durable power of attorney for health care and believes he would not want to be intubated, even though it might prolong his life for a few weeks or months longer.

29.3 Which of the following is an example of substituted judgment?

    A. A mother provides consent for her 3-year-old child to undergo a medically necessary surgical procedure.

    B. A man has experienced a severe traumatic brain injury and is not expected to recover. His wife thinks he would not want LST continued, and asks that he be made comfort measures only.

    C. A woman with advanced cancer develops septic shock due to a bowel perforation and if she is to be kept alive will require abdominal surgery. Her living will indicates clearly that she does not want any "aggressive" life-sustaining measures such as major surgery or prolonged mechanical ventilation. Her medical providers, on the basis of this document, decide to palliate her pain and make her comfort measures only.

    D. A 35-year-old gentleman has been severely mentally retarded all his life. His sister is his legal guardian. He develops renal failure and requires dialysis if he is to survive. His sister consents to hemodialysis.

ANSWERS

29.1 **B.** Beneficence suggests that the patient should be kept alive, at least for a time, because there is a reasonable chance that he will come to view life as a quadriplegic as acceptable. Respect for autonomy suggests that he should be permitted to refuse LST whenever he likes, as long as he has decision-making capacity. These principles are in direct conflict. Nonmaleficence is the principle of do no harm and does not seem to conflict with beneficence, nor does it seem to conflict with the principle of justice, which has to do with the fair or equitable distribution of limited resources.

29.2 **C.** This newly locked-in patient may well have the cognitive capacity to make decisions for herself, and since communication with her may soon be improved in the rehabilitation setting, an argument can be made to wait until she is in rehabilitation to make a decision to withdraw LST. The patients in A and B have permanently lost decision-making capacity, so surrogates will have to make any decisions for them. Answer D is a difficult case. Because the patient could potentially regain capacity if his pneumonia is treated, an argument might be made that he should be intubated in hopes that he can later decide for himself about LST. In his case, however, he has a known terminal disease, will not survive long in any case, and, knowing that his death was near, he assigned his daughter as his surrogate. It would be reasonable for the daughter to forgo intubation on behalf of this patient and for the clinicians to honor her decision.

29.3 **B.** Substituted judgment is exercised on behalf of an incapacitated patient when family or friends, who know something about their premorbid values and preferences, try to make the decision that the previously competent patient would have made. In answers A and D, the patients have never previously been competent, so one cannot try to estimate what they would have wanted on the basis of their previously expressed values and preferences. In those cases, a best-interests standard is used in which decision-makers try to pursue the course of actions that, all things considered, best serves the patient's interests. In answer C, caregivers are relying on the patient's advance directive (a living will), rather than exercising substituted judgment.

KEY POINTS

▶ Potentially competent patients should participate in important medical decisions, particularly when the decision being contemplated is irreversible and consequential.

▶ Whenever possible in the immediate aftermath of a devastating injury, decisions to discontinue LST should only be made in a deliberate fashion after the relevant parties have had time to adjust emotionally and learn more directly about what life will be like after the injury.

▶ Most ethicists and clinicians recommend a waiting period from a few months to a few years after a high cervical cord injury before discontinuing LST. Ideally, patients should learn about rehabilitation and should meet other survivors of high cervical quadriplegia.

▶ The principle of beneficence suggests that patients who have a reasonable chance of an acceptable recovery should be kept alive using LST, whereas the principle of respect for autonomy suggests that competent informed patients should be permitted to refuse LST.

▶ When ethical principles are in conflict, ethics consultation can be helpful in resolving the conflict.

REFERENCES

Beauchamp TL, Childress JF. *Principles of Biomedical Ethics*. 5th ed. New York, NY: Oxford University Press; 2001.

Bernat JL. *Ethical Issues in Neurology*. 2nd ed. Boston: Butterworth-Heinemann; 2002.

Cushman LA, Dijkers MP. Depressed mood in spinal cord injured patients: staff perceptions and patient realities. *Arch Phys Med Rehabil*. 1990;71:191-196.

Ditunno JF Jr, Formal CS. Chronic spinal cord injury. *N Engl J Med*. 1994;330:550-556.

Meisel A, Cerminara KL. *The Right to Die: The Law of End-of-Life Decision Making*. 3rd ed. New York, NY: Aspen Publishers; 2004.

Patterson DR, Miller-Perrin C, McCormick TR, Hudson LD. When life support is questioned early in the care of patients with cervical-level quadriplegia. *N Engl J Med*. 1993;328:506-509.

Sensky T. Withdrawal of life sustaining treatment. *BMJ*. 2002;325:175-176.

Whiteneck GG, Charlifue SW, Frankel HL, et al. Mortality, morbidity, and psychosocial outcomes of persons spinal cord injured more than 20 years ago. *Paraplegia*. 1992;30:617-630.

MG, a 58-year-old man, is hospitalized because he has glioblastoma multiforme (GBM), an incurable and advanced brain tumor, and has become less and less alert in recent days. He was diagnosed 2 years ago and has undergone several surgeries, radiation therapy, and chemotherapy regimens. There are no additional treatments available that would slow the progression of the tumor. Scans reveal that his GBM continues to progress and is so widespread that it is causing increased intracranial pressure, which is the likely explanation for his waning level of consciousness. Seizure, infection, and metabolic causes of his diminished mental state have been excluded with appropriate testing. He is being treated with high-dose corticosteroids in the hope that this will reduce the swelling; however, his situation has not improved after several days. He is now so somnolent that he cannot eat, and he is not adequately protecting his airway and is at high risk of aspiration of his secretions. MG is currently receiving intravenous (IV) fluids and has been fed by nasogastric tube for about a week. He would require gastrostomy to continue his nutrition, and, as his risk of aspiration increases, there is increasing pressure to intubate him for airway protection. If this were done, it would be a temporary solution that would eventually have to be withdrawn or replaced with a tracheostomy. MG's wife wants everything to be done to prolong his life, including gastrostomy for tube feedings, intubation, and mechanical ventilation, followed by conversion to tracheostomy.

▶ Would tube feedings and gastrostomy for MG be futile?
▶ Would intubation, mechanical ventilation, or tracheostomy be futile?
▶ If MG suffered cardiac arrest, would cardiopulmonary resuscitation (CPR) be futile?
▶ What should be done to resolve disputes about futility?

ANSWERS TO CASE 30:
Futility

Summary: A 58-year-old man is hospitalized with end stage and untreatable GBM, an incurable and advanced brain tumor, and has become more somnolent. He cannot eat, and is not adequately protecting his airway and is at high risk of aspiration. He has been receiving IV fluids and nasogastric (NG) feeds for 1 week. He would require gastrostomy to continue his nutrition, and, as his risk of aspiration increases, there is increasing pressure to intubate him for airway protection. Intubation would be temporary and would eventually have to be withdrawn or replaced with a tracheostomy. His wife wants everything to be done to prolong his life, including gastrostomy for tube feedings, intubation and mechanical ventilation, followed by conversion to tracheostomy.

- **Would tube feedings and gastrostomy be futile?** Tube feedings, even by gastrostomy, would not be futile for the purpose of providing nutrition and hydration and prolonging his life (even if only a little). But, if they are performed for the purpose of facilitating MG's recovery, they are futile. This difference points out the importance of defining the purpose for which an intervention is futile.

- **Would intubation, mechanical ventilation, or tracheostomy be futile?** Intubation, mechanical ventilation, and tracheostomy would not be futile for the purposes of airway protection, ventilation, and prolonging life. But, if they are done to pursue a cure or a recovery to an interactive and alert state, then they are probably futile. When the word futility is used in the medical context, always ask, "Futile for what purpose?"

- **If MG suffered cardiac arrest, would CPR be futile?** Likely, yes. One could imagine a type of arrest for which CPR would be physiologically futile. For example, if MG developed sepsis and severe acidosis that then resulted in cardiac arrest, it might be true to say that CPR will not succeed in restoring circulation. In that case, CPR should not be performed. On the other hand, it is more likely that he would suffer an arrest for which CPR would *not* be physiologically futile (eg, reversible arrhythmia). If CPR could restore circulation, even briefly, then it is not physiologically futile, but it might be normatively futile. There is some professional consensus, though it is not universally shared, that CPR for a patient who is imminently dying of an advanced cancer should not be performed because prognosis is so poor in these circumstances that it cannot achieve sufficient benefit.

- **How to resolve disputes about futility:** Disputes about futility usually boil down to disagreements about which goals are achievable and among the achievable goals, which are worth pursuing. A sensitive discussion with the patient can usually resolve this type of dispute. Facilitation by an ethics consultation service may also help and should be encouraged.

ANALYSIS

Objectives

1. Learn the different meanings of futility (physiologic futility and normative futility).

2. Acquire the ability to distinguish between the different types of futility in a clinical case.

3. Appreciate that normative futility judgments are value judgments, not strictly "medical" or "scientific" judgments. As such, some deference is due to patients or their surrogates when they do not share the clinician's values.

Considerations

When patients near the end of life, disagreements about which interventions are worth pursuing are common. In this case, the dispute seems to be about whether prolonging MG's life is a goal worth pursuing. If so, then a careful discussion must take place with MG's wife. Does she advocate prolonging MG's life because she believes it will result in improvement or a cure? If so, then she may need persuasion (and probably some more time) to understand that this is unrealistic (and "futile"). Does she advocate prolonging life because MG firmly believed that life should be prolonged, even unconscious life? If so, this would be a value judgment that ought to be given significant weight in the deliberations, and it would not be true to say that life-prolonging therapies would be "futile."

Whether the dispute is about the medical facts or about the values of the patient, the surrogate, and the clinicians, the first step is always discussion. Many institutions have ethics consultation services that can help in these complex and often emotionally charged conversations. Others may be of help, including social workers, psychiatrists, counselors, and spiritual leaders. If discussion and deliberation do not result in agreement, then procedures should be established for how to proceed. This might include offering transfer to another physician, or to another institution, or patients/surrogates might be offered the opportunity to seek legal recourse.

APPROACH TO:

Futility

DEFINITIONS

FUTILITY POLICY: Many institutions have policies regarding how to handle disputes about which goals should (or should not) be pursued. These usually begin with continued discussion and are often facilitated by an ethics consultation service or others. They usually include offering transfer to other clinicians or institutions in cases of protracted disagreement. When agreement cannot be reached, and transfer is not an option, patients and surrogates usually have the option of seeking legal recourse, asking the courts to order clinicians to pursue the interventions they advocate. Whether a court would agree with the patient/surrogates or the clinicians will depend on the individual case.

NORMATIVE FUTILITY: An action or intervention is normatively futile when it could potentially achieve the end that it is designed to achieve, but it is felt that those ends are not worth achieving. For example, for a patient who is dying of a brain tumor and is comatose, mechanical ventilation would prolong life, but many would judge that a slightly prolonged life in a comatose state would not be worth it, and, thus, futile with respect to goals that the patient would endorse as being worth pursuing. If a patient felt that a few more days of life in a comatose state were worth pursuing, then such a patient would not consider mechanical ventilation futile.

PHYSIOLOGIC FUTILITY: An action or intervention is physiologically futile when it will not achieve the end that it is designed to achieve (eg, chest compressions for a patient with a ruptured left ventricle). Clinicians are never obliged to perform any physiologically futile interventions.

CLINICAL APPROACH

Futility is a term frequently used and almost as frequently misused. It is important to be clear, if only in one's own mind, about what is meant by the term. Strictly speaking, an intervention should be said to be futile only when it cannot successfully perform the function it is designed to perform. For example, chest compressions are futile for a patient with a ruptured left ventricle because they will not generate circulation. This limited sense of futility is called physiologic futility. Clinicians are never obliged to perform interventions that, in their medical judgment, are physiologically futile. The interventions being discussed in the case of MG cannot be said to be futile in this sense—tube feedings would, in fact, prolong his life; airway protection and ventilation support would prolong his life.

More commonly, however, the word futile is used to denote situations in which clinicians think an intervention should not be performed even though it could successfully achieve the purpose for which it was intended. This is usually because the patient's overall prognosis is so poor that the patient's higher-level goals cannot be achieved. This sense of futility is called normative futility because it involves (or implies) an argument that ethical or moral norms call for not performing the intervention. Therefore, if a clinician said that intubation/tracheostomy or another procedure was futile for MG, then he or she would really be saying is that because MG's tumor cannot be treated, MG will not recover normal consciousness. And, because the interventions cannot postpone death indefinitely, artificial respiration, surgical procedures like tracheostomy, and even resuscitation are not worth the burdens or harms they might entail. Note that this is not a "medical" judgment per se; rather, it is a value judgment about the worth of the extra life that the interventions might provide. This is not to say that such a value judgment is wrong or that a patient or family would not agree with it—in many cases, they would. Rather, the point is to understand when the term futile denotes a medical judgment (very rarely) and when it denotes a value judgment (very commonly).

It seems clear from the analysis thus far that "futility," unless it is further specified, is not a helpful concept. To be useful, one must always qualify the term by indicating the purpose—an intervention is futile *for the purpose of* X. It is only after understanding *purpose* X that one can have a fruitful conversation about futility. One could easily imagine the following type of misunderstanding between MG's wife and a clinician named Dr M:

Wife: "If MG can't eat, then we need to give him tube feedings."

Dr M: "MG is dying of his brain cancer. Tube feedings would be futile."

Wife: "I don't understand. If he can't eat, then we need to give him nutrition."

Dr M: "We see this frequently. We know all about this type of cancer. When it reaches this stage, tube feedings are medically futile."

Wife: "I still don't understand. Is there some reason his tumor prevents you from putting in a feeding tube?"

This type of misunderstanding is all too common in end-of-life discussions. It occurs because the person using the term futile is not being clear about the specific objectives for which the intervention is futile. Dr M is not explaining what he means by futile, which is that tube feedings will prolong MG's life, at least a small amount, but it will not allow him to wake up or recover—which Dr M assumes are the goals most worth pursuing. MG's wife, hearing the word futile, thinks Dr M is saying that tube feedings cannot be physically implemented.

A much better way to proceed would be for Dr M and MG's wife to talk about what the goals of care should be first. Once they understand each other with respect to the goals, then the language of futility might be helpful in describing what can or cannot be achieved with a given intervention. Imagine a different conversation:

Dr M: "Because MG is unconscious, we have to make decisions for him. I need you to help me determine what he would want us to do."

Wife: "MG is a devout Orthodox Jew, and he has a strong belief that we must fight for every minute of life, even if it's of little value to us, since in the eyes of God our lives are gifts that we must treasure."

Dr M: "Would he want an invasive procedure like a gastrostomy, even if he knew that he wouldn't wake up or recover, and that he wouldn't live more than a few extra days or weeks?"

Wife: "Definitely. He gave a lot of thought to these issues and we had very detailed conversations with each other about feeding tubes and whatnot. He would definitely want his life prolonged, even if it's only a day or two."

For many readers who may have begun thinking that tube feedings would be futile for MG, a conversation like this may lend a new perspective. In this scenario, tube feedings, even by way of a gastrostomy, seem like they would indeed achieve this particular patient's goals. Because gastrostomy *in and of itself* is not a particularly painful or expensive or otherwise burdensome intervention, a strong case can be made that MG's wife's request for tube feedings is reasonable. Even though the goal of "every minute of life" is not one that many people would endorse, it is a goal that thoughtful reasonable people can endorse—and one that cannot be easily dismissed by referring to it as futile.

Now consider the following (different) scenario:

Dr M: "Because MG is unconscious, we have to make decisions for him. I need you to help me determine what he would want us to do."

Wife: "MG is a fighter. He'd want to keep fighting."

Dr M: "From everything you've told me about MG, I do get the impression he's a fighter. But the way to fight now is to fight for the end that he would want, because the end is coming and we can't stop it. We shouldn't just postpone it, we should fight for his comfort and his dignity."

Wife: "Okay, how do we do that?"

Dr M: "We should do everything in our power to make MG comfortable. If he's in pain, or if he's fighting for air, our job is to treat those symptoms the best we know how. Anything else, like ventilators or tube feedings, that doesn't help us achieve that goal of a good end for MG, we won't do those things."

Wife: "You mean you're not going to feed him?"

Dr M: "We're not, because tube feedings wouldn't help us achieve what we want for him. In fact, they might even be counterproductive. He's dying, no matter what we do. But if we feed him food and water up until the end, then the fluids can accumulate in his legs, his abdomen, his lungs. And that can be painful and distressing. We're only going to do things that make him comfortable."

Now MG's wife may or may not be persuaded at this point, but note that she and Dr M at least understand what the other is talking about. Food and fluids will not help achieve the goals that we have already discussed and settled on. If Dr M wanted to use the word futility at this point, it might work—or at least it would not be grossly misunderstood. But note that it is not really necessary. As long as the goals under discussion are clear, it is easy to consider various therapies and assess what their impact on achieving those goals will be.

Special Case of Resuscitation

Some special attention needs to be paid to the issue of when resuscitation (in particular, CPR and defibrillation) should be considered physiologically futile, when it is normatively futile but subject to legitimate disagreement, and when there is fairly widespread professional judgement that it is normatively futile and thus should probably not be performed.

It's clear that in the case of MG, resuscitation would not be physiologically futile unless some new condition develops. If he were to go into cardiac arrest at this moment, it would most likely be due to an arrhythmia, which in many cases would be reversible. If there is a reasonable chance that circulation could be restored with resuscitation, then resuscitation is not physiologically futile.

Rather, in the case of MG, one would have to argue that resuscitation is normatively futile. That is, while it could potentially restore circulation and prolong life, resuscitation should not be performed because it cannot achieve the goal of restoring consciousness. The preceding discussion has indicated that normative futility judgements are matters for legitimate debate, and not strictly a medical judgement. In most cases, normative futility judgements call for more discussion, preferably facilitated by an ethics consultation service.

However, resuscitation is a special case. There is widespread misunderstanding among laypersons about the success rate and role of resuscitation, and there is widespread expectation that it should always be performed whenever circulation stops. However, in some circumstances there is widespread professional agreement that resuscitation should not be provided. The clearest example of such a consensus is in patients imminently dying of advanced untreatable cancers—physicians are not obliged to perform CPR and defibrillation in such patients, and many hospitals have policies that permit physicians to write "CPR not indicated" orders. The American Academy of Neurology has taken the position that resuscitation is not required in patients who are permanently unconscious due to severe brain injury.

So, does this mean that physicians can refuse to provide resuscitation to a patient dying of advanced and untreatable cancer in spite of patient or surrogate insistence that it should be provided? In short, yes, but clinicians must take some care to explain the decision not to provide resuscitation. It is best if the unilateral decision to not provide resuscitation is only made after a thorough discussion facilitated by an ethics consultation service, and clinicians will have more institutional support if they work in an institution with policies that permit such a decision.

If a decision is taken to not provide resuscitation, then clinicians should not continue to ask patients or surrogates for their endorsement of that decision, but the decision not to attempt resuscitation should be explained carefully.

COMPREHENSION QUESTIONS

30.1 Which of the following is an example of a physiologically futile intervention?

A. A 66-year-old woman with severe cardiomyopathy and advanced dementia is placed on a left ventricular assist device (LVAD) in order to augment her cardiac output.

B. A neonate with anencephaly is given a tracheostomy for airway protection and is fed via gastrostomy.

C. A 36-year-old woman in the persistent vegetative state is kept alive using tube feedings through a gastrostomy.

D. A 45-year-old woman has suffered massive chest wall trauma in a motor vehicle accident, and arrives in the emergency department (ED) pulseless. Echocardiography reveals a large rupture of the ventricular wall. No surgeon is immediately available. ED physicians consider whether to continue chest compressions.

27.2 Which of the following statements is true of normative futility?

    A. If clinicians believe an intervention is normatively futile, they have no obligation to perform it.

    B. Saying that an intervention is normatively futile is equivalent to saying that, while the intervention would work in a physiologic sense, it would not work to achieve worthwhile goals.

    C. Normatively futile interventions do not work.

    D. Patients or their surrogates must get a court order if they want physicians to perform a normatively futile intervention.

ANSWERS

30.1 **D.** In a patient with a large rupture of the left ventricle, chest compressions would not restore circulation even temporarily, and are thus physiologically futile. An LVAD in a severely demented patient would indeed augment circulation and is thus not physiologically futile. Likewise, tube feedings for the anencephalic patient (who will never be conscious) and the patient in the persistent vegetative state (who is unlikely to regain any consciousness) would prolong life by providing nutrition and hydration. They are thus not physiologically futile.

30.2 **B.** Normative futility is a value judgement. It implies that while an intervention may work to achieve the physiologic ends of the intervention, those ends are not worth pursuing. If clinicians believe an intervention is normatively futile, they may or may not be obliged to provide it. If the ends that can be achieved by the intervention are endorsed by the patient (or by a surrogate on their behalf), on the basis of well-considered and firm value judgements, then, ordinarily, the intervention should be performed even if clinicians disagree with the value judgements. Normatively futile interventions do work in a narrow physiologic sense. Patients or surrogates may be able to persuade the clinician that the reasons for pursuing an intervention are good ones, and that those reasons are consistent with the patient's considered values. If they succeed, then ordinarily the clinician would be obliged to provide the intervention.

KEY POINTS

► There is an important distinction between interventions that are physiologically futile and those that are normatively futile.

► Physiologically futile interventions do not work and clinicians are never obliged to provide them.

► Normatively futile interventions work in a physiologic sense, but are considered futile because someone judges that the aims that the intervention could achieve are not worth pursuing.

► When clinicians and patients or surrogates disagree about normative futility, this is usually an argument about value judgments. Thus, clinicians should be circumspect about arguing that an intervention is futile when what they mean is that the intervention could work is *not worth* pursuing.

► In some circumstances (eg, patients dying of advanced untreatable cancer) clinicians are not obliged to attempt resuscitation even when patients/surrogates insist on it.

REFERENCES

American Heart Association; International Liaison Committee on Resuscitation. Guidelines 2000 for cardiopulmonary resuscitation and emergency cardiovascular care: an international consensus on science, part 2: ethical aspects of CPR and ECC. *Circulation.* 2000;102(suppl I):I-12-I-21.

Beauchamp TL, Childress JF. *Principles of Biomedical Ethics.* 5th ed. New York, NY: Oxford University Press; 2001.

Bernat JL. *Ethical Issues in Neurology.* 2nd ed. Boston: Butterworth-Heinemann; 2002.

Burt RA. The medical futility debate: patient choice, physician obligation, and end-of-life care. *J Pall Med.* 2002;5:249-254.

Ebell M, Becker LA, Barry HC, Hagen M. Survival after in-hospital cardiopulmonary resuscitation: a meta-analysis. *J Gen Internal Med.* 1998;13:805-816.

A 28-year-old gravida 1, para 0 is in early labor. Her prenatal course has been unre-markable. Her blood pressure is 110/70 mm Hg and her heart rate is 80 beats/minute. She is currently at 5 cm dilation and having regular uterine contractions every 4 minutes. The fetal heart rate pattern shows a normal baseline fetal heart rate of 150 beats/minute with decreased variability and persistent late decelerations, indicating significant fetal hypoxia. Various maneuvers, such as positional changes, oxygen, and intravenous (IV) fluid bolus, are attempted, and the decelerations persist. The obstetrician recommends cesarean delivery due to the fetal heart rate pattern. She explains to the patient that the persistent late decelerations and decreased variability are indicative of fetal hypoxia, which can progress to acidosis and possible long-term neonatal organ failure. The patient states she wants a natural birth and declines to accept the recommended cesarean delivery. The patient's husband is concerned, but he has left the decision to his wife.

▶ What is the best approach for the obstetrician to take?
▶ What are the ethical issues surrounding this case?
▶ Is there ever a circumstance in which a cesarean could be performed without patient consent?

ANSWERS TO CASE 31:
Maternal–Fetal Conflict

Summary: A 28-year-old primipara with uncomplicated prenatal course, in labor remote from delivery with nonreassuring fetal heart rate pattern, indicative of fetal hypoxia. Cesarean delivery is recommended for fetal indications but the patient is refusing the cesarean delivery due to her strong desire for natural delivery.

- **Obstetrician's best approach:** Continue to closely monitor the fetal heart rate pattern and progress in labor and discuss recommendations for delivery with the patient. Document all discussions with the patient and her family. Sometimes involving another physician such as a pediatrician or another obstetrician can be helpful. Make sure the patient understands what the outcomes might be if the cesarean delivery is not performed. Maintain a nonadversarial relationship with the patient, even though you may not agree with her decision.

- **Ethical issues:** Patient autonomy and informed consent are at play here.

- **Circumstances when a cesarean delivery can be done without patient consent:** In the case of a pregnant patient unable to give consent (unresponsive/unconscious) with no known health care proxy, and the cesarean delivery is considered the only intervention to prevent imminent harm to the mother, then performing the cesarean delivery would be considered acceptable.

ANALYSIS

Objectives

1. Describe common ethical issues involving maternal–fetal conflict.

2. List key steps in working through maternal–fetal ethical issues.

3. Describe some circumstances when interventions such as a cesarean may be performed without patient consent.

Considerations

This scenario illustrates one of the basic tenets of medical ethics, patient autonomy, which is the principle that patients can choose what is to be done with or to their body. A patient is considered able to give consent for treatment if they understand the medical condition, the recommended treatment(s), the risks and benefits of those treatments and the possible outcomes if any of those treatments are not performed. Patients may accept the physician's recommendations or refuse them, and the physician should respect the decision. Although we often consider the fetus as a separate "patient," a fetus, even at a viable gestational age, is not a separate individual from the mother until it is born. This leaves the responsibility of decisions that can influence fetal outcomes to the mother alone. In the event when the patient does not accept recommended interventions, as is the case with this patient, it is important to maintain open lines of communication and not create a hostile environment. Any frustrations or antagonistic words should not be voiced by the obstetrician, and attempts to "strong arm" the patient or family are often counterproductive. The patient's physical and mental stress while in labor, which can influence decision-making should be considered. Having other health care professionals such as a pediatrician or another obstetrician can also be helpful. By continuing the conversation with the patient and her husband at regular intervals, in an honest and respectful fashion, there is a possibility of finding a compromise or a solution that may satisfy both the patient, her family, and the physician.

APPROACH TO:

Maternal Fetal Conflict

DEFINITIONS

DECISIONAL CAPACITY: The ability of a patient to make his or her own medical decisions.

INFORMED CONSENT: The process by which a patient gives permission for a treatment after obtaining information including the risks and benefits about the treatment.

PATIENT AUTONOMY: The right of a patient to make an informed decision.

CLINICAL APPROACH

The field of obstetrics provides many instances where medical ethics plays a large part in patient management. Under current US law, the fetus is not considered a separate patient until birth; however, many obstetricians feel a need to consider the fetal well-being in all decision-making processes. In almost all instances, medical decisions are made based on maternal desires and consideration of possible harm or benefit to the fetus. There are some cases where decisions made by the mother might pose a significant risk on fetal outcome. These types of situations can test an obstetrician's ethical principles whether it is in a case of a mother refusing a recommended intervention or a patient who makes a deliberate decision to continue using alcohol or illicit drugs during their pregnancy.

The 4 founding concepts of medical ethics—patient autonomy, beneficence, nonmaleficence, and justice—are often intertwined with decisions made in obstetrical care. Some experts in bioethics suggest that patient autonomy is the concept that precedes the remaining 3 concepts, but in many clinical instances separation of the concepts is unrealistic. Patient autonomy often plays a major role in how we provide prenatal care in the United States.

The basic goal of prenatal care is to optimize the outcome of every pregnancy. There have been many attempts in the recent past to recognize the unborn fetus as separate patient but this can challenge the right of a mother's ability to make decisions on medical care. By considering the fetus as a separate individual, authorities are enabled to criminalize maternal behavior that might be associated with fetal harm or adverse outcomes. Sometimes health care providers find it difficult to accept patient's decisions, particularly when these decisions are not consistent with medical recommendations. Physicians may try to rely on the legal system to force compliance; however, the courts have upheld the belief that a pregnant patient can make her own decisions, as long as she has decisional capacity. Legal cases have come under scrutiny as they try to criminalize maternal behavior such as alcohol use, drug use, or refusal of recommendations for care. Despite this, no US court of law has found any indication where the mother's decision has been refused based on possible adverse fetal outcome.

As we develop better imaging and fetal testing and therapeutics, it can be easy to separate the fetus from the mother as independent patients. Societal influences also promote this thinking. This concept can allow inflammation of the divergent behaviors (eg, those decisions that the mother makes that may have potential harm to the fetus, rather than promote the positive/congruent behaviors by the mother that enhance the beneficial outcome of the pregnancy).

A physician has the ethical obligation to respect patient autonomy, and pregnancy is no exception to this obligation. The condition of pregnancy does not change the rights of patients to have informed consent and bodily integrity. If the patient is not willing to accept recommendations for care, then it is the obstetrician's goal to encourage the pregnant woman to develop health promoting behavior(s), not to criminalize or punish her actions. Coercive and punitive policies are counterproductive; they may discourage any prenatal care or treatment. Compliance to recommended treatments or interventions may be limited by medical judgment of individuals, and there is never an absolute guarantee of any outcome based on an intervention or lack of one. Medical knowledge has limitations and even accepted recommendations or discouraged behaviors often do not yield expected outcomes. Obstetricians need to present balanced evaluation and expected and possible outcomes with and without interventions, based on data.

In some cultures community, family roles, and religious background play a large part of the patient's identity and can question some of the fundamentals of medical ethics. Pregnant patients may allow the husband or family matriarch the ability to make decisions on medical care. Some obstetricians may feel frustrated with this situation, feeling that the patient is not allowing her wishes to be heard. However, one can view this as an expression of patient autonomy in the context of respecting cultural values—the right of the patient to give the decision-making to another member of their family. In certain settings, this is appropriate, not because the patient lacks the ability to make a decision, but because she willingly gives the authority to another person as a way of respecting her place in her family.

Other scenarios that are common with patients from different ethnic backgrounds are refusal of treatment or delays in treatment based on cultural beliefs. In pregnancy, this may take the form of delaying a test or procedure that is time sensitive or refusing an invasive procedure which can give information about the well-being of the fetus. It is important that physicians respect these wishes and work with the patient to discuss options and a possible compromise. However, a patient who requests testing or interventions that are not indicated or are futile should be discouraged and the physician is not obliged to act on those requests. Physicians and especially obstetricians must be aware if a patient is of the Christian faith of Jehovah's Witnesses as the devout followers may not accept blood transfusions even if faced with a life or death situation. This should be discussed early in the pregnancy to accurately document what interventions the patient will or will not accept in the case of hemorrhage (eg, albumin, platelets).

Many patients use the information given to them by their physicians as the basis of making their medical decisions, which puts the physician in a unique position of being able to interject their opinion in the discussion. Some physicians may not be aware that they do this, but some physicians use it as a method to get the patient to accept an intervention. Such paternalism is not consistent with the principle of informed consent, which should be as free from personal bias as possible. Honest discussions promote good relationships between doctor and patient, greater trust and confidence in the physician, and greater satisfaction with care from the physician. All of these are reflected in better compliance with medical care, which can optimize the outcome of any pregnancy.

Informed consent is mandatory for any invasive procedure, but in its widest context, it is what a physician does at every visit with every patient. The explanation of the condition, both immediate and future, what testing is recommended, the risks, benefits and alternatives, and then the decision-making and follow-up are all parts of a comprehensive patient visit. It is a key aspect to any therapeutic relationship and especially important in the field of obstetrics. This is due to the fact that the physician sees the patient for many visits in preparation for a known acute event (eg, delivery). The development of a durable trusting relationship helps with patient compliance, and in any pregnancy, there are many instances where a normal pregnancy can change to a high-risk situation. If the relationship between patient and physician is strained, then a management plan that is acceptable to both the obstetrician and the patient may be difficult to obtain. Collaboration between the doctor and patient is of utmost importance in achieving an acceptable plan and optimizing the prenatal care.

Patients have responsibilities in this equation also. Once a plan is agreed upon, they have to fulfill their piece of the arrangement (eg, adhering to medication regimens, alterations in diet, appointments with other physicians if needed). All of this is dependent on the patient being able to give consent or permission for treatment. There are many reasons why a patient is not able to make a decision about their medical care. Sometimes it is simply a language barrier, and an interpreter provided by the facility (eg, hospital, clinic) will suffice. However, the patient's family should not be used for primary interpretive service as you cannot be sure of their level of medical knowledge and if the translation is accurate. Other considerations when you are questioning a patient's ability to consent are the patient's ability to comprehend the situation based on intelligence, the emotional state and the medical condition of the patient. Age also may be a factor, and in some states, if a patient is pregnant, she is considered an emancipated minor and can make medical decisions for herself without parental involvement. Age of consent, which is the age after which a child can make decisions for themselves, varies from state to state, but it is usually 14 to 18 years of age.

Who can consent for treatment when a patient cannot? If the patient is deemed incompetent or lacking the ability to make medical decisions, a close family member or friend or an appointed proxy can be the patient's surrogate. There are cases where a patient is "unrepresented" or "unbefriended" and the institution has to appeal to the legal system to appoint a proxy to make health care decisions. In emergency situations, including obstetrics, if an intervention is the best life-saving measure for the patient, and there is no one to consent to this, the physician can act in the best interests of the patient and perform the procedure or treatment. In theory, this should be able to be done without much debate. In practice, there is much controversy when a situation like this arises. Who makes the decision regarding the best intervention? There are many unknowns in medicine and "expert opinions" vary based on individuals, institutions, and geographic regions. Life-saving measures apply to the mother, not the fetus, which can also question the decisions being made.

COMPREHENSION QUESTIONS

31.1 A 26-year-old gravida 1 para 0 patient at term is evaluated on labor and delivery and is found to be in early labor. The fetal heart tracing is reassuring and she has had an unremarkable prenatal course. Upon admission, she tells you she is a Jehovah's Witness and will not accept a blood transfusion. Which of the following is not a recommended step in her management?

A. Document your conversation in the patient's chart and inform the appropriate patient care team members.

B. Ask the patient if she will accept any blood or tissue products and, if yes, which ones.

C. Try to convince the patient that it can be detrimental to her or her baby and that she should reconsider.

D. Tell the patient that you respect her wishes, and ask her if she would like to be made aware if at any time a blood transfusion would be recommended so she has the ability to change her decision.

31.2 A 32-year-old woman arrives at your clinic for a first prenatal visit. She is accompanied by the father of the baby and her mother. They recently arrived to the United States from Pakistan and the patient and her mother have a very limited comprehension of English. The father of the baby has a better command of English but does not comprehend some of the medical terms. What is the best way to continue with this patient visit?

A. Secure a medical interpreter through the clinic either in person or by telephone.

B. Continue using the father of the baby as the interpreter.

C. Reschedule the appointment for another time when you can find someone to interpret.

D. Do a limited examination and give the patient some material to read and instruct her to look on the Internet for information about prenatal care in her native language.

31.3 A 15-year-old pregnant patient arrives by ambulance to labor and delivery after being involved in a motor vehicle collision. The patient receives prenatal care at your hospital and she is at 23 weeks 0 days gestation; she was dated by an early first trimester sonogram. She is unresponsive and is quickly diagnosed with a massive intra-abdominal bleed from an unknown source. Her vital signs are consistent with hypovolemic shock. The trauma surgeons are recommending immediate surgery to look for the injury and correct the bleeding, but there is no one with the patient and attempts at contacting the family are unsuccessful. There is also a question regarding how this type of procedure will affect the fetus. What is the next best step in management?

A. Proceed with the surgery as it is considered life saving for the patient.

B. Continue to seek out family members who can give consent for the patient.

C. Do not do the surgery as it may potentially harm the fetus.

D. Ask for a second opinion to see if there are any alternatives to the surgery.

ANSWERS

31.1 **C.** Patients who are followers of the Jehovah's Witness faith are aware of the risks involved with refusing transfusions, and trying to convince the patient to accept blood is rarely successful. It would be beneficial to support the patient's decisions and maintain a respectful and supportive relationship with the patient, with the possibility of acceptance of other blood products if that is recommended at any point in her care.

31.2 **A.** Family members should not be used as interpreters unless it is an emergency and there is no alternative. Hospitals and clinics have provisions for interpreting services for many languages and these interpreters are specific for medical interpretation. The accuracy of the discussion is maintained and you are assured the patient has gotten correct information.

31.3 **A.** If it is truly a life-saving measure, as in this patient, then surgery can proceed without consent because you are acting on behalf of the best interests of the patient. Consent is not necessary and the well-being of the fetus is not a factor in the decision. Waiting for another opinion or to seek out other family members who can make the decision may result in more serious outcomes for the patient and cannot be justified.

> ## KEY POINTS

> ▶ Patient autonomy allows a competent patient the ability to consent for treatment or refuse treatment, and this should be respected by the physician. Pregnant patients are no exception and the mother can act on behalf of the unborn fetus. The fetus is not recognized as a separate individual until it is born.

> ▶ The patient's cultural and religious beliefs often are part of the medical decision-making process, in addition to the recommendations made by her physician.

> ▶ Informed consent should be a process that is as free from physician bias as possible.

> ▶ It is of utmost importance for physicians to maintain a good communicative relationship with a patient, even if the recommended medical treatment is refused by the patient. Collaboration and compromise may be a solution to maintain a level of medical care that is acceptable by both parties.

> ▶ In life-saving situations, if the patient themselves cannot consent for treatment and there is no other person to speak for the patient, the medical team can provide treatment and interventions in the best interests of the patient.

REFERENCES

American College of Obstetrics and Gynecologists. Ethical decision making in Oobstetrics and gynecology. ACOG committee opinion no. 390. *Obstet Gynecol.* 2007;110:1479-1487.

American College of Obstetrics and Gynecologists. Maternal decision making, ethics, and the law. ACOG committee opinion no 321. *Obstet Gynecol.* 2005;106:1127-1137.

Annas G, Elias S. Legal and ethical issues in obstetrical practice. In: Gabbe S, Niebyl J, Simpson J, et al. eds. *Gabbe: Obstetrics: Normal and Problem Pregnancies.* 6th ed. Philadelphia, PA: Saunders; 2012:1200-1211.

Minkoff H. Teaching ethics: when respect for autonomy and cultural sensitivity collide. *Am J Obstet Gynecol.* 2014;210:298-301.

Patient preferences. In: Jonsen AR, Siegler M, Winslade WJ. eds. *Clinical Ethics: A Practical Approach to Ethical Decisions in Clinical Medicine.* 7th ed. New York, NY: McGraw-Hill; 2010.

BJ, a 2910-g male infant, was born at 38 weeks of gestation. His mother is a healthy married woman aged 34 years. During this pregnancy, polyhydramnios was found, but ultrasonography did not reveal evidence of an upper gastrointestinal obstruction. The parents were also counseled that the condition could result from a neurologic abnormality or condition resulting in diminished swallowing during fetal life. The parents themselves had also researched the possible causes on the Internet before birth. At birth, BJ emerged with a weak cry, profound hypotonia, and limited spontaneous movement. His respiratory status deteriorated and it was determined that he would probably require intubation and mechanical ventilation. The care team indicated to the parents that they were going to intubate the baby. They explained that they were very concerned about severe neurologic injury, such as an intracranial hemorrhage or malformation, and were embarking on evaluation. The parents disagreed with the plan to intubate. They had been worried about the cause of the polyhydramnios since the diagnosis had first been made weeks earlier, and they were convinced that it was wrong to put their son through invasive medical care if his neurologic outcome was going to be poor. They asked that intubation not be performed, that intensive support be withdrawn, and that their son be allowed to die peacefully and comfortably. The care team expressed understanding of the parents' worries but strongly made the point that there was, in their opinion, not yet enough evidence to make a decision of this sort. They explained that many of the causes of neonatal hypotonia are not fatal and are compatible with a reasonable if not normal quality of life. They asked the parents to delay a decision to forego life support until a full evaluation was completed. The attending physician made it clear that if the evaluation revealed a cause that was incompatible with a meaningful life, the care team would then be willing to limit care to comfort alone and withdraw life support. After some deliberation, the parents agreed to this plan. BJ was intubated but only required mechanical ventilation for a few hours, but he continued to have poor tone and minimal suck. A few days later chromosome analysis confirmed Prader-Willi syndrome, which is characterized by short stature and variable degree of intellectual disability (moderate to severe). The hypotonia and poor feeding in early infancy usually resolve. Patients usually develop hyperphagia, frequently resulting in obesity. Life expectancy can be normal and intellectual function is variably diminished. Once the diagnosis was established, the care team again met with the parents, who reiterated their desire that supportive care, including fluids and nutrition, be withdrawn and all efforts be focused on comfort alone.

▶ Would it be permissible to withdraw or withhold life support from BJ?
▶ How do we decide about care for patients who lack the capacity to speak for themselves?
▶ What are the limits of parental authority regarding the care of newborns?

ANSWERS TO CASE 32:
Neonatal Intensive Care Unit (NICU) Ethics

Summary: BJ is born at term gestation, with polyhydramnios noted, and found to have a weak cry, profound hypotonia, and limited spontaneous movement. Several hours after birth, his respiratory status deteriorated and he required intubation and mechanical ventilation. The physicians were concerned about neurologic injury. The parents refused, because "it was wrong to put their son through invasive medical care if his neurological outcome was going to be poor." The care providers explained that many of the causes of neonatal hypotonia are not fatal and are compatible with a reasonable if not normal quality of life. BJ was intubated but only required mechanical ventilation for a few hours. He continued to have poor tone and minimal suck. A few days later, chromosome analysis confirmed Prader-Willi syndrome. Once the diagnosis was established, the care team again met with the parents, who reiterated their desire that supportive care, including fluids and nutrition, be withdrawn and all efforts be focused on only comfort measures.

- **Would it be permissible to withhold or withdraw life support from BJ?** Likely not in this case. Put another way, does a diagnosis of Prader-Willi syndrome portend such a compromised life that allowing BJ to die might be the kindest, most compassionate or reasonable thing to do? It is broadly accepted that there are circumstances in which allowing death is the best option. Typically, however, these are conditions in which death is likely in any case, or conditions in which no hope of a meaningful life exists. This cannot be said of Prader-Willi syndrome. Although the cognitive limitations in Prader-Willi syndrome can be severe, they can also be moderate, and there are many individuals with Prader-Willi syndrome whose lives are well worth living. Given the uncertain prognosis in the case of BJ, it would not seem to be permissible to withhold or withdraw life support.

- **How do we decide about care for patients who lack the capacity to speak for themselves?** In adults who were previously competent, we usually try to exercise *substituted judgment* by looking for information that gives us the best sense of what an individual might choose. This information is gained from how they have lived their life, and any wishes, or opinions they have expressed about what they might want in different clinical situations. Obviously, there is no such information or accumulated life experience for newborns, who have never been competent, and we must rely on a best interests standard, for example, what would be in the best interests of BJ, all things considered? Because parents usually have the best interests of their children in mind, we tend to rely heavily on parental judgment, usually deferring to the wishes of the parents.

- **What are the limits of parental authority regarding the care of newborns?** Although we usually defer to parents about the best interests of their children, parental authority is not limitless. Although parental autonomy is an important principle, it can conflict strongly with the principles of beneficence and non-maleficence. Certainly respect for autonomy does not require that clinicians honor a request for something that is clearly harmful to the patient.

ANALYSIS

Objectives

1. Understand that in making decisions about the care of compromised newborns, the same basic ethical principles of autonomy, beneficence, nonmaleficence, and justice apply as in adults.

2. Recognize that parental role and rights in making decisions for their newborn are not limitless.

3. Understand the differences between "substituted judgment" and a "best interest" standard in decision-making, and the circumstances in which each is appropriate.

4. Develop a framework through which one can analyze the conflicts that may exist between autonomy, beneficence, and nonmaleficence and use it in understanding decisions about care and support.

5. Understand that the goal in decision-making is not always to find an absolute answer, but rather to allow all stake holders to explore decisions and work together to find a best answer and approach.

Considerations

In the case of patients who lack the capacity to speak for themselves, such as newborns, decisions must often rely on substituted judgment based on information about the patient's own ideas and conclusions about what they would want done in a particular situation. As for older children and adults, the decisions that are made are guided by the same four fundamental principles: respect for autonomy (recognizing and supporting the individual's right to choose), beneficence (offering care with the potential to do good for the patient), nonmaleficence (to the greatest extent, avoidance of things that are harmful, or harmful without potential benefit), and justice (the provision of care that is fair to all patients and reflects the most reasonable distribution of resources. The special challenges in the care of newborns include the fact that no patient has the capacity to speak for himself or herself, and, indeed, infants lack any life experience that might help us discern their wishes or shape their choice. In general, caregivers look to the parents of the newborn for guidance in these decisions, and almost always they are the most appropriate surrogate decision-makers. We recognize that most parents are deeply invested in ensuring the "best" for their child, and that the views of children are in general driven by or patterned after those of parents. At the same time, caregivers are bound by the obligation to serve as advocates for their patient, and in so doing may reach different conclusions or decisions than do the parents. Most often, these differences can be resolved by sharing information and facts pertinent to the case and engaging in an on-going dialogue through repeated conversations. When this fails, consultation by the hospital ethics service is often helpful. Only if no conclusion can be reached is it necessary to engage the legal system for resolution.

In the approach to this case, we recognize that we do not have this information for a newborn with no accumulated life experience or capacity to speak or make decisions. We instead look first to parents as a guide for what an infant might want, but we maintain impartial advocacy for the patient himself; therefore, we must test such parental decisions against basic ethical principles and societal norms, while considering if such decisions are defensible when viewed against a best interest standard.

APPROACH TO:

Forgoing Life Support In Newborns

DEFINITIONS

BEST INTERESTS STANDARD: Medical decisions are made by deliberating about what is in the best interests of the patient, all things considered, in patients who have never had decision-making capacity. For newborns and children, parents are usually considered the best judges of what the best interests standard requires.

FUTILITY: A futile action or therapy is one that will not ever result in any benefit. Because there are many uncertainties in clinical medicine, it is rarely possible to absolutely define an action as futile, and the closest one may get is to determine that something is "most likely" or "overwhelmingly likely" to have no benefit.

SHARED DECISION-MAKING: A process of clinical decision-making that relies on the joint participation of caregivers and the patient or surrogate. It is recognized that the caregivers are expert in the medical care and are best able to offer a determination of prognosis and likelihood of various outcomes. For newborns, the parents are recognized to have the expertise and framework to interpret the medical information in terms of what it will mean for their child and what impact the different outcomes will have for their child.

CLINICAL APPROACH

Determining the best or right thing to do for a particular patient begins with the accumulation of as much factual information as possible. Simply put, good ethics depends on good facts. In a case such as this, this meant a concerted effort to determine the diagnosis and prognosis. Multiple consultants were approached for help in determining the underlying cause of hypotonia. Rapid genetic testing using fluorescent in situ hybridization quickly identified a deletion in 15q11, making the diagnosis of Prader-Willi. Once the diagnosis was made, several consultants familiar with Prader-Willi syndrome were asked to provide an expert opinion about the prognosis in BJ's case. All of the clinicians and consultants involved concluded that no definitive predictions could be made about the severity of BJ's cognitive limitations.

Because prognosis was uncertain, and because the range of uncertainty included a significant chance of a good-quality life for BJ, the clinicians all felt that it would be inappropriate to withhold or withdraw life support. Ethics consultation was requested, and the ethics consultants agreed with this conclusion. They felt that the principles of beneficence and nonmaleficence obliged the clinicians to continue life support, even though this arguably required over-riding parental autonomy.

Once this decision was reached, the remainder of the case involved helping the parents to understand the ethical and moral reasoning behind this conclusion. Frequent frank and open discussions with the family were conducted. The main purpose of these discussions was to help their understanding and acceptance, but alternatives such as legal recourse and attempts to transfer to another institution were discussed.

ANALYSIS AND DISCUSSION

The approach focused on frank and open discussions with the parents and their family members. Given the difference of opinion over the right thing to do, it was critically important for everyone to realize that a single discussion was unlikely to be sufficient. Everyone needed to realize that different people reach conclusions at different rates. Oftentimes, caregivers reach a conclusion more quickly than do families, largely because they have the benefit of experience and a ready understanding of the evolving facts of the case.

In this case, the parents had a prolonged period during the latter part of the pregnancy to read about and understand the possible causes of the polyhydramnios and limited fetal movement. They had already decided that, if the diagnosis entailed severe cognitive limitations, then they would not want their child to undergo life-sustaining measures such as mechanical ventilation or artificial hydration and nutrition. However, in BJ's case, the prognosis did not clearly indicate that he would have severe cognitive limitations and instead included a significant probability of a good quality of life, despite moderate cognitive limitations. This was a possibility they had not fully considered prior to delivery, and they would need some time to better understand what the diagnosis of Prader-Willi syndrome entailed.

Although the clinicians and the family disagreed, they committed to keep meeting and discussing the options. This ensured that the avenues of communication were open and that each group understood the position of the other. In this way, the therapeutic relationship was maintained and discussion could continue in the hopes of reaching a mutually satisfactory conclusion.

Early in the discussions, the family asked about their legal rights. The attending physician made it clear that they could pursue a legal course of action, but he discouraged it for a few reasons. First, he believed that continued discussions among the people close to the case (caregivers and family) could result in a conclusion with the help of the ethics consultants. Second, he felt that leaving the question in the hands of the court would actually further remove the parents from the process. Finally, he believed that no court could fully appreciate the points of view of those close to BJ.

The care team offered to search for other neonatologists who might agree with the family that it would be ethically permissible to forgo life support. The family favored this, but despite widespread efforts over a large geographic area no such neonatologist could be found. The team offered to attempt to transfer BJ's care to another institution if the parents wished, but they declined. The care team reported on discussions about prognosis with consultants from several specialties familiar with patients with Prader-Willi syndrome. The care team and family had hoped that there might be something about BJ's presentation that might reliably predict the degree of his ultimate impairments. Unfortunately, the consultants had no additional insight or information that would allow for a confident prognosis about BJ's future disability.

At the end of these multiple meetings it was clear that the impasse could not be resolved, that transfer to another institution was not desired, and that no clinicians could be found who would agree to forgoing life support. The care team explained that all avenues had been exhausted and still they could not agree with the parents' desires. The attending physician told the parents that their only alternative to continued life support was to petition the court. They also had the option to relinquish their son to the care of another family.

Hydration and Nutrition in the Newborn

Although some believe that hydration and nutrition must always be continued, most acknowledge that some circumstances are associated with such a poor prognosis that it is preferable to forego all life support, including medically administered hydration and nutrition. Cases in which death is imminent regardless of the treatment provided are perhaps the most straightforward, as in those instances there is no therapy that is effective. Cases in which life could continue indefinitely but which are associated with terrible quality of life are somewhat more contentious, but there is widespread consensus that competent patients have the right to forego hydration and nutrition and that incompetent patients have that same right, only it is exercised through surrogates.

Hydration and nutrition is just like any life-prolonging therapy; it is associated with benefits and harms. The basic principle of beneficence suggests that a therapy or intervention must offer some benefit (good) for the patient or its use is not justified. Similarly, the principle of nonmaleficence guides us to avoid harm. What matters is the balance of harms and benefits when deciding which therapies should be offered, but it is not always clear what should count as a benefit or a harm. Should continued life always be considered a benefit? Many would claim that continued life in an unacceptably poor state should count as harm. This evaluation of whether prolonging life counts as a benefit or harm is usually left in the hands of parents, but there are limits when prognosis includes the possibility of states that cannot reasonably be considered "not worth living in."

In this case, it was clear that continuing nutrition and hydration would almost certainly result in BJ surviving into adulthood. He and his family would suffer the consequences of his disorder—the hyperphagia and behavioral problems of childhood, and the profound strain on him and his family as they attempted to control his eating. However, although the condition is difficult and stressful, individuals with this disorder can thrive and are not generally unhappy. In adulthood he would face intellectual disability of unpredictable severity, but it is still unlikely that he would be unhappy.

These factors led the care team to conclude that the only ethically defensible course was to continue to support him with nutrition and fluid. Although his life would have limitations, they were not at all certain to end up so poor that most reasonable persons would opt to end their life instead. Even the argument that the possible need for a temporary gastrostomy tube meant undue pain and harm was more than balanced by the clear benefit it would offer and its temporary nature. The balance of beneficence and nonmaleficence seemed to clearly favor continuing life support for BJ.

These concepts are usually mirrored in societal positions or mores regarding similar conditions. For example, children with Down syndrome (Trisomy 21) face limitations and uncertain prognosis, but the societal view is that the presence of Down syndrome alone would never justify limiting or withholding care. Indeed, current society strives to actively support life-prolonging therapies for those with Down syndrome. Because the cognitive prognosis Prader-Willi syndrome spans a range of disabilities that is not dissimilar to that for Down syndrome, there seems to be societal support for the conclusion that BJ should be kept alive.

An objection might be made that the clinicians in this case unacceptably infringed on parental choice or autonomy in the case of BJ. As touched upon earlier, parents are generally regarded as the reasonable choice to act as surrogates for their newborn. This assumes that the parents are able to assess all the information about their child's case, and also to understand the guiding principles around in what circumstances a choice about continuing care exists. Parental choice does not automatically supersede the caregivers' responsibility as advocates for the child, and parents cannot choose a harmful or unreasonable program of care for their child.

It is rare that parents would deliberately chose something bad or wrong for their child, but surrogacy for newborns is impacted by several nuances unique to this area of medicine. Parents cannot be guided by information about what the newborn would himself or herself want because the baby has no life experience on which to draw. Even surrogates for adults find it difficult to separate their own wishes from the wishes of the patient; this is even more problematic in a newborn who has never had or expressed wishes of his or her own.

Moreover, just as parents are dealing with the crisis in their newborn, they are at some level grieving the loss of the perfect child they had hoped and dreamed for. Complex decisions are more complex in the midst of grief, and it is difficult to overcome the hopelessness that accompanies this loss, making it difficult to seize onto the positive parts of prognosis. This is exacerbated by a lack of a framework or personal life experience for dealing with an ill or compromised newborn. Most people have had no experience with this, indeed may not even be aware of the conditions that affect newborns until it happens to them.

Finally, parents may see each of their children and, indeed, their future children as a part of their entire family unit. It is impossible for them to separate the impact of a disease or disorder on the whole family from its impact on the single child alone. As a result, they naturally factor this impact into their thoughts about care choices. The support of a compromised child might take all their energy and resources, and it is hard to ignore the negative impact this could have on their lives and the lives of their other children. This consideration is natural and in many ways appropriate—it reflects the basic ethical principle of justice and fairness to all.

Were these parents selfish or bad in wishing to withhold fluid and nutrition from BJ and allow him to expire? This hardly seems likely. They had spent weeks researching the possible causes of polyhydramnios before he was born, and their research convinced them that a life with Prader-Willi syndrome was so awful that it was not worth living. They were not looking for an easy way out for themselves, as it was clear that the anguish they brought to their decision would burden them for their entire lives. They initially rejected the idea of adoption, because they believed so strongly that BJ's life anywhere would be terrible and unacceptable, and their desire was to prevent having him go through the life they deemed to be bad.

In the end, they understood that the care team was not simply opposing them reflexively or dogmatically, but rather had reached the societally supported position that this was not a case where limiting care to comfort alone was indicated or acceptable. They in fact took some solace from the fact that everyone devoted so much time to BJ and to them, and struggled with them in trying to determine the best thing to do.

In the end they changed their minds about seeking a directive through the courts. They feared that they would be misunderstood there, and that their relationship with their older daughter would be jeopardized. Thus, the stakes seemed too high to them in their already stressed situation and the option of placement for adoption was chosen.

COMPREHENSION QUESTIONS

32.1 Parents are usually considered as the best surrogate decision-makers for a new-born. In which of the following situations, is it reasonable to question their authority when what occurs?

A. They disagree with caregivers.

B. They base their decisions on religious beliefs.

C. Their decision appears in conflict with the best interests of the infant.

D. Never; they can make whatever decision is their choice.

32.2 In addition to autonomy, which principles of ethics are most important in arriving at a clinical decision?

A. Beneficence and nonmaleficence

B. Justice and honesty

C. Compassion and cultural concerns

D. Futility and dignity

32.3 When parents or surrogate decision-makers disagree with caregivers, what is the best approach in attempting to reach a resolution?

A. Defer to parents because they have ultimate decision-making power.

B. Override the parents because they do not understand the medical issues.

C. Engage in ongoing discussions and attempt to engage family members or family advisors.

D. Immediately seek legal recourse.

ANSWERS

32.1 **C.** As is true for adult patients who lack capacity, decisions for compromised newborns must be made using the best available information about what is best to do. In most cases we accord parents with the right and responsibility to guide these decisions because they usually represent the best source of information, and they are presumed to have the best interests of the newborn at heart. It does not matter whether they agree with caregivers or whether their decisions are based on religious or secular beliefs. At the same time, their power is not limitless, and they must be held to a best interest standard. If the parental choices appear contrary to these interests, then they must be questioned and, in some cases, rejected.

32.2 **A.** The three most important principles in decision-making are autonomy, beneficence, and nonmaleficence, along with the principle of justice. Rarely can these concepts be totally separate, and in attempting to apply one we might of necessity compromise another to some extent. For example, we do in general respect the autonomy of the patient or their surrogate in making decisions, but we must weigh those decisions against the magnitude of possible harm or the injustice of treating one patient completely differently than we would treat others. As an even simpler example, we strive for nonmaleficence, but every therapy or treatment has some inherent risks of harm. If they are counterbalanced by the potential to provide benefit, then we accept this as an acceptable balance.

32.3 **C.** When there is a disagreement or impasse, it is most important to attempt to keep and open dialogue between parents and caregivers. This can often be aided and facilitated with the help of ethics consultants, and, frequently, several discussions are needed to help break down the impasse, with the commitment of all participants to keep listening and honestly offering their opinion. These discussions can often be aided by engaging additional family members, family advisors or clergy (as the parents may wish) or by including other medical consultants. Neither should caregivers simply defer to parental wishes without considering whether those wishes are correct or ethically defensible nor should they override such wishes.

Seeking an opinion through the legal system is the only recourse in some cases; however, this is usually a late resort. Such action can be disruptive to the therapeutic relationship at a critical time and may add barriers or result in a decision that no one is able to fully accept.

> ## KEY POINTS

> ► Decisions about the care of newborns are based on the same core ethical principles that guide decisions in adults.
>
> ► Newborns lack capacity to make or communicate decisions, and this responsibility falls to surrogates. In nearly all cases, parents are appropriate surrogates.
>
> ► As substituted judgment is impossible, most decisions are based or judged on a best-interest standard.
>
> ► Decisions about withholding nutrition or fluids in newborns are based on the same principles that guide such decisions in older children and adults.

REFERENCES

Hagen EM, Therkelsen ØB, Førde R, Aasland O, Janvier A, Hansen TW. Challenges in reconciling best interest and parental exercise of autonomy in pediatric life-or-death situations. *J Pediatr.* 2012;161:146-151.

Harrison H. The offer they can't refuse: parents and perinatal treatment decisions. *Semin Fetal Neonatal Med.* 2008;13:329-334.

McHaffie HE, Laing IA, Parker M, McMillan J. Deciding for imperilled newborns: medical authority or parental autonomy? *J Med Ethics.* 2001;27:104-109.

Porta N, Frader J. Withholding hydration and nutrition in newborns. *Theor Med Bioeth.* 2007;28:443-451.

Wilkinson D. How much weight should we give to parental interests in decisions about life support for newborn infants. *Monash Bioeth Rev.* 2010;20:13.1-25.

A 3-year-old child is brought into the pediatric emergency department (ED) with a 2-day history of fever, headache, and a 1-day history of emesis. On examination, temperature is 102°F and the child appears lethargic. Blood pressure is 80/40 mm Hg and heart rate is 140 beats/minute. There is neck stiffness and a positive Kernig's sign. Computed tomography of the head is normal. As the ED physician, you recommend lumbar puncture with prompt antibiotic treatment for possible meningitis. The parents of the child refuse lumbar puncture due to concerns about dangers of neurologic injury or chronic paralysis. You and the patient's primary pediatrician both discuss the risks and benefits of the lumbar puncture with the parents, but they continue to refuse.

▶ What is your next step in the management of this child's condition?
▶ Are parents allowed to refuse treatment for their child?

ANSWERS TO CASE 33:
Parental Refusal

Summary: A 3-year-old child with fever, altered mental status, and signs of meningeal irritation is suspected to have bacterial meningitis. Lumbar puncture for collection and analysis of cerebrospinal fluid (CSF) is the standard of care for establishing the definitive diagnosis of meningitis. In addition, the results of the CSF culture are helpful for guiding the appropriate antibiotic treatment of the child.

- **Next step in the management of this child's condition:** Start empiric parenteral antibiotics. Bacterial meningitis in children carries a significant risk of both morbidity and mortality. The mortality rate for meningitis in children ranges from 4% to 10%. The early initiation of empiric parenteral antibiotics directed at the most likely organisms is the mainstay of treatment. Although lumbar puncture is useful for diagnostic and therapeutic purposes, it should not delay the initiation of antibiotics. In this case, because of the risk of severe neurologic damage and dying from untreated meningitis, it would be prudent to start antibiotics instead of continuing to convince the parents to consent to lumbar puncture.

- **Are parents allowed to refuse treatment for their child?** The authority to refuse treatment for a child is generally over-ruled if the child is at risk of significant harm or death as a result of the refusal.

ANALYSIS

Objectives

1. Define the principles of parental consent and distinguish it from child assent.

2. Recognize the developing capacity of children for participating in medical decision-making.

3. Describe the process of consent by health care proxy for pediatric care.

4. Recognize the conditions that qualify a minor to be considered an emancipated minor.

5. Utilize appropriate communication skills to facilitate shared decision-making and to resolve conflicts.

Considerations

This 3-year-old child does not have the capacity to make decisions about his own health care. Thus, his parents are charged with this responsibility. In most instances, pediatric health care professionals and parents have the best interest of the child in mind and come to a shared agreement about the best plan of action for diagnostic and therapeutic interventions. Many practitioners believe that they have responsibility for advocating for the best interests of the child even if this is opposed to the parents' wishes. In this case, the parents are concerned that the child may be at risk for harm from the lumbar puncture and refuse to allow it. The physician feels strongly that it is in the child's best interests to perform lumbar puncture. Failure to do so would put him at risk for untreated meningitis or if treatment is initiated without a spinal tap, the child is at risk for receiving the incorrect therapy or therapy of a duration that is longer than would be needed if a diagnostic lumbar puncture was performed. The parents should be made aware that a presumptive diagnosis of bacterial meningitis is being made. A more definitive diagnosis with a specific etiologic organism cannot be determined in the absence of CSF analysis. There-fore, the child will likely need broad-spectrum parenteral antibiotics for a full 14- to 21-day course to ensure that even the "worst-case scenario" is treated appropriately. In other words, by not performing lumbar puncture prior to initiation of antibiotics, the child may need a broader and longer course of antibiotics.

Under common law and the statutes of most states, parents or legal guardians assume the responsibility for making decisions about all aspects of their child's health care, including diagnostic and therapeutic interventions. The authority to consent to treatment also implies that parents or legal guardians may refuse treatment for almost any reason, such as religious or cultural beliefs. However, the authority to refuse treatment for a child is generally overruled if the child is at risk of significant harm or death as a result of the refusal. The courts or other state welfare agencies for children's services should be involved in such situations to mediate the dispute between the health care team and the parents.

APPROACH TO:
Medical Decision-Making In Pediatrics

DEFINITIONS

ASSENT: An expression of agreement or willingness to accept a proposed medical intervention.

CAPACITY TO CONSENT: The legal ability to form a valid contract and the psychological or developmental ability to make sound decisions.

CONSENT BY PROXY: The process by which the person with the legal right to consent to medical treatment for a minor delegates that right to another person, such as another family member or caregiver.

EMANCIPATED MINOR: A child who is younger than 18 years of age but who is treated as an adult with regard to medical decision-making because of a special circumstance.

INFORMED PARENTAL CONSENT/PERMISSION: Approval of the parent or legal guardian for medical interventions related to the child. "Informed" implies that the parents or guardian have been provided appropriate information of the interventions and have an adequate understanding of the information. This is not necessary once a child turns 18 years of age and is considered an adult by the medical profession in the United States.

CLINICAL APPROACH

Principles of Parental Consent and Child Assent

In general, pediatric patients are unable to make informed health care decisions for themselves. Under common law and the statutes of most states, parents or legal guardians are given the authority to make decisions about the minor's medical care. In turn, pediatric providers are required to seek the permission of a parent or legal guardian before rendering medical care. The Committee on Bioethics of the American Academy of Pediatrics affirms the following: "Physicians have an ethical, as well as legal, obligation to obtain parental permission to perform the recommended medical intervention of a pediatric patient." This obligation pertains to routine matters of health care such as preventative care and to nonemergent medical care for a child. For emergent medical issues, pediatric providers should attempt to seek consent from a parent or guardian; however, if obtaining consent would cause a delay that would likely put the child in danger of death or significant harm, then the provider should proceed with the recommended medical intervention.

Although most children are not able to make binding decisions about their own health care until they reach they age of majority, most experts would agree that older children and adolescents should be involved in the medical decision-making process as an active participant. Including children in the discussion of medical care honors the ethical principle of "respect for all persons" and empowers children to engage in the discussion to the extent of their capacity or developmental capability. Research has shown that children aged 14 years and older are as competent as adults in making informed treatment decisions. However, age alone is not sufficient to determine a child's capability to understand. It is important for the pediatric provider to consider factors such as knowledge, developmental status, experience making prior decisions, and cultural and religious beliefs prior to ascertaining the child's capacity for understanding. When asking for a child's assent, the health care professional should explain the medical condition and proposed intervention at a developmentally appropriate level, assess the patient's understanding of the situation, and solicit an expression of the child's willingness to accept the proposed care. A child's assent is recommended but not necessary to proceed with medical care.

Consent by Proxy

In some situations, a parent or legal guardian may not be able to accompany a child to routine or nonurgent medical visits. It is not unusual for another family member like a grandparent or a baby sitter to accompany a child to such visits. The parent or guardian has the ability to delegate to another adult the legal right to consent for the minor as long as that adult is legally and medically competent. The provider should have written documentation for the consent by health care proxy. It is also imperative for the health care professional to understand the state laws that dictate specific regulations around consent by health care proxy.

Emancipated Minors

Certain adolescents have the legal right to make decisions about their health care when younger than 18 years of age. State legislation designates the settings in which minors have the authority to make such decisions. Specific qualities of the adolescent may determine emancipation, such as self-supporting or not living at home, marriage, pregnancy or parental status, military status, or declaration of emancipation by the court. In addition, in certain states, minors are able to consent for their own health care if they have a specific medical condition that requires treatment. These conditions include sexually transmitted infections, pregnancy, and substance abuse. When diagnosing or treating these medical issues, pediatric providers may encourage minors to discuss the situation with a parent as a means to provide additional support to the child, but parental involvement or consent is not necessary prior to the initiation of medical services.

Communicating With Pediatric Patients and Families

Communicating in the pediatric encounter is a complex process usually involving physician, patient, and parent(s), which demands sensitivity to the perspective of the child as well as the parents. The patient- and family-centered care approach has been adopted by the American Academy of Pediatrics as the preferred model for pediatrics to "capture the importance of engaging the family and the patient in a developmentally supportive manner as essential members of the health care team." It is based on the principle that the family is the major source of strength and support for the pediatric patient. Incorporating the patient and family's preferences in decision-making is an important part of patient- and family-centered care.

Shared decision-making requires a conversation in which the physician elicits the patient's perspectives, shares his or her own perspective, and then negotiates a solution. More than one management option exists for most medical decisions and, thus, engagement of the family through shared decision-making is usually possible. Core physician competencies of informed, shared decision-making have been defined as follows:

1. Developing a partnership with the patient.

2. Establishing the patient's preferences for information (amount and format).

3. Establishing the patient's preferences for role in decision-making.

4. Eliciting and responding to patient's ideas, concerns, and expectations.

5. Identifying choices and evaluating the research evidence in relation to the patient.

6. Presenting evidence, taking into account patient's preference for information and role in decision-making.

7. Making or negotiating a decision in partnership with the patient.

8. Agreeing on the action plan and making arrangements for follow-up.

The model above can be adapted for pediatrics by considering family members as well as the patient. Furthermore, additional factors to consider are the child's developmental stage, engaging the parent so as not to undermine the parent-child relationship, motivation of the child in making decisions, and parental attitudes and beliefs about the child's involvement. In deciding on the plan, the clinician must balance giving the responsibility and control of decision making to the parents with giving his or her personal opinions as the voice of authority.

Most pediatricians consider advocacy for the child, their patient, to be their primary responsibility. Thus, if the pediatrician perceives that the parent's perspective is not in the patient's best interest, then he or she will negotiate a solution with the parent on the patient's behalf. In this type of negotiation, it is critical that the clinician identifies shared interests and whether there is any flexibility in either viewpoint. The case of suspected meningitis in which the parents refuse the diagnostic lumbar puncture at the start of this chapter demonstrates that if parents adamantly refuse an important diagnostic procedure, then another path could be chosen. The clinician must find a solution that addresses the shared interests of treating the child and ensures that this is done quickly. In this case, the alternative solution was to treat the child without lumbar puncture, a less optimal but adequate decision negotiated with the family.

COMPREHENSION QUESTIONS

33.1 A 10-year-old girl presents to your office with her mother with upper respiratory symptoms. Upon examination you notice that she has multiple petechiae all over her body. You explain the need for a complete blood count to her mother and she readily agrees; however, the child refuses to have her blood drawn. You consider leukemia versus immune-mediated thrombocytopenia in your differential. What do you do next?

A. Because this is a potentially life-threatening situation you get a court-ordered health care proxy to make a decision to draw the blood.

B. Negotiate with the child to do the blood test the next day.

C. Explain to the child that you need to draw her blood today and will need to do it whether or not she agrees.

D. Do not speak further with the child and call in your nursing staff to hold her down for the blood test.

E. Because the child refuses, you cannot draw her blood.

33.2 Your 12-year-old patient presents with his fifth asthma exacerbation in 6 months. You suspect he is not compliant with his controller medications. You decide to try shared decision-making to more fully engage him and his father in developing a treatment plan. Communication strategies you will use include all of the following except:

A. Eliciting the patient's motivation for developing a management plan.

B. Assessing his maturity and capacity to understand his illness.

C. Exploring alternative options to your recommended treatment, which may be more acceptable to the patient.

D. Exploring the family's views on how much autonomy the child should have with respect to taking his medications.

E. Using an empathic tone to tell the patient that you know that it is hard to take controller medications but that you have experience with asthma management and he must take the medication in the way in which you have prescribed them.

33.3 A 15-year-old girl presents unaccompanied by her parents to the ED with severe abdominal pain. She is sexually active. A work up reveals a negative pregnancy test, with no evidence of pelvic inflammatory disease on pelvic examination. Ultrasonography confirms a diagnosis of ovarian torsion. You consult the surgeon who recommends that she undergo urgent surgical procedure. The patient gives assent for the procedure but you are unable to contact her parents. What do you do next?

A. Get informed consent from the patient because she is sexually active and therefore an emancipated minor.

B. Inform the surgeon that he cannot operate before you get informed consent from the parents and admit for observation.

C. Document your attempts to contact the parents, notify a hospital administrator, and take the patient to the operating room as soon as possible.

D. Contact her 19-year-old boyfriend for consent.

E. Discharge the patient home with adequate pain medication and clear instructions on follow-up.

ANSWERS

33.1 **C.** The child's assent is recommended but not necessary to proceed with the evaluation of this potentially life-threatening condition. The parent has given her consent, so a court-ordered proxy is unnecessary. Deferring the evaluation until the next day may put this child at risk of harm; therefore, this would not be in the patient's best interest. This 10-year-old child does not have the capacity to make decisions about her health care; thus, her refusal should not be upheld. Attempts to negotiate with the child and to involve her in shared decision-making should be made prior to restraining her for the blood test.

33.2 **E.** All of the above communication strategies are consistent with informed, shared decision-making adapted for the pediatric encounter except for answer E, which represents the "kind but paternalistic approach." Informed, shared decision-making is somewhere on the continuum between paternalism, in which the doctor makes all decisions without involvement of the patient, and complete patient autonomy, in which the patient takes the entire responsibility for medical decision-making.

33.3 **C.** This adolescent female has a condition that requires emergent surgical intervention to preserve the function of her ovary. Although she is sexually active, the ovarian torsion is not related to sexual activity or a result of a sexually transmitted infection. Therefore, because she is a minor, it is necessary to obtain parental consent for the procedure. Her parents did not accompany her to the visit. The ED physician did not obtain parental consent prior to the work-up in this sexually active girl because it was reasonable to suspect that her abdominal pain may have been secondary to her sexual activity. In most states, adolescents can consent for their own reproductive health care. After recognizing that the medical problem was not related to sexual activity, the physician is obligated to contact the parents to obtain consent for the remainder of the medical care. If the parents are not available, then the risks of delaying the procedure to obtain parental consent must be considered. In this case, the potential loss of ovarian function is high if the torsion is not surgically corrected. It is in the patient's best interest to go to the operating room in a timely manner. The physician should document the details of the case and the attempts to reach the parents. The physician should also notify a hospital administrator about the situation. Contacting her boyfriend would not be of any use in this situation and would breach her confidentiality if she did not give you consent to discuss this with him. It would be a gross deviation from standard of care to discharge a patient with ovarian torsion prior to definitive treatment.

KEY POINTS

▶ Ideally, the pediatrician is able to obtain both the parents' consent and the child's assent in developing a management plan; however, the child's assent is not a requirement.

▶ Parental consent is required for pediatric care; however, many states allow teens to seek care for issues related to sexual activity and substance abuse without the consent of a parent.

▶ If a parent's decision about the health care of their child could result in death or significant harm, then a court-appointed health care proxy may make decisions on the child's behalf.

▶ Shared decision-making engages the patient and family with the pediatrician in developing the management plan when multiple options exist.

REFERENCES

Barry MJ, Edgman-Levitan S. Shared decision making – the pinnacle of patient-centered care. *N Engl J Med.* 2012;366;780-781.

Butz AM, Walker JM, Pulsifer M, Winkelstein M. Shared decision making in school age children with asthma. *Pediatr Nurs.* 2007;33:111-116.

Chavez-Bueno S, McCracken GH. Bacterial meningitis in children. *Pediatr Clin N Am.* 2005;52:795-810.

Committee on Bioethics of the AAP. Informed consent, parental permission and assent in pediatric practice. *Pediatrics.* 2012;130:2 e467-e468.

Committee on Hospital Care and Institute for the Patient- and Family Centered Care. Patient- and family-centered care and the pediatrician's role. *Pediatrics.* 2012;129:394-404.

Kon AA. Answering the question: "doctor, if this were your child, what would you do? *Pediatrics.* 2006;118:393-397.

McAbee GN. Consent by proxy for non-urgent pediatric care. *Pediatrics.* 2010;126:1022.

Richards EP, Rathbun KC. Law and the Physician: A Practical Guide. New York, NY: Little Brown and Company; 1993.

Rozovsky FA. *Consent to Treatment: A Practical Guide.* 3rd ed. Aspen, CO: Aspen Publishers; 2004.

Towle A, Godolphin W. Framework for teaching and learning informed shared decision making. *BMJ.* 1999;319:766-771.

Weithorn LA, Campbell SB. The competency of children and adolescents to make informed treatment decisions. *Child Dev.* 1982;53:1589-1598.

A third-year surgery resident, KE, on the trauma service has been assigned to scrub on a case of a 32-year-old man who has a gunshot wound in his right leg. The resident informs her team that she will not scrub on the case but does not give a reason. After the chief resident meets with KE in private, KE admits that she noted that the patient is HIV positive, and that is very concerning to her. She states that she has discussed this with her fiancé, and they have decided that the possibility of a needle stick or other exposure in a patient who is HIV positive makes them uncomfortable.

▶ What should be the response of the chief resident?
▶ What are the ethical responsibilities of physicians in the care of patients infected with HIV?

You are counseling a 20-year-old pregnant woman, gravida 1, para 0, about her positive HIV test, which has been verified by a confirmatory test. Recently, she emigrated from another country to the United States. The patient is very tearful. She says she cannot tell her husband because he will beat her, and she is considering moving back to her home country where no one will know of her diagnosis.

▶ What should be your response to the patient?
▶ Is the physician ethically obligated to disclose?
▶ Is the patient ethically obligated to disclose?

ANSWERS TO CASE 34:
Caring for a Patient Infected with HIV

Summary: A third-year surgery resident refuses to scrub in on a trauma case because she is concerned about the patient's HIV-positive status. She has discussed the issue with her husband and decided the risk of infection from a possible exposure is higher than she is comfortable.

- **Response:** The chief resident should first ensure that the resident is informed about the true risk of infection after needle-stick exposure (0.3%) and explore any other perceived barriers impeding the resident from caring for this patient. After exploring the subject together, the chief resident should try to accommodate the preferences of the resident, if possible, and inform the attending faculty physician.

- **Ethical responsibilities:** Congruent with the ethical responsibilities of physicians in the care of all patients, the care of patients with HIV infection should uphold the principles of confidentiality, respect, autonomy, justice, and beneficence. Keeping the patient's best interests as a priority and treating them fairly (eg, not denying care) define beneficence and justice.

Summary: A 20-year-old pregnant woman is counseled about her HIV-positive status, and she expresses concern about informing her husband. She also expresses a desire to return to her home country.

- **Response:** First, the patient's knowledge, attitudes, and fears must be explored and addressed by the physician. She should also be counseled on the course of the disease and available treatments necessary to improve outcomes for her and her child. Counseling on the prevention of transmission is also essential in discussing her decision to return to her home country.

- **Ethical obligations of the physician:** The patient is ethically obliged to encourage at-risk contacts to be tested, to disclose information about their infection to partners, and to maintain appropriate preventive behaviors. The ethical obligations of the physician include confidentiality, respect, beneficence, and social responsibility. The physician must also be aware of and abide by any reporting requirements and state laws addressing the duty-to-warn at-risk partners or contacts. The latter point creates an ethical tension between respect for patient confidentiality and the duty to warn.

- **Ethical obligations of the patient:** The physician is obliged to promote safe behaviors that promote prevention and reduce the risk of transmission of disease.

ANALYSIS

Objectives

1. Describe the ethical obligations of health care professionals in treating patients with HIV infection.

2. Describe the ethical dilemma of duty-to-warn versus patient confidentiality in caring for patients with HIV infection.

3. Describe key principles in working through disclosure, duty to warn persons at risk for infection, and counseling of patients with HIV infection.

4. Describe societal and access issues that patients infected with HIV may face in other countries.

5. Describe key principles in international research in HIV and the role of medical students.

Considerations

The physician in the first case has been confronted with the decision to treat a patient who is HIV positive. This is not an uncommon situation, as there are currently 1.1 million persons living in the United States infected with HIV. Given that HIV is an infection that affects multiple organs and systems, physicians across specialties may be called on to care for these patients. This implies that physicians must be aware of their responsibility toward the care of patients infected with HIV and explore their willingness to treat and address any attitudinal or other personal barriers to their treatment. Beyond the physician's willingness to evaluate and treat, there are other major ethical considerations involved in the care of patients with HIV infection. The second case presents a commonly encountered dilemma. Patients who refuse to disclose their HIV status to their partners due to fear of rejection or misconceptions of the consequences. This requires the physician to balance her duty-to-warn (patient safety) and principle of patient autonomy and confidentiality. This decision is guided by other principles that include justice, social responsibility, and beneficence. The reporting requirements may also dictate certain decisions for the physician. HIV is a reportable public health disease in the United States, although state laws vary with regard to duty-to-warn.

APPROACH TO:

Patient Infected with HIV

DEFINITIONS

BENEFICENCE: An ethical principle that obligates physicians to act in the best interest of their patients.

DUTY-TO-WARN: A physician's duty to inform unknowing partners of individuals infected with HIV or other infectious disease about their risk to encourage testing.

NONMALEFICENCE: An ethical principle that obligates physicians to do no harm.

CLINICAL APPROACH

Overview of Ethics in HIV

HIV is a sexually transmitted illness that affects multiple organ systems, and physicians across specialties are involved in the care of these patients. Despite the increasing array of drugs available for the management of HIV infection, many patients still progress to AIDS. Moreover, HIV is considered a reportable public health disease within the United States, as it comes with a high risk of infection following the exchange of bodily fluids, such as sexual intercourse and sharing needles. In addition, needle-stick accidents, which are not uncommon occurrences in the health care setting, also present a small risk for infection recorded to be 0.3%. The perceptions of HIV and the associated social implications vary by region, country, and by cultural traditions or practices. These realities of HIV create several ethical considerations for students, physicians, and patients.

Duty to Treat

With regard to the physician, the willingness to treat patients infected with HIV is the foremost consideration. Physicians are responsible for treating all patients without prejudice to any race, age, or social factors. However, an individual's perceptions may at times influence their decision to treat. In the case of patients with HIV, treating physicians may have biases against certain social behaviors exhibited by the patient. These biases may present as attitudinal barriers to the duty-to-treat and may include homosexual bias, negative attitudes toward drug users, and discomfort with dying patients for those with HIV/AIDS. In addition to this, there may be structural barriers that influence the decision to treat. Physicians may lack certain knowledge to adequately care for patients with HIV infection and they may perceive excess time demands in their care. These barriers can be addressed through physician education, involving discussions that openly explore these themes. Following all attempts to discuss perceptions and barriers, a physician may still choose to transfer the care of a patient if his or her condition is chronic with no acute concerns, and other physicians are available to provide the necessary care.

Tension Between Confidentiality and Duty to Warn

Medical information is always confidential; however, in the case of HIV additional precautions are taken to ensure patient confidentiality. An HIV-positive status is still often associated with social stigma and implications, and, hence, the sensitivity of disclosing this information, even if among the public health community.

Within the United States, health care professionals are obligated to report any HIV case to the public health authorities. At this point, there are countering ethical principles that create ethical dilemmas. The decision to disclose information is then dictated by weighing the benefits and risks of a given situation. In the case of reporting requirements, the need for constant disease surveillance—including demographic patterns—outweighs confidentiality responsibilities toward the patient. With the duty to warn patient's partners, the ethical arguments become more complex. The risk of infection for active sexual contacts is significant, especially when no protection is used. Health care professionals have a social responsibility that challenges their confidentiality to the patient. This allows for certain exceptions to be considered when appropriate. When the ongoing risk for a contact are high, and the patient refuses to share information about the risk with their partner and to take appropriate measures to reduce the risk of infection, than the physician may consider informing the contact of the risk. Furthermore, some states may have laws regulating the exceptions to confidentiality in the case of HIV. When confidentiality is breached, all measures should be taken to minimize the adverse implications of the breech, and the patient should be made aware of it.

HIV Infected Health Care Workers

Another exception to confidentiality exists when the patient with HIV infection is a health care professional. Even though US federal laws allow some flexibility with regard to disclosing information about the HIV-positive status of health care professionals to their patients, state laws are more clear. Some states require that patients of health care professionals with HIV infection be informed of their care provider's status, and this must be included in the informed consent of any procedure. Some states also limit the clinical activities of health care professionals with HIV infection to limit the risk of infection of patients. Other states weigh the risk of discrimination toward the health care professional to be greater than the benefit of disclosure to the patient, especially because the risk of infection has been shown to be low in the health care setting.

Therapeutic Alliance

Building a strong therapeutic alliance—as the foundation of the physician–patient relationship—is essential throughout the process of exploring these ethical dilemmas. Involving the patient at each step and ensuring adequate communication will minimize conflict and improve outcomes.

Global Perspective

Worldwide, there are currently more than 35 million people living with HIV infection. Two-thirds of these cases are in Sub-Saharan Africa. The heavy disease burden of HIV infection in developing countries, coupled with the limited resources in these settings, makes for several additional ethical considerations. In the setting of limited resources, health care systems will often lack adequate infrastructure to cater for follow-up services for patients with HIV infection, especially in rural areas. One ethical debate concerns testing for HIV status and obtaining true informed or implied consent. When there are insufficient resources to manage patients who are HIV positive, what will the diagnosis contribute to the lives of the patients? Moreover, careful attention must be given to pre- and post-test counseling, as health literacy and medical information may be very different than in developed countries.

In the pretest phase, informing the patient about the purpose of testing, its implications, and the possible outcomes is important. Post-test counseling should involve discussions about the course of the disease, health posts where management is available and disclosing information to partners at risk. These considerations are particularly important when testing the status of patients is associated with a potential for conflict of interest. Health care professionals may be looking to report on HIV prevalence or recruit patients for clinical trials. In these situations, the intention for testing should be clarified and patients should be made fully aware of the details of their participation in any study.

Global frameworks may also affect the ethical tension arising from the principles of the duty-to-treat and duty-to-warn. Depending on societal values, certain ethical principles may hold more weight. For example, social responsibility may be emphasized over an individual's confidentiality. Foreign health care professionals in these settings should also be informed about reporting requirements and aware and respectful of the cultural differences in evaluating ethical situations.

Moreover, visiting medical students to international sites will more than likely be asked to care for patients with HIV infection. Being prepared, emotionally and clinically, to deal with these patients is important. Students may be placed in situations where the must exercise their ethical judgment. Recalling the ethical principles of respect, justice, beneficence and non-maleficence will aid students in their decisions. These principles will help balance considerations of the patient's autonomy in medical and nonmedical decisions, seek justice through fair treatment of all patients, and emphasize avoiding causing harm.

COMPREHENSION QUESTIONS

34.1   A male patient who is sexually active and HIV positive has 2 current partners and is refusing to disclose any information about his HIV status to them. Which of the following would not be an acceptable justification for the physician to breach physician–patient confidentiality?

   A.   The patient has more than 1 sexual partner.

   B.   Breaching confidentiality is done to protect a known person from significant harm.

   C.   The patient is not competent—as measured by guidelines—to decide about disclosure.

   D.   The physician has exhausted all possible options in working with the patient to reduce risk of infection to other known persons.

34.2   In outreach programs that aim to screen large populations for HIV infection, which of the following actions or services should be considered?

   A.   Distributing condoms to all participants.

   B.   Disclosing information to partners and families of persons who are HIV positive.

   C.   Pre- and post-test counseling services.

   D.   Providing Enzyme Linked Immunosorbent Assay (ELISA) tests and other confirmatory tests on-site.

34.3 A medical student is asked to scrub in on a caesarian delivery where the patient is known to be HIV positive. The student is reluctant to scrub in. What ethical principle is best demonstrated by this case?

A. Confidentiality
B. Duty to treat
C. Respect
D. Duty to warn

34.4 A third-year medical student is completing a research elective in Haiti. As part of her studies, she is assisting a team that is investigating the prevalence of HIV in the community. She has intermediate French language skills. One afternoon, due to shortage of team personnel she is assigned the task of reporting laboratory test results, including the HIV rapid test results to the patients. She has not had any experience or training in reporting HIV results, and she is not aware of any pretest counseling or follow-up services. The manager of the team gives her a list of patients to call. How should the student respond?

A. Do some research on the Internet regarding how to give this news and follow the published protocol.
B. Discuss her concerns with her senior or supervisor at the medical camp.
C. Use a mobile phone application to translate for her.
D. Proceed to counsel the patients because they will require only a fifth-grade level of language.

ANSWERS

34.1 **A.** There are certain exceptions to the general principle of patient confidentiality that may justify informing sexual partners about their risk against the patient's wishes. If the physician fails to convince the patient of the importance of notifying sexual partners of their risk, and of acting to minimize risk of transmission to partners, then a breach to confidentiality may be considered when the harm to others is significant, or if a patient is clinically judged to be incompetent in making medical decisions. The number of partners is not relevant as a sole determinant for breech in confidentiality.

34.2 **C.** In settings in which screening of many individuals is simultaneously performed, there are important considerations to ensure that adequate care is given to all patients. In areas with limited access to health care resources, pre and post-test counseling are vital in assisting patients in their decisions to be tested, as well as to follow-up on the test result. Confirmatory testing, distributing medications, and ancillary services are provided by secondary or tertiary health care centers.

34.3 **B.** The student's reluctance to scrub in may be due to several factors, including personal prejudices or misconceptions. The student should recall that, first and foremost, as a physician she has a duty to treat all patients. The other principles are also applicable as the student should respect all patients and keep their information confidential.

34.4 **B.** The student is not familiar with breaking bad news in this cultural context and should avoid the task of reporting to patients. She should discuss her concerns with her senior or supervisor at the medical camp. There are major ethical issues. Because one of the student's goals is to assist with a research project that involves reporting on the prevalence of HIV infection, she may experience a conflict of interest to assist in the disclosure of results. For example, she may wish to impress her team to garner a good evaluation or to contribute substantially to the research in order to be a named author in a study publication. This setting for disclosing HIV rapid test results is different from and would not likely be appropriate at her home institution. Her actions should be driven by shared ethical principles, including equity, justice, and nonmaleficence, especially given that no pre- or post-test counseling and follow-up services are noted.

KEY POINTS

▶ HIV is a reportable public health infection in the United States, with varying reporting requirements by state.

▶ When balancing the duty to warn versus maintaining patient confidentiality, the key guiding ethical principles are beneficence, justice, social responsibility, and autonomy.

▶ Breach of confidentiality in cases of duty-to-warn should only be considered when (1) attempts to reason with the patient have failed, (2) identifiable high-risk contacts are noted, and (3) the patient has been informed of the intention to disclose this information.

▶ A physician's willingness to treat patients positive for HIV infection should be explored with attention to the attitudinal barriers and misconceptions about perceived risk that may influence decision-making.

▶ Physicians have an ethical responsibility to treat all patients without prejudice, with nonmaleficence, and with justice.

▶ In international settings with limited resources and a high prevalence of HIV infection, there is a need for pre- and post-test counseling, education about follow-up services, and attention to patient confidentiality and autonomy in informed consent for testing and in disclosure of HIV status.

▶ From a global perspective, some differences in ethical frameworks may exist, especially regarding the principles of autonomy and social responsibility.

REFERENCES

Barthwell AG and Gibert CL. Legal and ethical issues. In: *Screening for Infectious Diseases Among Substance Abusers*. Rockville, MD: US Department of Health and Human Services; 1993.

Gerbert B, Maguire B, Bleecker T, Coates TJ, McPhee SJ. Primary care physicians and AIDS. Attitudinal and structural barriers to care. JAMA. 1991;266:2837-2842.

Huprich S, Fuller KM, Schneider R. Divergent ethical perspectives on the duty-to-warn principle with HIV patients. *Ethics Behav.* 2003;13:263-278.

Wolf LE, Lo B. *Ethical Dimensions of HIV/AIDS*. San Francisco: UCSF; 2001. http://hivinsite.ucsf.edu /InSite?page=kb-00&doc=kb-08-01-05. Accessed June 1, 2014.

TM, an 18-year-old woman with insulin-dependent diabetes and anorexia nervosa, was discharged from an inpatient psychiatric unit following a suicide attempt in which she took an overdose of her insulin and citalopram, which had been prescribed for anxiety and depression. She had stabilized during a 2-week hospital stay in which she was switched from citalopram to lamotrigine, a mood stabilizing medication. Her eating had improved, her blood sugar levels were normal, and she was back on her insulin as prescribed. She was referred to an outpatient psychiatrist for medication management and supportive counseling to help her comply with her treatment plan. At the first appointment, TM reports that she still periodically has suicidal thoughts and urges, but no intention or plan to harm herself. She states that she frequently writes about her feelings on her blog and her Facebook page. She also uses Twitter to share her feelings with more than 250 followers. The psychiatrist, who is Internet savvy and maintains Facebook and Twitter accounts for professional purposes, wonders if he ought to monitor TM's online posts to assess her psychiatric stability and safety.

▶ What are the pros and cons of monitoring online posts by patients with medical/psychiatric illness and risk factors for suicide?
▶ Should the physician obtain informed consent from the patient before engaging in such monitoring?
▶ What ethical and legal considerations come into play in these scenarios?

ANSWERS TO CASE 35:
Social Media Ethics

Summary: An 18-year-old woman has been recently discharged from an inpatient psychiatric unit following a suicide attempt. She reports periodic suicidal thoughts and urges, but has no intention or plan to harm herself. She states that she frequently writes about her feelings on her blog, her Facebook page, and Twitter with more than 250 followers. The outpatient psychiatrist, who is Internet savvy and maintains Facebook and Twitter accounts for professional purposes, wonders if he ought to monitor TM's online posts to assess her psychiatric stability and safety.

- **Pros and cons of monitoring online patient posts:** This kind of monitoring might enhance patient safety, but doing so can also compromise patient privacy and limit patient self-expression.

- **Should the physician obtain informed consent before monitoring?** This issue deserves careful reflection and decision-making on a case-by-case basis.

- **Ethical and legal considerations:** In the absence of clear legal guidance, physicians must balance competing requirements so that they are able to provide safe clinical care and respect patient privacy.

ANALYSIS

Objectives

1. Understand the possible role of social media technologies for gathering clinical information on patients.

2. Consider the clinical/ethical question of whether to search for patient information online or to monitor online posts.

3. Develop a framework for determining whether it is ethical to use social media to monitor patient clinical status and safety issues.

Considerations

The scenario presents a patient at risk for suicide. She reports to posting her feelings on online sites such as her blog, Facebook page, and Twitter account. The treating psychiatrist is contemplating whether to monitor the patient's online postings. Although the intention may be good, perception of invasion into privacy may harm the physician–patient relationship. Physicians today can use social media to optimize treatment outcomes; however, at the same time they are required to respect their patients' fundamental rights to autonomy, free expression, and privacy. Several clinical and ethical considerations come into play when a physician is challenged with the question of whether to search online for patient information or to monitor a patient's online posts. On one hand, searching online might help to identify patients who are at risk for self-harm or violence toward others. On the other hand, patients may deserve privacy to express themselves freely online without unwanted monitoring by their physicians. A structured, pragmatic thought process could help clinicians to determine the optimal course of action in these situations.

APPROACH TO:
Social Media Ethics

DEFINITIONS

AUTONOMY: Self-determination; the freedom to make decisions on one's own.

BENEFICENCE: Action that is done for the benefit of other people.

PATERNALISM: Protective action that limits another person's liberty.

PRAGMATIC: Dealing with matters realistically and on the basis of practical (rather than theoretical) considerations.

CLINICAL APPROACH

In accordance with the ethical precept of beneficence, physicians may use social media to benefit their patients and enhance clinical care. The case discussed above might involve the physician's learning critical (potentially life-saving) information about a patient via social media or other online searching. At the same time, physicians ought to respect their patients' autonomy and freedom to express themselves online without unwanted attention or reprisal from medical professionals. In this scenario, paternalism would involve the physician's deciding to monitor online information about patients who are potentially dangerous to themselves or others on the basis of a psychiatric condition. Before engaging in such online monitoring, the physician should engage in a structured, pragmatic thought process on a case-by-case basis to determine whether such action is ethical and clinically warranted.

ANALYSIS AND DISCUSSION

The explosion of social media and Internet technologies presents both opportunities and ethical dilemmas for psychiatrists and other physicians. Internet search engines and social media sites have become incredible sources of information about medical and psychiatric conditions. Physicians can quickly and easily access information about cutting-edge research and treatment approaches that might be clinically useful. It is widely considered a major advance for clinical care when physicians have computer access to peer-reviewed medical journals, the *Physicians Desk Reference*, and other electronic sources of up-to-date knowledge in medical science.

Increasingly, physicians can also access useful information about individual patients whom they treat. Many states, for example, empower physicians to check online via secure websites whether their patients may be receiving prescriptions for controlled substances from other physicians. This information can indicate to the physician that a substance abuse disorder may be present and allow him or her to take appropriate action in the patient's best interest. Electronic information of this kind from pharmacies generally has not been considered a breach of the patient's privacy rights. Rather, it is essential data that might lead the doctor to avoid prescribing a drug of abuse and to refer the patient for substance abuse treatment. In addition to the individual clinical benefits this might bring, this information can help enhance public health by reducing the number of people in the population with access to drugs of abuse.

But what about other kinds of computer-based searches for information about patients? Is it acceptable, for example, for physicians to search online on a real estate site for information about where a patient lives and the value of his or her home? Is it appropriate to read online news accounts about a patient's arrest for a misdemeanor or felony? Should a physician research whether a patient is a registered sex offender? Such information is easily obtainable on publicly available websites, and such information might be clinically relevant. If the physician learned that a patient is a registered sex offender and is coming to office visits at a practice located around the corner from an elementary school, then the physician could inform the patient of this fact and make a referral to another practice. On one hand, that intervention could help to protect the patient from being arrested and having further legal action against him. On the other hand, there is real concern that this Internet snooping may be a privacy violation and the patient may experience it as intrusive, discriminatory, and detrimental.

What happens to a sense of safety and confidentiality in the physician–patient relationship when patients know that their doctors may be combing the Internet for personal information? Does this erode the trust that is so essential to establishing an effective physician–patient relationship in which patients can receive respectful and nondiscriminatory clinical care? Is it unduly paternalistic for doctors to decide on their own that the benefits of this kind of online searching outweigh any risks? Should information about patients, even if publicly available online, only be obtained and used by doctors if patients disclose it to them? The traditional physician–patient relationship, which privileged face-to-face communication between the 2 parties, is seriously threatened by this ready availability of online information.

In the case vignette presented above, the physician learns that clinically relevant (and potentially life-saving) information about the patient is available via online searches for the patient's blog or her Twitter and Facebook accounts. The physician could find and read the blog, usually without the patient knowing about it. Likewise, the physician could look at her Twitter postings without her knowing (although she would know the doctor was looking if he or she decides to follow her on Twitter). With regard to Facebook, the physician may or may not be able to view the patient's posting without her knowledge, depending on her user settings. On a site such as LinkedIn, a person can usually see whether someone else has viewed his or her profile unless the viewer has arranged to be anonymous (in the case of LinkedIn, by becoming a paid subscriber). The bottom line here is that this physician could find ways to read the patient's online posts about her mental state either with or without her knowledge that he was searching for her online information.

Discovering online information about this patient's suicidality risk could be clinically beneficial, but it could also violate her privacy and autonomy. What if the doctor's Internet search revealed embarrassing photographs of the patient that she never wanted him to see? Aside from the risk that she could feel ashamed, there is a risk that her doctor could unintentionally infringe upon her fundamental right to privacy. Does she have a right to express her thoughts online without fearing that her doctor might read her online posts? What if the doctor read suicidal statements she made online and then had her hospitalized involuntarily on that basis? His action might save her life and it would be based on publicly available information, but doing so might also compromise her right to free expression. We must grapple with the specter of a "police state" when a patient who blogs or tweets about her feelings lives in fear of an unwanted, paternalistic reprisal by a well-meaning but overly intrusive physician.

Will your answer change if the patient has previously given informed consent to the physician to engage in online searching about clinically relevant information, or if the physician simply informs her beforehand that he does this kind of Internet searching at his own discretion and without necessarily obtaining consent from the patient? There are no laws to guide the physician in how to handle these situations, although the physician may be on firmer ground if he or she has permission from the patient to monitor her online activity. Some hospitals and health care systems have begun to formulate social media policies, but those policies are often vague and ambiguous with regard to the questions posed here, and physicians in private practice are entirely on their own in navigating these dilemmas. They need to develop awareness of the challenges by familiarizing themselves with both the opportunities and risks posed by social media and Internet search engines. Consulting with trusted colleagues, an ethics committee, a risk management team, and/or legal counsel might be warranted in some circumstances.

No absolute rule applies here. In some cases, the physician should possibly engage in an online search for patient information, and, in other situations, he or she certainly should not. If a patient requests that the physician do so (or gives informed consent upon request of the physician), then Internet searching is probably justifiable and potentially helpful in certain cases like the one presented at the beginning of this chapter. Of course, this begs the question of whether the physician has adequate time to keep up with online blogs, tweets, and other online information sources. The information to be monitored may be voluminous. Because this is uncompensated time and effort for the physician, time constraints and financial realities probably make it unlikely for doctors to do a great deal of online searching for patient information anyway.

Rather than have an overarching rule, doctors need to have awareness of the issue and knowledge of how Internet search engines and social media sites work. Medical students, residents, and young physicians are "tech savvy" by and large, and many older physicians are utilizing Internet technologies as well. But mere technical know-how can only get us so far in addressing the questions at hand, which are ethical and age-old at their core: How are physicians to balance beneficence and respect for patient privacy? Should physicians make critical decisions on their own or only with the consent of their patients? In addition to being familiar with social media and Internet search technologies, physicians need a structured thought process to grapple with the ethical dilemmas that arise when they consider whether to monitor their patients' online activity.

In a paper on the ethics of patient-targeted googling, my colleagues and I delineated structured thought process may be used to address this issue. Physicians must ask themselves the following 6 ethical and pragmatic questions before they conduct an online search for patient information:

1. Why do I want to conduct this search?

2. Would my search advance or compromise the treatment?

3. Should I obtain informed consent from the patient prior to searching?

4. Should I share the results of the search with the patient?

5. Should I document the findings of the search in the medical record?

6. How do I assess the ongoing risk/benefit profile of searching?

The answers to these questions do not necessarily tell the physician exactly how to proceed, but they help to ensure that he or she will consider the major factors at stake and not make a knee-jerk, impulsive decision. This is essential in an era when so many people, including medical students and physicians, are constantly accessing computers and smart phones engaged in Internet searching and social media use. By slowing down and considering the questions posed above, we position ourselves to make a reasonable, judicious decision that respects our patients' privacy and their clinical best interests at the same time.

What would you do in the case described at the beginning of this chapter? Because the physician knows that the patient has made a suicide attempt, continues to experience suicidal ideation, and writes online posts about her mental state, he or she may be duty bound to pay attention on a regular basis to what she is writing. If he or she has all of this information about her and does not monitor her online activity, would he or she be medicolegally responsible if he or she failed to discover and act upon a suicide plan that she posted online and then acted upon 1 week later? One could imagine a scenario in which her family might sue the physician for failure to protect this suicidal patient by keeping an eye on the blogs and social media activity of which he or she was well aware. Legal issues aside, could this physician be held morally and ethically responsible for this patient's death? Had he or she harmed the patient by not following her online activity prior to completing a planned suicide?

It would be advisable to get ahead of the issue by having a direct and honest discussion about the issue with the patient during the first office visit. The doctor could ask her more about her online posts and whether she would agree to sharing them with him even before they are posted online, especially if they have suicidal content, or the doctor might request that she stop posting online about her suicidality at all and get in touch with him to discuss these safety concerns more directly. An open dialogue about the physician's dilemma might lead to a deepening of trust and the clinical bond, which could promote her safety and further recovery. Bringing family members or close friends of hers into the discussion might also be helpful. They not only could provide her with emotional support, but they could also serve as the people who monitor her online posts and report any concerns to the physician.

In the end, however, the physician may not be able to escape a difficult decision about whether (and how often) to monitor her online posts. As long as he or she deliberates thoughtfully about how best to respect both her privacy and her clinical safety, the physician stands on reasonable ground. He or she should, of course, carefully document his or her reasoning in the medical record in case of medicolegal issues that might arise later. Social media and Internet technology will continue to evolve in unforeseen ways in the years ahead. Physicians today must learn how they can use the new technologies to optimize treatment outcomes while respecting patients' fundamental rights to autonomy, free expression, and privacy.

COMPREHENSION QUESTIONS

35.1 Which of the following ethical dilemmas must physicians consider when deciding whether to monitor a suicidal patient's online blog?
   A. Beneficence versus nonmaleficence
   B. Justice versus autonomy
   C. Beneficence versus privacy
   D. Paternalism versus quality of life

35.2 Which of the following questions should physicians consider before deciding to engage in an online search for information about a potentially suicidal patient?
   A. Does this patient know about suicide hotlines that provide online chat services?
   B. Should I seek informed consent from the patient for the online monitoring?
   C. What law applies to the question of whether I can read the patient's online posts?
   D. Will the patient's family sue me for negligence if I do not monitor the patient online and take necessary steps to prevent suicide?

ANSWERS

35.1 **C.** The key dilemma is whether the physician should respect the patient's online privacy, or prioritize safety and potential clinical benefits by monitoring online posts.

35.2 **B.** Considering informed consent issues is critical before conducting online searches for patient information. The availability of suicide hotlines is not relevant. There is no definitive legal or regulatory guidance regarding what the physician should do in these situations. The physician should not decide what to do to prevent a lawsuit, but rather to care for the patient while also respecting privacy and other fundamental rights.

KEY POINTS

► Social media and Internet search engines allow physicians to obtain information quickly and conveniently, including possible pertinent data about their patients.

► Acquiring information about patients online may be clinically beneficial, but doing so also runs the risk of causing privacy violations and other ethical concerns.

► Physicians should think carefully and systematically before searching online for patient information or monitoring their online posts.

► The prime consideration should always be practical and ethical: avoid harm to patients and optimize treatment outcomes.

REFERENCES

Brendel DH. Monitoring blogs: a new dilemma for osychiatrists. *Virtual Mentor.* 2012;14:441-444.

Clinton NK, Silverman BC, Brendel DH. Patient-targeted googling: the ethics of searching online for patient information. *Harv Rev Psychiatry.* 2010;18:103-112.

Guseh JS II, Brendel RW, Brendel DH. Medical professionalism in the age of online social networking. *J Med Ethics.* 2009;35:584-586.

Medical Ethics Advisor. Social media changing MD-patient relationship. *Med Ethics Adv.* 2013;29:129-130.

St-Laurent-Gagnon T, Coughlin KW. Canadian Paediatric Society Bioethics Committee. Paediatricians, social media and blogs: ethical considerations. *Paediatr Child Health.* 2012;17:267-272.

A 30-year-old gravida 0 woman presents to you for an evaluation of her headaches. Over the last 6 months, her headaches have increased in intensity and frequency, leaving her experiencing intense, pounding, right-sided headaches associated with nausea and occasionally vomiting. During the headaches she is unable to tolerate head movement, bright light, or sounds of any sort. They typically last up to 8 hours. She tried over-the-counter nonsteroidal anti-inflammatory analgesics with some relief but only if the headaches are not severe at the onset. Her neurologic examination was normal as was the magnetic resonance imaging (MRI) of her brain with and without contrast and basic laboratory tests. You diagnose her with chronic migraines and prescribe prophylactic medication. Over the next 3 months, you prescribe for the patient numerous migraine prophylaxis agents, including topiramate, propranolol, and amitriptyline. Despite adequate trials, these medications were not particularly effective. Finally, you prescribe divalproex sodium (Depakote) 750 mg by mouth twice daily, and this medication successfully reduced her migraine frequency to twice per month. You also prescribe a course of amoxicillin for the patient at that visit because you suspect she has an infection. At your next follow-up visit, the patient complains of fatigue and nausea, so you perform a pregnancy test. The results of that test are positive. The patient was surprised because she had been taking the same low-dose estrogen oral contraceptive pill daily for years without ever becoming pregnant. After she returned home, she spent hours on the Internet researching the teratogenicity of divalproex and the interaction between antibiotics and her oral contraceptive pill. Later that week, you receive an angry e-mail accusing you of malpractice. She promptly transferred her medical care to another physician.

► Is this a likely case of medical malpractice?
► What steps should you take now that you have received the patient's e-mail?

ANSWERS TO CASE 36:

Risk Management

Summary: A 30-year-old gravida 0 woman was started on divalproex sodium for migraine headache prophylaxis (a pregnancy category X for migraine headache prophylaxis but category D for seizures) and becomes unexpectedly pregnant despite taking oral contraception regularly. The pregnancy is the result of a drug interaction with an antibiotic that reduced the efficacy of the oral contraception she was taking. The patient is upset by both the unplanned pregnancy and the potential for iatrogenic fetal harm. You receive an e-mail from the patient accusing you of malpractice.

- **Is this likely a case of medical malpractice?** Yes.

- **What steps should you take now that you have received the patient's e-mail?** You must discuss the issue with your risk management team and consider an apology and disclosure of the medical error.

ANALYSIS

Objectives

1. To understand the basic theory behind medical malpractice lawsuits.

2. To understand how the legal system understands the duties of physicians to their patients.

Considerations

In the present case, the physician prescribed a teratogenic medication to a woman of reproductive age and simultaneously prescribed an antibiotic known to cause decreased efficacy of oral contraceptives without recommending a backup form of contraception. This is an example of medical malpractice. All of the elements of a malpractice suit are present: The physician owed the patient a duty of care, the physician breached this duty, the patient was harmed, and the physician's actions were the cause of the harm. This is also an example of medical error, and the physician should consider full disclosure to the patient with an apology.

APPROACH TO:

Medical Malpractice

DEFINITIONS

INFORMED CONSENT: A patient with decision-making capacity has the right to accept or refuse medical interventions. The informed consent process consists of several steps: (1) the physician introduces the concept of the informed consent process as one of mutual decision making, (2) the physician elicits the patient's current understanding of her condition and alternatives for management, (3) the physician provides additional information about the patient's condition and alternatives for management, including the option of doing nothing (4) the physician assists the patient in understanding the material presented, (5) the patient articulates her decision to the physician, and (6) after further discussion and agreement, the management decision is carried out by the physician.

MEDICAL MALPRACTICE: The negligent or improper provision of medical care by a licensed health care professional.

MEDICAL NEGLIGENCE: A plaintiff must prove the following four elements to prevail in a medical negligence lawsuit: (1) the physician owed the plaintiff a duty of care, (2) the physician breeched that duty (deviated from the standard of care), (3) the plaintiff suffered an injury, and (4) the physician's actions were the proximate cause of the plaintiff's injury.

PREPONDERANCE OF THE EVIDENCE: The evidentiary standard in medical negligence cases requires that the plaintiff prove the facts by a preponderance of the evidence. This requires demonstrating to the jury that the facts the plaintiff alleges were more likely than not to have occurred.

PROXIMATE CAUSE: But for the physician's action, the plaintiff would not have suffered harm. The proximate cause does not have to be the immediate cause, but the physician's allegedly negligent actions must have set up a series of events that led to the harm.

STANDARD OF CARE: Based on expert testimony, a jury is asked to determine what a reasonably prudent medical specialist in the same specialty as the defendant physician would have done in the same circumstances as the defendant physician. Typically, the standard of care is based on a national, not a local, standard.

CLINICAL APPROACH

Malpractice Basics

When filing a malpractice lawsuit in civil court, the patient alleges that the treating physician cared for the plaintiff in a manner that deviated from nationally accepted norms and resulted in injury. To win a medical malpractice claim, the plaintiff must demonstrate each of the 4 elements of a negligence claim. The elements are as follows:

1. The plaintiff must show that a physician-patient relationship existed, thus creating a duty of care. The physician–patient relationship inherently imposes this duty.

2. The plaintiff must prove that the physician's actions were negligent, in that they deviated from nationally accepted professional standards, by proffering expert testimony that a reasonably prudent physician would have acted differently under the same circumstances.

3. The plaintiff must demonstrate that he or she suffered physical, emotional, and/ or financial injury.

4. The plaintiff must establish that the physician's action was the proximate cause of the injury.

Unlike the more familiar "beyond a reasonable doubt" standard of criminal cases, in a medical malpractice case, the plaintiff must prove the 4 elements "by the preponderance of the evidence" (51% certainty), a much more lenient evidentiary standard.

ANALYSIS AND DISCUSSION

A variety of actions, if found to deviate from the standard of care, may form the basis of a negligence lawsuit. Negligent actions may reflect poor quality medical care including misdiagnosis, mismanagement of a disease process, or an improperly performed procedure. Allegations of negligence may also arise from unprofessional behavior. In addition, negligence may arise from a physician's failure to obtain adequate informed consent for a treatment. Under this theory of negligence, the plaintiff claims that the physician did not provide either the patient or the patient's surrogate enough information about the risks and benefits of a treatment to make an informed decision about whether to accept or reject a proposed intervention.[1]

In this case, the patient may have 2 theories of negligence on which to base a malpractice lawsuit: inadequate informed consent and poor quality medical care. Valproate-containing medications present a particularly heightened risk of adverse effects to the developing fetus. If the fetus experiences an adverse outcome, then the physician's liability exposure will depend, in part, on how thoroughly the physician discussed with the patient the risks and benefits of taking divalproex sodium, which is a known teratogen. Ideally, the physician discussed the teratogenic potential of the medication at the time the medication was offered and documented this discussion in the medical record. A woman of childbearing potential may reasonably expect to be informed about the heightened potential fetal harm should she become pregnant while taking a particularly potent teratogen. Thus, a physician who does not know enough to discuss the risks and benefits of a therapy or forgets to do so is providing poor medical care and inadequate informed consent.

Another complication of this case is that the patient became pregnant around the time that the physician prescribed her an antibiotic known to reduce the efficacy of her oral contraceptive medication. The physician's liability exposure depends on whether and how the patient was counseled about the drug–drug interaction. The physician may have missed the fact that the patient was taking an oral contraceptive pill. Alternatively, the physician may not have been aware of the drug–drug interaction and thus did not know to counsel the patient to take extra contraceptive precautions during the time of antibiotic use. These errors in either procedure (medicine reconciliation) or knowledge (ignorance of drug–drug interactions) may also form the basis of a malpractice lawsuit for negligence.

This case also raises the question of apologies for medical errors. Although a thorough review of the topic of apologies for medical error is beyond the scope of this case, physicians should be aware that states approach the admissibility of

---

[1]Cases in which the quality of informed consent is in dispute may rely on either a "reasonably prudent medical professional" or a "reasonably prudent lay person" standard, depending on the jurisdiction. The plaintiff in a jurisdiction operating under the first standard must demonstrate that the defendant physician failed to disclose what reasonably prudent physicians typically disclose to patients under similar circumstances. Plaintiffs in jurisdictions employing the second, more common standard must demonstrate that the defendant physician failed to disclose what a reasonably prudent patient would want to know in order to assess the risks and benefits adequately.

apologies during a medical malpractice lawsuit differently. Ethically, physicians are expected to offer some type of apology for a medical error. The current legal protections for physicians are inadequate in most states to facilitate free communication with patients and families after a medical error has been committed. Although some states have no law in this area, the majority of states have apology laws. Apology laws typically protect only the actual expression of sympathy but not the expression of fault that may accompany the expression of sympathy. A minority of states has disclosure laws. These laws mandate disclosure of certain unanticipated outcomes and may protect the communication from being used against the physician in a legal or administrative action. Knowing the law and working with local risk management personnel is advisable in these difficult situations when a medical error has been made.

COMPREHENSION QUESTIONS

36.1 A patient visits his primary care physician (PCP) with the complaint of difficulty sleeping. The physician conducts a thorough history and physical examination, depression screening, and laboratory evaluation but can come up with no explanation for the difficulty. After extensive counseling, the PCP prescribes a sleeping pill, only providing 14 tablets and requiring the patient to come in for follow-up in 2 weeks. The patient goes home and takes all 20 tablets and is found dead by family members later that day. His family members sue the physician for medical malpractice. Which element of the medical malpractice claim will it be most difficult for the patient's family to prove?

   A. Duty
   B. Breech of duty
   C. Injury
   D. Causation

36.2 A patient presents to you for her yearly annual examination. You review her results from the previous year prior to entering the room, and you see that you never reviewed her mammography result from the previous year. The mammogram was abnormal. You send the patient for repeat mammography, the results of which shows evidence of growth of the abnormality in the intervening 12 months. Breast biopsy reveals breast cancer. You disclose to the patient your failure to review the mammography results, and you offer an apology. Which of the following statements is true?

   A. You owed this patient a duty of care, but you did not breach this duty.
   B. Your disclosure of medical error and apology will not be admissible in court as evidence against you in a malpractice claim.
   C. Your disclosure of medical error and apology may be admissible in court as evidence against you in a malpractice claim depending on the law of the state in which you live.
   D. You should not have disclosed the error to the patient.

ANSWERS

36.1 **B.** In this case, the physician owed the patient a duty of care, but it is unclear whether the physician breached his duty to the patient. The physician screened the patient for depression and found no suggestion that the patient would be at increased risk for suicide. The physician also counseled the patient extensively before prescribing the medication. Finally, the physician prescribed only 14 tablets and requested a follow-up visit.

36.2 **C.** You owed this patient a duty of care and you breached that duty. Ethically, disclosing an iatrogenic error is the action you ought to take; however, not all jurisdictions offer legal protections to physicians who choose to disclose iatrogenic error and apologize. It is important to become familiar with the laws of your state and the recommendations of your institution.

KEY POINTS

► Medical malpractice claims for negligence require the patient/plaintiff to establish all of the following:

  ► Physician duty to the patient

  ► Physician breach of that duty

  ► Injury to the patient

  ► The physician's actions were the direct cause of the injury

► Ethically, when an iatrogenic error is committed, the physician should consider disclosure to the patient in addition to an apology.

REFERENCES

Kapp MB. The interface of law and medical ethics in medical intensive care. *Chest.* 2009;136:904-909.

Kass JS. Epilepsy and pregnancy: a practical approach to mitigating legal risk. *Continuum (Minneap Minn).* 2014;20:181-185.

Mastroianni AC, Mello MM, Sommer S, Hardy M, Gallagher TH. The flaws in state 'apology' and 'disclosure' laws dilute their intended impact on malpractice suits. *Health Affairs.* 2010;1612:1611-1619.

Clinical Cases

Case Listing by Topic (Alphabetical)